THE ENDANGERED
MEDICAL RECORD

THE ENDANGERED MEDICAL RECORD

ENSURING ITS INTEGRITY
IN THE AGE OF INFORMATICS

VERGIL N. SLEE, MD
DEBORA A. SLEE, JD
H. JOACHIM SCHMIDT, JD

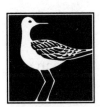
Tringa Press
Saint Paul, Minnesota

©2000 Tringa Press

Tringa Press
Saint Paul, Minnesota
help@tringa.com
http://www.tringa.com

Cover illustration: detail from *Erasmus Writing* by Hans Holbein the Younger. Oil on panel, 42x32cm, Louvre, Paris, France. Giraudon/Art Resource, NY.

Library of Congress Cataloging-in-Publication Data

Slee, Vergil N., 1917–
     The endangered medical record: ensuring its integrity in the age of informatics / Vergil N. Slee, Debora A. Slee, H. Joachim Schmidt.
          p. cm.
     Includes bibliographical references and index.
     ISBN 0-9615255-2-5
          1. Medical records. 2. Nosology. I. Slee, Debora A. II. Schmidt, H. Joachim (Herbert Joachim), 1948–   III. Title.
          [DNLM: 1. Medical Records—standards. 2. Classification methods. WX 173 S632e 2000]
     R864.S57   2000
     651.5'04261—dc21
                                                                99-020388

Table of Contents

Section 4: Coding Systems

Section 5: Other Resource Materials

List of Figures

Foreword

FLORENCE NIGHTINGALE would have demanded that everyone read this book.

While Nightingale is popularly remembered as the "the Lady of the Lamp," ministering to British soldiers wounded in the Crimean War, she was also an ardent and early advocate of what we would call information-based medicine.

"To understand God's thoughts, we must study statistics, for those are the measure of His purpose," Nightingale pronounced. As part of her effort to improve sanitary conditions in hospitals, Nightingale campaigned tirelessly for reliable data on outcomes. "There is a growing conviction that in all hospitals, even in those which are best conducted, there is a great and unnecessary waste of life," she wrote, "[but] accurate hospital statistics are much more rare than is generally imagined."

Some 150 years after Nightingale penned those words, Vergil N. Slee, Debora A. Slee and H. Joachim Schmidt have compellingly laid out the causes and effects of the crisis that afflicts hospital statistics in our time. Their argument is simple, yet has profound implications: our healthcare system is built on information from the medical record. That information, in turn, is constructed from a series of codes that are designed to condense a complicated clinical narrative into a simple and consistent set of numerical values. Unfortunately, those codes are neither as comprehensive nor as precise as they should be. Moreover, it's not just that the same code can be interpreted differently by different physicians or members of the hospital records department. Worse, the same code in different years may actually be describing separate clinical conditions, thanks to coding updates and revisions.

The result is an edifice "built on sand," flawed at every step.

The ramifications of this design defect may not be immediately apparent to the average clinician who still relies on his or her handwritten notes. Indeed, when the American College of Surgeons met in 1923 to discuss the need for a common patient record, it faced objections that still resonate today. On the one hand, doctors confidently insisted that they kept all the important information about their patients in their head. On the other hand, physicians worried about the privacy implications of sharing the records of "their" patients with the entire hospital staff. Not to mention the nagging "dearth of adequately trained record librarians."

In our time, too, clinicians have tended to view the official medical record with some suspicion. Coding has been warily regarded as primarily a financial, rather than clinical, exercise. This suspicion has been given credence by the proliferation of vendors promising to help hospitals and physicians wring the maximum reimbursement out of each episode of illness — within legal limits, of course. Other legal concerns have also contributed to the jaundiced view of medical record-keeping. Apart from the traditional worries about documenting potential malpractice, clinicians have fretted about writing down comments the patient might someday see — for example, comments related to the patient's mental state or lack of cooperativeness.

Yet as medicine has moved from a quill-and-pen sensibility (albeit with such modern conveniences as ballpoints and electric typewriters) to the era of the microchip, the importance of the properly coded medical record has grown exponentially. Coding is being transformed from a reimbursement mechanism and rudimentary clinical review tool to the basic byte of information needed to manage the healthcare system. Coding provides the lens through which we view everything from illness prevalence to quality improvement effectiveness to financial trends. Yet as this book disturbingly details, that lens is pockmarked with distortions.

We don't know the true size of the AIDS epidemic some 19 years after the first case appeared in the United States. We can't properly track Gulf War syndrome. We have rendered the personal medical record unreliable. And, perhaps worst of all, the advent of the electronic medical record (EMR) is likely to only imbed the inherent weaknesses of our current system even deeper into the very fabric of medical transactions.

The authors argue persuasively that a rethinking of the basic architecture of medical coding is long overdue. But instead of rethinking fundamentals, the entrepreneurs of the age of informatics are frantically building ever bigger and more ostentatious electronic structures whose wiring and plumbing are outdated and dangerous.

Hints of that danger occasionally pop into public view. When Medicare coding patterns showed a sudden increase in the prevalence of serious bacterial pneumonia, as opposed to the less serious viral variety, the Centers for Disease Control and Prevention sounded the epidemiological alarm bells. Further investigation uncovered an etiology more related to coding creep than clinical patterns, and the Department of Justice launched an investigation of its own.

Then there's the Internet site that purports to give Web surfers free access to risk-adjusted clinical outcomes information on every hospital in the country. The problem is that those outcomes are based on Medicare claims data, a source whose flaws are thought by some to be uncorrectable by any *ex post facto* form of risk adjustment.

As disturbing as these problems are, they may yet prove to be a blessing in disguise. As a rule, Americans do not address infrastructure problems until they are forced to, whether the problem is disintegrating highways, lack of readiness training in the military or public health preparedness. The growing need of the provider community for accurate information about the practice of evidence-based medicine, the growing need of purchasers for data on the value of what they are buying, and the growing need of policymakers for precise tracking information all provide the basic ingredients for a full-blown crisis. Given the entrenched investment in the current system, and the investment of time and money it will take to bring about change, a crisis is manifestly what is needed to transform this issue from a wonk concern to a White House one.

Fortunately, Vergil and Debora Slee and Joachim Schmidt have provided us with not only a call to arms but with suggested solutions, as well. In doing so, they have managed to produce a book that is both written in astoundingly plain English, yet backed by blue-ribbon technical sophistication. That accomplishment is due in large part, one suspects, to the sterling credentials of the authors. Vergil Slee is a renowned medical informatics pioneer. He not only developed the first hospital discharge abstract system, he also led the team which modified the International Classification of Diseases, Ninth Edition, for use by U.S. hospitals. Vergil's daughter, Debora, an attorney and writer, is both an information systems consultant and a contributor to the literature on medical record terminology. Schmidt, meanwhile, is both an attorney and software applications engineer.

Whatever the looming potential of information-driven 21st century medicine, the mundane truth of "garbage in, garbage out" remains an immutable law of computing. We must improve the "front end" of our information-gathering system in order to take advantage of budding technologies such as neural networking, which offer the hope of the kind of large-scale quality improvement studies so critical to improving the efficiency of clinical interventions. The promised payoff is delivery of care that is as consistently as possible the best we know how to make it.

Too bad Florence Nightingale never got a chance to read this book. It would make her proud.

Michael L. Millenson

Michael L. Millenson is the author of *Demanding Medical Excellence: Doctors and Accountability in the Information Age* (University of Chicago Press), a consultant, and a visiting scholar at Northwestern University's Institute for Health Services Research and Policy Studies.

Preface

THIS BOOK is coming off the press early in the year 2000, a year in which important decisions may be made about the management of the diagnostic information in medical records. As a part of the Health Insurance Portability and Accountability Act (HIPAA) rulemaking process, consideration will be given to introducing the *International Classification of Diseases, 10th Revision, Clinical Modification (ICD-10-CM)* to replace the *International Classification of Diseases, 9th Revision, Clinical Modification (ICD-9-CM)*, which has been used to code diagnoses for virtually all purposes since it was released in 1978.

On the face of it, this substitution of a more modern version of the classification ought to be a step forward — the twenty years of experience between the two versions should have led to a better system. There has indeed been a great deal of medical progress in these twenty years, and there is an overdue need to accommodate that progress in disease classifications for both statistical and clinical studies.

But the coding change under consideration, and for which the federal government has made preparation, does not improve our healthcare information system. This is because our system fails to conform to a fundamental concept which is at the heart of all observational sciences: *keep data at the most discrete level possible.*

And there are other problems with our system, as well. This book is intended to shed light on these "flaws", to provide a solid grounding in the history and concepts of healthcare coding, and to offer concrete methods to solve the problems.

If you have just five minutes, please read the Abstract on page 2. If you can devote an hour or two, look at the first chapter, "Four Serious Flaws in Our Health Information System," page 3, which is designed to provide an overview of everything else in the book.

For more leisurely study, or for reference, see Section 2, History & Background (page 43), which covers medical records, coding, and healthcare classification, and Section 3, Problems & Solutions (page 223).

Resource materials include Section 4 (page 345), covering a number of coding systems, Section 5 (page 513), which has other materials, an extensive Bibliography, and an Index.

Many dedicated people have contributed in myriad ways to the knowledge the book contains, including the kind obtained through the "trial and error" (or maybe better said, "live and learn") method. Just a few are listed here; many more are noted throughout the book.

The authors thank Gordon Briggs, Bruce P. Brown, Susan DesHarnais, Marjorie Greenberg, Fay Hemphill, John Horty, Kathy Jamerson, J. M. Juran, Henk Lamberts, Jack Lewin, Michael Millenson, Richard G. Rockefeller, David Rothwell, Robert Seeman, Henry Vaughan, Clarence Velz, Myron Wegman, Karel Weigel, Kerr L. White, Kenneth Williams, Maurice Wood, George Zajdel, and Marjorie Zernott.

By far the largest supporting role was played — with great patience — by Beth Ellen Stoke Slee. Thanks, Beth; thanks, Mom.

We would especially like to acknowledge the constant support for this effort from Richard Remington, PhD (1931-1992). This support began when Doctor Remington was completing his doctorate in biostatistics at the School of Public Health of the University of Michigan. He gave valuable counsel throughout his career, as a faculty member in the School of Public Health and later its Dean, and it continued after he had left the University of Michigan to become Vice President for Academic Affairs and Dean of Faculties at the University of Iowa, and later its Interim President.

His last letter to the senior author is reproduced on the following page.

This book is dedicated to Richard Remington.

THE UNIVERSITY OF IOWA

COLLEGE OF MEDICINE

August 13, 1991

Dear Vergil:

I have read with interest your proposal for the conversion of the present one step disease coding and classification operation based on the International Classification of Diseases to a system based on entity coding, and your description of entity coding's advantages and disadvantages.

It is hard to believe that entity coding was not put in place long ago. The principle that coding should retain, to the greatest possible degree, the detail present in the original observations seems unarguable. Most if not all scientific disciplines adhere to this principle, sometimes without even realizing it. The combination of classification and coding into a single step must inevitably lead to a loss of detail and to accretion of error. When this is applied in a setting in which classifications are periodically changed, chaos, or at best near-chaos results.

If it were possible to return to original records and recode, the problem would not be so bad. However, in using clinical or even many types of research records, this is not feasible. Even in the relatively simple environment of the death certificate, the present system leads to elaborate "concordance" experiments involving multiple coding, whenever we move from ICD-X to ICD-(X+1).

Entity coding clearly offers the possibility of avoiding these and the other shortcomings of combined coding/classifying operations outlined so clearly in your description. You wisely stop short of stating that no new problems will be created by entity coding. Surely there will be problems, some foreseeable and some not. The point is, I think, that entity coding is a concept firmly based in logic and all observational science, and it is certainly worth exploring in detail for application to health statistics.

Thanks again for sharing your thoughts with me.

Sincerely,

Dick

Richard D. Remington
Distinguished Professor and Director
Department of Preventive Medicine and Environmental Health

Section 1: Overview

Abstract

The medical record is the nucleus of our healthcare system — for the care of the individual patient, reimbursing providers, and providing intelligence for tasks ranging from the operation of individual facilities, to developing national healthcare strategies, to participating in international health affairs.

There are serious, real threats to the truthfulness and completeness of medical record content. These spring from biasing influences such as the power of coded information to control reimbursement, the power of regulations to enhance or inhibit proper recording, the fear of loss of confidentiality in the computer, human resistance to change, and purely technological problems of data management.

The technological problems considered most serious are those which stem from the fact that, in an information world which is irreversibly "code-dependent," we do not code the essential clinical information. We code diagnoses, procedures, and other information directly to the pigeonholes of classifications, using a process called category coding. Unless we *also* code the precise diagnoses — the "clinical entities" — we throw away forever the detail which should be preserved permanently.

The solution to this problem is to code every clinical entity and keep it permanently with an unalterable code. This can be done by adding a new "front end" in the medical record, both paper-based and electronic. From the entity-coded information, the cases can not only be retrieved unambiguously, but also can easily be placed in the categories of any classification, past, present, or future.

The other major, technical problem is that our healthcare codes are ambiguous. They have no intrinsic identification, and their meanings change from time to time. This can lead to errors in statistics and make longitudinal studies almost impossible. We need to "tag" each of our healthcare codes with a *key* identifying that code and providing information essential to decoding it.

Both the medical record itself and the systems which use its information externally — billing, statistics, research, quality management, policy — will be better able to serve their purposes.

1

Four Serious Flaws in Our Health Information System

YOUR PERSONAL MEDICAL RECORD is a crucial element of your personal healthcare. Its primary function is to assist healthcare providers in caring for you, and for this it must contain a complete and accurate record of your health problems, their management, and your response.

And our national health information system begins with the medical record. Information collected from individual records provides the basis for most of our knowledge about our nation's healthcare — who gets sick, what they get, how they're treated, how they respond. These records — several billion each year — contain priceless information, which could provide a depth to our collective medical knowledge impossible before now.

But we can't get at all of this information, nor can we rely on what we do get. That's what this book is about.

Background | **The medical record: an irreplaceable tool for medical care**

Medical records were invented by physicians and nurses in order to make sure that they remembered all the facts about each individual patient, and so that all the people concerned in the care — consultants, other physicians, nurses on other shifts, specialized technicians, referral institutions — would have the same information.

Your personal, individual medical record (sometimes you have more than one) should contain information about your past and present problems, diagnoses, care provided, and the results. At any time you come into contact with healthcare providers, information should be added by all the individuals involved (including you). Your record also collects information from the laboratory, X-ray department, pharmacy, and other sources.

> Your medical record is a living, growing resource for your health and healthcare. As, over time, more and more caregivers become involved in your care, it is increasingly important that your record be able to function as the source of memory and the center of communications.

There have been problems for decades with our "system" of recording and retrieving health information, and it's time to give these problems immediate attention. We hope to convince you why it's imperative to fix these problems now — and how it can be done.

Of course, they are many kinds of information, and many "routes" into the information system — death certificates, reports of diseases, health surveys, and so forth — but in this book we focus on the huge segment of information which starts with medical records. Just looking at these, we're dealing, at the beginning of the 21st century, with about 33,000,000 hospitalizations, 100,000,000 emergency room visits, 350,000,000 outpatient visits, 700,000,000 visits to physicians, and 300,000,000 home care visits each year in the United States — each of which generates either a new medical record, or new information added to an existing one. There is also an unknown number of encounters in the alternative healthcare community, perhaps one-third to one-half as many as in the mainstream system, and many of these will also be documented in medical records.

Background

Our national health information system

Well, there isn't one.

We don't have a national *healthcare* system, either.

What we have in the United States is *what we have* — in other words, the sum total of whatever's out there is included in the term "system." We are a large flotilla of various sized boats, each with its own captain, following diverse and ever-changing maritime laws.

The "flotilla" includes hospitals and other health care facilities, health professionals, and others who make up an informal network across the country through which care is provided. Insurance companies are part of the fleet, as is the government (federal, state, and local), drug companies, equipment manufacturers, and patients — everyone involved in delivering, receiving, or paying for healthcare, or for research or prevention of disease.

A number of factors compete to give (or force) direction: the marketplace, reimbursement, federal and state regulations, professional standards, institutional standards, and so forth. Many individuals and organizations have helped to make our healthcare excellent and ensure its availability. What we've never had, however, is a single, cohesive plan which encompasses this vast "network."

And all of this pertains to our national health *information* system, as well, which is really just an inextricable part of the healthcare system itself. So when we talk about the "system" in this book, we are simply referring to what is there, now, and how things are done, now.

Your Personal Medical Record

You probably assume that all essential information has been recorded in your medical record, and that as you visit providers for care, that information will be available to them. Unfortunately, this assumption is increasingly shaky. There are elements of our present healthcare system, and of our information technology, which interfere with both the accurate recording of clinical information and its retrieval. Let's imagine some real-life scenarios.

Examples

What if ...

... your physician went to your medical record to help his memory with your physical problem, which he had felt was partially due to stress, but the details were vague in his mind. Then he remembered that he had left out critical facts about a family problem because he was afraid that the computer would not keep them confidential — although he had been assured that security was higher in the electronic system than in his old paper-based records. This sometimes happens.

What if ...

... your physician consulted your medical record about your illness last year, and found only that you had "some other disease of the respiratory system." Your former doctor is not available, so your new doctor looks up the code for "some other..." She finds 30 pages of things you didn't have, but is still no closer to what you actually had. This happens today.

What if ...

... you had served in the Gulf War and when you returned you thought your symptoms were the result of something that happened over there. So did your doctor, and he tried to record Gulf War syndrome. He was instructed to put in your record codes for "late effects of war" and "fatigue" — there was no way to put down what he actually wanted to. This is still true in 2000, and the war has been over for years.

Secondary Uses of Medical Record Information

As our healthcare system has become more complex, medical records have been called upon to serve many "secondary" purposes, beyond direct patient care. These range from individual case billing, to quality management, research, and formulating national health policy, to exchange of international health statistics. Many of these uses are vital.

Imagine again some scenarios, and what might result if we can't rely on our data:

Examples

What if ...

... you were writing a newspaper story and tried to back-track on the AIDS epidemic as it had been treated in your state. You got figures, and asked where they came from. You learned that they came from the coding in medical records and on bills submitted from hospitals and doctors. You also found that there had been a half dozen or more ways that AIDS cases might have been coded since the first cases in 1981, but that no one could tell you how they actually had been coded. Sometimes they were coded as diseases of the immune system and sometimes as infectious diseases. And no one was really sure whether or not all the codes that could have been used were actually looked up in compiling the statistics. *And* your state was not unique — all states had the same fuzzy data.

What if …

… you were doing research on the history of heart attacks (acute myocardial infarction (AMI)). Of course you had to look up AMI by finding its code, but you found that its codes had changed in mysterious ways. Before 1948, AMI was lumped into a group of different kinds of arteriosclerotic heart disease. In 1962 it was separated out pretty well with its own code, but in 1965, in one coding system you couldn't separate it from "arteriosclerotic heart disease of over 8 weeks duration," while in another you had to look in two codes, "AMI with hypertension" and "AMI without hypertension." In still another system, you could also find out which artery was involved. Of course, all these codes had different numbers. Hopeless. Medicine knew a lot about AMI before 1948 — it was well known and diagnosed, including which artery. But the codes — the only kind we still use today — get between us and the detail we are looking for.

What if …

… you wanted to look at healthcare data to help in managing a hospital, and then at another time wanted to look at the same data as the base on which to develop public policy. You'd want quite different views, neither of which could be met very well from data whose primary use is to code for the bills submitted for care.

The Four Flaws

The problems illustrated in the scenarios above are the result of four "flaws" in our health information system:

1. **"The System"[1] Encourages Distortion of Information**

2. **The System Can't Capture Enough Clinical Detail**

3. **We Use Codes That Are Ambiguous**

4. **Our "Single Classification" System Can't Serve All Needs**

Underlying the last three of the flaws, and part of the first flaw as well, is the fact that our system for retrieval of information, and increasingly for

---

1.   See "Our national health information system," page 4.

putting information into the medical record, is based on coding — our system is "code-dependent." We must learn how to live with this code-dependency.

So before we talk specifically about the flaws, we need some background on coding and classification in health information.

Code-Dependency in Health Information

Since the first "secondary usages" of medical records, their information has been coded. Hospitals and the larger clinics, which have greater demands on medical record information, found it more convenient and trustworthy to file and retrieve the records and the information in them by the use of codes, rather than by using narrative terms or phrases.

This was simply the adoption of the methods used elsewhere in society. One doesn't order a car part by giving a long description of the part; one asks for it by giving its unique part number. Hospitals gave patients numbers and filed their medical records ("charts") by these numbers. Physicians were also given numbers, both for convenience and confidentiality. Diagnoses, operations, and other treatments were given code numbers.

Background   **The first "secondary" uses of medical records**

Early on, hospitals began using medical record information internally, for statistics on groups of patients. Hospitals wanted to know what their case loads were, and the trends, so they could intelligently plan their facilities. Physicians wanted to know the rates of success and failure with the care their hospitals provided and the success they achieved as individuals (quality measurement). Each statistic was, of course, developed by aggregating data from individual records.

The next demand for detail on the individual patient was external, and it began when healthcare insurance appeared on the scene. Payment was made (or denied) based on the clinical information (diagnoses and treatments) in the individual medical record.

It is a given today that retrieval of diagnoses and procedures is on the basis of their codes — not the language in which the diagnostic and procedure terms are expressed in the record itself prior to coding. This "fact of life" has resulted in some problems, but that doesn't mean we can't live with it. In fact, we need codes — they serve a number of essential purposes.

"Category Codes" — and Why They're Essential

Not only do we need codes, but we need codes which will place patients into groups. Collecting diagnoses into categories is essential. No one could dispute the necessity, for some purposes, of classifying cases according to their demographic characteristics or on the basis of their problems, diagnoses, management, and outcomes. We need this information for:

- Billing & healthcare financing — a million different diagnoses would be unmanageable
- Quality review — displaying patterns of care
- Administration, including staffing & facilities planning
- Clinical research
- Epidemiological studies
- Evidence-based medicine
- International statistics
- Public policy, planning
- Actuarial analyses

Coding diagnoses according to their categories (where they belong in a classification), rather then their identity (what the diagnoses are) is called "category coding."

Background   ### Where we got our first clinical codes

When coding of diagnoses and procedures first began, a source was needed for the codes themselves. The most prominent source of codes in the 1930s was the American Medical Association's *Standard Nomenclature of Diseases and Operations* (SNDO), which attempted to introduce a standardized, "controlled" language for physicians to use to describe what the patient presented, what they found, and what treatments they employed. SNDO was a "Nomenclature," not a coding system. But each term was preceded by a number used for sorting the terms, and quite naturally, this sorting number was immediately used as a code to be exchanged for the term.

Our diagnosis codes today originate from the *International Classification of Diseases*[2] *(ICD)*, used universally in this country since the mid-1960s for management of medical record information. Each revision of *ICD* has required modification for use in the U.S., to give it additional specificity for clinical use. The current edition is *International Classification of Disease, 9th Revision, Clinical Modification (ICD-9-CM)*.

The codes of *ICD-9-CM* are for some 13,000 *groups* of diagnoses — not for individual diagnoses. These diagnoses are collected into *categories*, and it is the rare category, indeed, which contains only one diagnosis. Decoding only gives the name of the *ICD-9-CM* category. The code doesn't know what the original diagnosis was, only that it was one of the group of diagnoses within that category at that time.

For hospital reimbursement, we further aggregate the various diagnoses (after they are coded to *ICD-9-CM*) into about 500 "Diagnosis Related Groups" (DRGs). That has been proven to be a large enough list of "products" for which to develop prices.

---

2.   A classification with periodic, numbered *Revisions*, published by the World Health Organization (WHO). See "The International Classification of Diseases," page 155, and the appendices, page 347.

How we got into category coding

There are just entirely too many diagnoses to always deal with individually. *ICD-9-CM* lists the names for roughly 100,000 different diagnoses. Indexes to medical textbooks and publications add several hundred thousand more. And the language actually used by both caregivers and patients adds another few hundred thousand. With so many diagnoses, there are likely to be many diagnoses (or diagnostic terms) for which there are only a few patients. We could never make significant statistics or develop a reimbursement scheme without grouping the patients.

SNDO was abandoned in the 1950s as our source of diagnosis and procedure codes because it was unable to retrieve medical records in the fashion that they were called for. The demand made on the indexing system was for groups of patients — the diagnostic picture of the patients in each clinical service of the hospital, all patients having appendectomies, death rates for patients with heart attacks, and so forth. The ultra-specificity of the SNDO approach was worse than no coding at all; it actually interfered with assembly of the desired groups.

The codes of the *International Classification of Diseases (ICD)*, which we began using in the 1950s, automatically grouped patients in clinically useful ways. They also used language much closer to that of medicine rather than the artificial, imposed set of modular terms found in SNDO.

Category coding evolved from the need to group cases, and has simply grown, over time, without serious analysis. The information system began with the manual systems used within individual hospitals, where individual medical records were always available if the exact diagnoses were required. As computers entered the picture, they simply picked up what was being done manually.

And almost imperceptibly, we transferred our *retrieval* of information to the computer as well — and it uses the codes instead of the original narrative. We are now beginning to realize the handicap we have created for ourselves by using *only* category coding in our information system.

The "Four Flaws" — Where the Problems Are

With this background, let's take a closer look at the "flaws" in the system.

Flaw 1:   The "System" Encourages Distortion of Information

The information that caregivers put in the medical record is being influenced more and more by the healthcare world. There are several elements in our system today which undermine, rather than support, truthful recording of clinical information. These include factors which tend to bias the information, and factors which interfere with the accuracy of information.

"Biasing" factors include reimbursement, federal regulations, and security fears.

"Interfering" factors include limitations on and inhibitions to getting accurate information into the medical record. Specifically, the emerging electronic medical record can seriously constrain what gets recorded.

Reimbursement

Medicare and other payers only cover specific diagnoses, procedures, and services. The provider must submit the correct codes to obtain payment. Software is available to assist in optimal coding. Sometimes, the software will warn the provider against using "unacceptable" codes (codes which may set off alarms in the payment system) — even if they are the accurate ones.

Background   **"Gaming" the system**

Medical record information needed for billing is submitted in the form of codes. At first, billing coding was only detailed enough to find out if the case was entitled to benefits. Initially this was determined by asking for codes from a limited list (even though many codes were for things *not* covered).

The list contained, for example, an item entitled "mental illness" which, if present (i.e., if it was recorded or coded), could be denied. At this point the first "gaming" of the information system appeared. An acceptable primary diagnosis such as pneumonia was listed first, and the unacceptable but "actual" diagnosis, perhaps "alcoholism," was listed as secondary. This gaming worked as long as the billing system was simple and payment was determined only on the basis of the first diagnosis listed.

Federal Regulations

Medicare requires specific documentation of the service for which payment is claimed by the provider. Software to handle this, and to achieve "bullet-proof bills," is available. This software tends to influence what is recorded.

Security Fears

Concerns about confidentiality, exacerbated by the advent of electronic medical records, are — with or without justification — inhibiting the recording of essential information.

Technological Constraints

The electronic medical record (EMR) is becoming a reality. Over 200 vendors are offering EMR products (sometimes called the computer-based medical record (CPR)). While the EMR carries a vast amount of — and easily accessible — information, it can also serve to constrain the information which it "absorbs."

Background

The electronic medical record (EMR) — are we there yet?

There is no agreed-upon definition of an EMR, and the products range along a continuum of attributes. At the "low" end of the spectrum are what Peter Waegemann calls "automated medical records," which are essentially paper-based records (though roughly 50% of the information has been placed in the records by computers). At the other end are far more sophisticated products which have much more information, including laboratory reports, physicians' orders, drugs administered and known interactions, images of such record elements as electrocardiographic tracings, and other data. Some EMRs can collect the information from multiple sites, such as several hospitals and physicians' offices.

Soon the EMR will span a lifetime, and become known simply as the "electronic health record" (EHR). Everyone will probably carry a card, similar to a credit card (usually called a "smart card"), which carries their entire health history in electronic format.

The EMR can present information at the touch of a finger, with legibility and helpful display techniques. Time series of laboratory values, for example, can be shown graphically, abnormal values can be color-coded — features not practical with paper-based records. Patient education can be both triggered and provided within the sophisticated systems. Patient and physician reminder notices — health check points — can be generated automatically. Medical care can be made much more efficient and less error-prone.

Despite its many real advantages, adoption of the EMR has been slow, largely because it has required changes in the habits of physicians and other caregivers, and because the input methods have slowed down the care process (at least initially). Physicians have been loath to devote learning time. Time saved later in care — the promise of "delayed gratification" — has not been enough to overcome these problems.

For example, in the interests of making the EMR "user friendly," its designers are coming up with fast and easy ways for clinicians to record information. Perhaps the most common device is the "pick list," the computer-age version of the pencil-and-paper checklist. A pick list has a drop-down menu of "possible" terms. The user selects the appropriate term with a click of the mouse, and that term is then placed into the medical record. The pick list, however, has two inherent problems: (1) the terms which *are* on the list, and (2) the terms which are *not* on the list.

What is offered on the pick list The only practical sources of terms for such lists of diagnoses have been the categories in *ICD-9-CM*, the "Disease" module of *SNOMED*,[3] and some proprietary "nomenclatures." Since it is *ICD-9-CM* which is involved in the payment system (because its codes are used in allocating cases to their DRGs), all EMRs on the market appear to offer the *ICD-9-CM* list.

---

3. *Systematized Nomenclature of Human and Veterinary Medicine.* College of American Pathologists, 1993. See page 85 and the appendices, page 429.

What is not on the pick list It is impossible for any pick list to include *everything* a patient may present with. And, of course, it is almost inevitable that EMR vendors will in fact *prune* the list so that users are not offered codes which may give trouble in the payment system (whether they would be useful in describing the patient or not).

The physician can, of course, record what each diagnosis really is in a narrative note (by typing it in, or perhaps dictation). But this is more time consuming, and perhaps impossible to retrieve. It's much easier (perhaps, in some cases, mandatory) to use the list, even if it means selecting only the "closest thing." Also, lawyers advise that nothing in medical record comments should be in conflict with the coded entries, because nothing is more damning than an internally "inconsistent" document.

Prognosis

If nothing is done to reverse this trend toward distortion of information, the medical record will lose more and more of its value for the physician and patient in the delivery of care to the individual, and will also lose more and more value as the source for many information needs in our society. We might even see the physician try to keep "two sets of books" — one for clinical care and one for reimbursement.

Flaw 2:   The System Can't Capture Enough Clinical Detail

Over the years, a problem arose silently. No one called what we did "category coding" — it was simply called "coding" of diagnoses and procedures. We thought we were asking of a diagnosis, "What is its code?" — when we were really asking, "Where does it go?"

A category code tells us only *where the case goes:*

      (1) its category, in

      (2) the specific classification (e.g., *ICD-9-CM*)

It can never tell us more than that. It can't tell us *what the diagnosis was.*

Detail is lost, because the label (and code for) a category in the classification is substituted for the diagnosis which was recorded in the original record. Decoding brings back the category label; it can never bring back the detailed term. More than 10,000 diagnoses, for example, are crammed into 100 categories in *ICD-9-CM*. The total number of diagnoses in the universe of diagnoses is unknown, but the alphabetical index to *ICD-9-CM* has about 100,000 terms. Valid synonyms, local variations in usage, and expanding knowledge would increase that number greatly and continuously, perhaps by an order or more of magnitude.

Example

> ## The Guillain-Barré story, part I: what caused the epidemic?
>
> In the 1970s, there was a sudden, sharp increase in the U.S. in the incidence of Guillain-Barré syndrome (GBS), a rare type of paralysis.
>
> Naturally, a cause was sought. Swine Flu vaccine had been recently developed and a large-scale immunization program was carried out. Investigators suspected the vaccine, and began searching for connections.
>
> They ran into immediate trouble because Guillain-Barré syndrome had lost its identity during the coding process, when it was dropped into the category called "Polyneuritis and polyradiculitis." Since retrieval was via the code, the investigators could only find out whether there were or were not any cases in this group, not their specific diagnoses.
>
> The needed specificity could only be determined by consultation of the original medical records, a task which would have to be carried out wherever the records were filed — that is, in each of thousands of individual hospitals, a task so enormous that it was never undertaken.
>
> As a result of this experience, Guillain-Barré syndrome thereafter was given its own category, 357.0, in *ICD-9-CM* (and in *ICD-9*, its parent volume from WHO). But most diseases and diagnoses have not been so fortunate. And of course, this measure was taken only after the pig had left the pen.

The lack of specificity in coding is surprising, an aberration from the detail we demand elsewhere in clinical records. Drug administration, for example, is recorded as to the specific drug (not a group, such as antibiotics), along with its dosage, administration schedule, and duration of treatment. Under some circumstances, we can even find the manufacturing batch of the drug.

With patient age, we record the date and time of birth. Immediately after birth, age must be known to the minute, a bit later to the hour, then to the day, and only considerably later, to the year. It would be almost useless to record only the decade of a person's age.

Example

The Gulf War syndrome

In 1992, following the Gulf War, veterans complained of symptoms which they attributed to their war service. Much effort has been expended in an effort to decide whether or not there is actually such a condition, commonly called the Gulf War syndrome (or Persian Gulf illness).

Because of the medical debate on the issue, and because of the limitations of the coding system, no code has yet been offered for it (as of January 2000). Instead, coders are directed to transform the term Gulf War syndrome to the code for "Late effects of war" plus a second code to record the symptoms, e.g., "fatigue."

It will never be possible to reconstruct the cohort of persons who have presented with this possibility.

Lack of detail presents problems for both patient care and secondary uses.

Category Coding and Patient Care

In our traditional paper-based records, the exact diagnoses are recorded by the physician, either by writing them directly or by dictating and having them transcribed. The paper record can readily be consulted.

When electronic medical records replace the actual, detailed diagnosis with a category code, only that code's label is retrievable. And often the EMR offers only codes "immune" to challenge in the payment process. In these EMRs even the original medical record would not have the actual diagnosis — the clinical detail would be lost forever.

Example

Category coding "cyst of the pleura"

As an example of the this loss of information by category coding, "cyst of the pleura," a diagnostic term which labels a "clinical entity," is put into a category which transforms it into "Other diseases of the respiratory system, not elsewhere classified" (code 519.8). If this code were the total diagnostic information in the individual patient's record, as it might be in some electronic medical record systems, it would be of almost no help to the physician.

There are over 200 other categories of respiratory diagnoses — the physician would have to consult nearly 30 pages in *ICD-9-CM* to know what it (code 519.8) wasn't, and he would still not know what the patient's diagnosis was. And if someone wanted to search records to find patients with cyst of the pleura, the category code would return only whether or not there were any patients which fell into the "waste-basket" group where it would have been filed.

The developing electronic medical record (EMR) systems typically record only category codes. This diagnosis would, therefore, be absolutely unretrievable in a typical EMR, unless the physician had taken the time to record additional "comments" — and these would have to be laboriously searched.

Category Coding and the Bigger Picture

Every conclusion we reach from statistics developed from medical records will be futile if we gather only untrustworthy or useless information. We must make sure that the records tell the truth about the exact problems presented by the patients and give adequate detail about the care given. Without correct input, it will be meaningless to attempt to assess the successes and failures of our care, to accurately picture health and illness in the population, or to determine the resources needed to maximize health in the community.

Flaw 3:   The Codes We Use Are Ambiguous

Classifications change, and so do their categories and the contents of the categories. Biomedical progress is such that these changes cannot be avoided. Causes of diseases are elucidated. New diseases appear.

Progress in our knowledge of genetic abnormalities is an excellent example. In 1975, *ICD-9* provided 186 categories, nine of them for chromosomal abnormalities. In *ICD-10* (published in 1992, prior even to the vast explosion in knowledge in this field), the category number had grown to 709 categories, with 77 allocated for chromosomal abnormalities. No one has attempted to estimate what the counts would be if the classification were to be revised in the year 2000.

Why Category Codes Have No "Fixed Meaning"

As categories change, their "code" numbers often change with them. The categories are numbered (are given category codes) for the purpose of putting them in the sequence demanded to make the classification orderly; the codes are actually "sorting" numbers. Naturally, they change when new sorting and sequencing demands it — it is no surprise that the same category codes are used for categories with different labels, different contents, or both.

Background	**How classifications are created**
	The creation of a classification, say of diseases, is done by an "author" following a schema. For example, the author decides that the desired sequence is: (1) infectious diseases, (2) cancers, (3) metabolic diseases, and (4) injuries. Here, these numbers in parentheses are the same thing as category codes. If a category for obstetrical conditions is then added, and the author thinks it belongs in the middle of the list, it may become number (4), which displaces injuries into being number (5). Neonatal conditions probably should follow the obstetric, and become number (5), with injuries now number (6). We have taken these sorting (sequencing) numbers to use as our codes — and so the codes change as the schema changes.

"Leaving Room" Doesn't Work

The fact that there are inevitable changes in classifications is recognized and anticipated, so designers of classifications postpone the periodic major change by "leaving room" for new things. But this can't handle the kind of unpredicted explosion seen in genetics, for example, let alone changes in thinking as to how the various kinds of entities should be grouped. AIDS was first thought to be (and classified as) a disease of the immune system. Later it was moved into the infections disease section of the classification. Never has "leave room" provided a permanent solution to the "space" problem, nor has it solved the problem of the need for outright changes in where, in the schema of a classification, a given entity belongs.

Background   **"Decennial" revisions of *ICD***

ICD is intended to be revised every ten years, but this time frame has not been generally followed. For example, it was 17 years between *ICD-9* and *ICD-10*.

However, modifications are introduced *each year* in *ICD-9-CM* in the United States. Although they are relatively few, their effect is not trivial.

Annual modifications introduced in October, 1998, for example, added 81 new codes to the roughly 13,000 codes in *ICD-9-CM*. Of these 81, 30 are "V" codes, added to the chapter entitled "Supplementary Classification of Factors Influencing Health Status and Contact with Health Services." (Some insurance carriers do not recognize V codes, although Medicare allows a few of them to be used.) Fifteen codes were deleted.

In describing these changes, a coding advisory publication warned the users to immediately make changes in their coding reference materials, but that carriers might vary in their dates of implementation. But of course, not all who should do so will even read the modifications list.

Trails Are Lost

It is impossible to maintain an information trail from one classification to another. Data once aggregated cannot be disaggregated. Statistics developed under one classification cannot be fairly compared with another, unless the grouping is so broad as to be of little value for most purposes — as, for example, "cancer" or "heart disease" or "injuries."

Example   **The Guillain-Barré story, part II: how big was the epidemic?**

Guillain-Barré syndrome (GBS) is not a reportable disease, so another source of information was sought. Its victims are invariably hospitalized, and a poll of hospitals was suggested as a method to to quantify the actual situation. Had there been an actual increase, and, if so, how large was it?

At the time, the code for classification of Guillain-Barré was *ICD-8* code 354.0, "Polyneuritis and polyradiculitis." A reasonable assumption might have been that changes in the size of the group of cases in this category would be a strong clue that the incidence of GBS had increased, although it would still have been necessary to "look inside the group" to be sure.

But prior to 1968, the classification in use was *ICD-7*, in which code 354 meant "migraine." After 1978, code 354 meant "Mononeuritis of upper limb and mononeuritis multiplex" *(ICD-9-CM)*.

It was impossible to determine *with any precision* the incidence of the syndrome prior to the perceived increase, because there was no inherent way to tell which generation of a given classification had been used for coding — the codes all look alike. A coder could, without detection, have simply continued to use the 7th Revision even after the 9th Revision appeared.

In fact, the senior author learned that one developed nation had simply skipped the 8th Revision of *ICD* in its national statistics, going directly from the 7th Revision to the 9th (in violation of the international treaty to which it was a party). One can only speculate on the undetected effects of this violation on any international statistical comparisons in which it was included during that decade. For example, was its neonatal death rate really that high? Or were we comparing apples with oranges?

Flaw 4: Our Single Classification System Can't Serve All Needs

At present, because we are using only category codes, we are restricted to using only one diagnosis classification for all purposes. But a single classification can't serve all masters. It is much better to use classifications specifically tailored to their purposes, for example, for billing, evidence-based medicine, policy making, planning, epidemiology. Plus, a researcher should be able to custom-tailor data collection to get the optimum case grouping for the study.

Background

Purposes of *ICD*

ICD originated as simply a classification to serve a single purpose — to present statistical comparisons of mortalities of nations for public health purposes. The first expansion, still for public health, was to include morbidity, which meant adding pigeonholes for non-fatal conditions and events.

Even these early uses of *ICD* reflected competing demands on the classification: was the purpose to classify the causes or the effects of processes? Infections and trauma, especially, were of concern because they often could be prevented — an argument for the causes. Infections could be classified by organism or by disease. For trauma, an "External Cause" chapter was provided, so that an injury could be classified under both its physical effects and its external cause.

Then came hospital indexing, followed by efforts to make *ICD* useful for a wider array of activities, such as quality measurement, billing for care, establishing health policy, studying office and ambulatory care, facility planning, and evidence-based medicine. Not only did these changes in the organization and content of the classification complicate the construction of and learning to use each successive generation, but they also made the product — the classification itself — less useful for *any* of the different purposes. Common sense would suggest that a classification for billing would have different attributes than one for quality assessment, which in turn would differ from one designed to compare health and healthcare among nations.

Using Only One Classification — and Coding Process — Has Enormous Consequences

If we stick to only one kind of coding — category coding — we must change the entire system periodically, with serious results. The effects of making the change are far greater than most realize:

- Information quality slumps

- Continuity is lost

- Large amounts of money are spent

Background | **ICD coding in the United States**

More than half a dozen published classifications, based on three generations of *ICD*, have been used in the United States since we first used category coding, which began with a few pioneer hospitals using modifications of *ICD-6* in the mid-1950s. In addition, for the past twenty years there have been periodic "minor" changes.

WHO published *ICD-7* in 1955 and the United States Public Health Service's adaptation for indexing hospital records and operations (PHS 719) went into use in 1960. *ICD-8* was published in 1967 and the two competing clinical modifications, *ICDA-8* (*ICD Adapted for Hospital Indexing*, United States Public Health Service publication 1693) and *H-ICDA* (*Hospital Adaptation of ICD*, Commission on Professional and Hospital Activities) appeared in 1968. As noted, *ICD-9* (1975) led to *ICD-9-CM*, put in use in 1978. *ICD-10* was published by WHO in 1992, and its clinical derivative is now essentially completed (although not yet implemented).

Information Quality Slumps

Decisions based on faulty information are one serious result of periodically changing classifications. With our present, single-code coding system, a change from one classification to another causes a serious deterioration of information quality during the changeover period, deterioration which typically lasts two or three years.

The introductory period of any new classification creates less accurate information, because any new process has to be learned and corrections made in light of actual experience. Less apparent are the problems of timing of the adoption of the new system. In the hospital, for example, are the new codes to be used for patients on the basis of their admission or their discharge dates? Individual institutions will be ready for the change at different times.

Intermediaries and carriers have similar readiness problems. Their solutions and responses are difficult or impossible to police or trace. In the 1960s some carriers, for example, had not allowed for enough digits in the diagnosis fields in their databases for the longer codes used by *ICDA-8* and *H-ICDA* as compared with their predecessors. Without detection, some of the carriers and intermediaries simply truncated the incoming data (a situation similar to the Y2K problem, and to the problem noted above of the country which simply skipped one revision of *ICD*). Many of these problems have widespread impact.

Continuity Is Lost

Another substantial effect of a category coding change is on the research which can be conducted and the validity of inferences which may be drawn from the data. Vitally important longitudinal studies — those which span a time period including two or more classifications — often cannot even be attempted.

It is essential that we know what is going on in health and in healthcare over periods longer than the nominal decade between revisions of *ICD*. Are genetic defects really increasing or declining? We might be able to judge a question that broad if we could aggregate all the kinds of genetic defects. But we may be completely thwarted if we wish to pinpoint the specific kinds of defect which are increasing or declining. And the explosion in knowledge in this field compounds the issue.

Example

What happened with AIDS[a]

AIDS presents a real-life example of the longitudinal study problem, even within a single generation of the classification *(ICD-9-CM)*. AIDS was first described in 1981. There was no agency to which coders could turn in order quickly to find where to classify it so, in order to keep the paperwork flowing and reimbursement coming in, they simply made their own decisions — and we don't know *where* they put it.

In October 1982, an official coding decision was published in the Journal of the American Medical Record Association (of course, we don't know how many coders read this issue). The Journal gave, as preferred, code 279.19, "Other deficiencies of cell-mediated immunity," and thus it was put into a "waste-basket category" — not a classification specific to AIDS. Alternative codes were also given: 279.10, "Immunodeficiency with predominant T-cell defect, unspecified," and 279.3, "Unspecified immunity deficiency" (more waste-baskets).

Because of these classification decisions, prior to October 1982 retrieval of AIDS cases would have required searching countless classification pigeonholes, and even after that date, one would still have had to go back to all of the original medical records having any of the three codes suggested.

Unique coding for AIDS did not begin until late in 1986, when an addendum to *ICD-9-CM* was issued assigning the unused codes 042, 043, and 044 to AIDS — a jump from the " ... Immunity" chapter to the "Infectious ... " chapter in the classification. This addendum contained nearly five pages of instructions as to how to classify AIDS cases, AIDS-like syndromes, and HTLV-III/ LAV infections, taking into consideration various symptoms and "with" and "due to" relationships with other conditions. Further changes occurred two years later when the nomenclature of HIV infection and the diagnostic criteria were revised.

The delay in uniquely identifying AIDS in the data system was due in part to debate over just how to classify it, but also to administrative and bureaucratic factors — in the words of one nosologist, a "political/resource consumption quagmire."

a.   For more about this, see "Coding AIDS," page 263, and "The Definition of AIDS," page 271.

Large Amounts of Money Are Spent

Making the change is very expensive.

Outside the immediate healthcare setting — hospitals, clinics, physician's offices — a sizeable industry has grown up for teaching and supporting healthcare coding. A new classification requires this industry to develop training materials and training facilities, and prepare consultation and reference services. New coding software for use in clinical sites must be written, installed, taught, and supported. A tremendous amount of resources go into this (raising the costs of coding and, therefore, of healthcare).

Then there are far-reaching effects for the coders themselves. Replacing one entire classification with another requires many steps. Preparation of the coders usually takes time away from productive work during the educational process. Meanwhile, the daily coding with the old system must go on. Something must be compromised. There is an inevitable decline in productivity as familiarity is being gained in actual coding.

And perhaps greatest of all, the change disrupts the reimbursement/ payment system; this is discussed further below.

The Solutions: Living With "Code-Dependency"

Solution 1: Support the Truth

✗ *Response to Flaw 1,"The System Encourages Distortion of Information"*

It's time for our society and the healthcare industry to support and encourage the truth.

We have to set up the reimbursement system in such a way that frankness is not "punished." It is essential that payment accurately covers necessary care, so that no one is tempted to "fudge" the information. People should be rewarded for doing the right thing.

Measures taken to "ensure" honesty — such as the federal regulations requiring specific information supporting payment — must be carefully considered. First, are they really necessary? If so, how can the situation best be handled so as not to perpetuate the very "evil" we're trying to avoid?

These are difficult problem areas, but they must be addressed.

Luckily, the other constraint on information — technology — is much easier to tackle. We can design the electronic medical record so that it does not force expedient codes at the cost of information distortion. We can find ways so that, in fact, we get much more, and much more accurate, information than ever before. The other solutions proposed below will directly contribute to our meeting this challenge.

Solution 2: Introduce "Entity Codes" to Capture Detail

✗ *Response to Flaw 2, "The System Can't Capture Enough Clinical Detail"*

Flaw No. 2 — lack of clinical detail — is due to the fact that we presently have no way to capture individual diagnoses in our code-dependent system. Since retrieval of clinical information for both patient care and secondary uses is almost exclusively via codes, it should be clear that, if clinical entities such as exact diagnoses are ever to be retrieved, the clinical entities themselves must be coded.

We need to add to our medical records a feature called "entity coding." Entities are defined as the "most detailed information available" — for example, diagnostic entities are the exact diagnoses as recorded by the physician. If the diagnostic entity is as crude as "heart disease," so be it.

If the record contains anatomic detail as to the branch of a coronary artery involved in an occlusion, that level of detail is also an entity.

Entity coding tells us what the original diagnoses are, and does it with permanent, unalterable codes which, when decoded, give us the physician's statements verbatim.

Implementing entity coding requires adding a new "front end" to our medical record system to incorporate the necessary detail. A master database of clinical diagnostic entities and codes is needed, and the medical record information system must be modified to properly accommodate them.

The "Entity Coding" system must have the following essential features:

- The database must contain all diagnoses, no matter how long the list.

- There must be only one master database (list) of entity terms and entity codes for each type of information (diagnoses, for example). Competing lists would defeat the entire purpose.

- Each diagnostic entity must have its own permanent, unalterable, never-to-be-reused code.

- Each code must be identified, just as the category codes will be identified, to show it is an entity code (this might be as simple as "IHEC-", for "International Healthcare Entity Code").

- The system, once begun, must remain permanently available.

- Entity codes must be instantly available to any coder.

We don't have an entity coding system yet — the tool has not been built. A master database of entity codes must be compiled. Software must be written, and technical issues resolved, so that entity coding can work. "Someone" must create and service the entity coding system. For lack of a better word, let's call this institution the "secretariat."

The first job of the secretariat would be to establish the master diagnosis entity database. Populating it would initially be done by simply taking the diagnostic terms found in the various classifications in use (*ICD-9, ICD-9-CM, ICD-10, ICD-10-CM, SNOMED,* MeSH, NHS Codes, and others), and from textbooks and standard publications as has been done with its Unified Medical Language System (UMLS) by the National Library of Medicine. Several hundred thousand terms would probably result from such an initial search. This starting list would be relatively easy to compile, and it would be expected to handle a very high percentage of the demands.

Once initially populated, the master database would simply grow by acquisition of new terms as they appear in the literature and as they are presented to the secretariat by coders requesting entity codes. Each diagnostic term encountered would automatically be an "entity," with no argument. It would be entered in the master entity database, and it would be given its own unique, permanent "entity code." This would essentially be an accession number (the next number).

It is essential to capture the language used by the clinician, which of course varies with the physician's medical school, graduate training, cultural background, and geographic area of practice. Biomedical progress is often enhanced by the fact that various investigators and research centers use their own terminology, reflecting subtle differences in concepts. And history tells us that, except in highly controlled and motivated situations (such as in academic medicine and specific research projects), the clinician cannot be constrained to use a "prescribed" language.

No one should even *try* to tell the physician (or patient, or anyone on the team) what to say. The entity code must be essentially just an accession number. No effort should be made to decide whether or not the term is the "preferred" term, a controlled term, a synonym, an alternate spelling, a new entity, or even whether it is a "legitimate" term at all. The secretariat should simply capture the terms actually used in medical records and assign codes to them. It should not make judgments about them.

To compromise on this issue and expect entity coding to change the language actually used in healthcare would, we contend, prove fatal to its implementation.

Background

The language of healthcare can't be "prescribed"

Attempts to control clinical language — for example, that of the American Medical Association with *SNDO*, and later with its "Current Medical Information and Terminology" — have been abandoned. Other "languages," such as *SNOMED*, have never been widely adopted except within such settings as the pathology laboratory — and even here the changes in codes with successive generations of *SNOMED* have been frustrating.

However, SNOMED's "compromise," the provision of a module entitled "Diseases/Diagnoses," is being offered by some vendors of electronic medical records as an answer to the specificity problem. But that module offers (1999) only about 41,000 terms (and 4,000 of these are for veterinary use only). This isn't even close to the hundreds of thousands of terms used in real clinical life.

At the same time the master database is being created, we can prepare the medical record — both paper and electronic formats — to incorporate tagged entity codes, as well as tagged category codes.

Today's medical records, electronic as well as paper-based, are only prepared to handle, as codes, the category codes (dictated by reimbursement). In the case of paper-based records, these codes are recorded for transfer to the bills. In the EMR, there may be only the codes, without any supporting language. (Except as that language is generated "in reverse," because the computer knows what the label is for the code recorded, and it can print that, or a truncated version of it to fit the space allowed. Truncation usually, of course, further distorts the meaning.[4])

System designers for both paper-based and electronic records will have to accommodate the needed flexibility of input. This requires physical space, in both the paper-based and electronic records — but this is a technical problem which can be solved. In the individual medical record, there is likely to be essentially a one-to-one correspondence between a

---

4. For example, the record contains the code for "Meningitis due to gram-negative bacteria not elsewhere classified." What it prints out may look like "MENINGITIS DT GR-NEG NEC."

given entity and the category into which it is to be classified. The fact that a category may contain ten or a hundred entities does not mean that each patient has that many entities; the likelihood is that one patient has only one entity belonging in one category. Thus the additional space demand in the medical record to accommodate entity codes would be minor. In any case, room is no longer a problem in this age — see "The Luxury of Space," page 312.

The other major task is "deployment" of the codes (and coding system). This will initially involve publicity to announce the concept, question-and-answer type sessions, and then specific education and training for those using the system.

Finally, getting the codes to those who need them will be almost a "snap." Access to the master list can be in hard copy and CD-ROM. Terms not available in those formats could be sought via an "800 number" or the Internet (where, on a web site, the list is updated in real-time). Instant response is possible because either the entity would have been encountered earlier, in which case it would already have its code, or it would be accepted and given its code without any delay, since the code will be just the next available number on a list of code numbers (it has no inherent meaning).

Background   **Why category coding can never be updated immediately**

In today's category coding system, there is nothing resembling an instant response service for answering coding questions. When an entity new to the system (or a configuration of entities for which there is no precedent) is encountered, an "official ruling" often takes months or years (see the examples of AIDS, page 24, and Gulf War Syndrome, page 17).

And of course, with category coding, the decision is *where* to put the new entity along with others. Rarely is an entire new category offered for a newly encountered entity.

Entity coding does not require a decision on the classification of an entity before it can be coded and placed in the information system (both in the original medical records, and in the secondary records derived from them). Classification decisions require a *separate step*.

Of course, coders will have to learn the new "front end." But entity coding has a distinct advantage over category coding. To do category coding, one must learn to classify — a process requiring a good deal of knowledge, training, experience, and judgment. With entity coding, the coding process — substituting a code for a term — is essentially as simple as looking up a telephone number or calling for directory assistance. Of course, computers will be immensely helpful in looking up codes.

Over time, we may expect the health information system to evolve to the point where the category coding (the classifying process) is also delegated to the computer. The computer would take the entity codes for a given case, pick up the other information needed from the rest of the medical record, and classify the case. Classifying would become more uniform, and costs would be lowered. Most importantly, health information professionals — not having to deal with the "morass" of coding anymore — would have the time to practice their profession, concentrating on the *uses* of information.

Solution 3: "Tag" All Codes

✗ *Response to Flaw 3, "The Codes We Use Are Ambiguous"*

It is time to add to every code in all our code series, both those series coming from classifications and from the entity code master lists, a key which tells:

- The name of the "code series" to which it belongs, e.g., *ICD-9-CM*, *ICD-10*, "International Health Entity Codes" (IHEC), etc., and

- The specific version of the classification, e.g., 1997 modification, and

- Any further correction or modification of the series.

Once a category code is combined with its key, that "key + code" *combination* will become unique, and we will always be able to accurately decode it. To illustrate:

With the *ICD* series, the key would tell at least

ICD + Revision Number + "Edition" (e.g., U.S. Clinical Modification) + Version Number (e.g., "1998") + Perhaps, to cover errata, "corrected"

Thus keys could have solved the swine flu vaccine incidence problem in the earlier example, in which the investigator was trying to find at least which category would contain the condition. The "key + code" combinations would have uniquely identified each category. See "Tagging Healthcare Codes," page 309.

Permanently identifiable, unique codes is not a new idea. The number 355-34-3222 means nothing, until we prefix it with SSN to denote a social security number. If we order a car part, we usually have to give both the car model number (MN) and the part number (PN), and sometimes even the SN — serial number. And the book world depends on the ISBN number.[5]

Example	**ISBN numbers**
	The International Standard Book Number (ISBN) is used internationally to identify each edition (and within that edition, each binding) for every book published. It is a unique, unambiguous code.
	Each number identifies just one book, forever. The number includes "ISBN" as a prefix to denote the kind of code it is. This book is ISBN 0-9615255-2-5.
	The number itself contains some information about the book. For example, the number 0-9615255-2-5 tells us:

    0 - the book originated in an English speaking country
    9615255 - identity of the publisher
    2 - the particular title and edition (hard or soft cover) of book
    5 - a check digit, used to verify the accuracy of the other digits.

If an ISBN were — like a category code — not unique, it would be useless. We would not tolerate a book identification system, for example, in which an ISBN number pointed to a shelf (or shelves!) full of books rather than to a specific volume. Nor could we be expected to buy all the books on the shelf, just to get the one we really wanted.[a]

    a. For more about ISBN numbers as codes, see page 307.

---

5.   Since the initialism ISBN stands for "International Standard Book Number," saying "ISBN number" is technically redundant. However, it tends to flow from the tongue more smoothly that way, so we beg your forgiveness for this transgression and will occasionally repeat it.

Solution 4: Use "Tailored" Classifications

✗ *Response to Flaw 4, "Our Single Classification System Can't Serve All Needs"*

We must work toward changing the "system" so that cases can be allocated to more than one classification — each tailored to a specific use.

Especially important would be classifications truly appropriate for billing under a variety of circumstances, e.g., inpatient vs. home care. Our acknowledged problems with DRGs are primarily due to the compromises which had to be made in DRG design because of the limitations of *ICD-9-CM*, the only available source of input at the time the DRGs were created.

We can't have multiple classifications in the "system" today because, with the data already aggregated (into the *ICD-9-CM* categories), it can only be placed in broader, rather than different, groups. It can never be disaggregated so that one can start over and classify it another way.

With entity coded information available, however, each case can be coded to any classification, past, present, or future.

Example	**Wouldn't it be great if** …
	… we had classifications which were:
	(1) broad, to be used for public policy,
	(2) clinically-based, for evidence-based medicine,
	(3) designed for billing in various settings
	(4) etiologically oriented, for epidemiologic surveillance,
	(5) "product line" style, for facility planning,
	(6) custom-made for *your* needs ?

The Time Challenge

We must remedy flaws 2 and 3 — the "coding" flaws — as soon as possible. This will go a long way in helping to cure the other flaws. The remedies will require us to:

1. Tag all codes.

2. Develop and implement entity coding.

Obviously, creating and implementing these solutions, especially adding entity coding to the medical record and its information system, cannot be accomplished overnight. It will take several years and a good deal of developmental work.

In the meantime, there is pressure for the entire United States healthcare industry to "switch" from *ICD-9-CM* to the clinical modification of *ICD-10* (the latest *ICD* revision). The leading force spurring the change is that it would make it easier for the federal government to meet its obligations to use *ICD-10* in the international exchange of healthcare information.

Background

About ICD-10

The International Classification of Diseases and Related Health Problems, Tenth Revision (ICD-10) was published by the World Health Organization in 1992. By treaty agreement, the United States must submit certain statistics to WHO, using the standard classification. Most other countries also submit statistics in the same manner.

In creating *ICD-10*, WHO made far-reaching changes from *ICD-9*. The new classification has 13,000 codes, whereas ICD-9 had just 7,000. Also, *ICD-10* is physically much larger, as can be seen by the increase in the number of pages:

Volume	Pages in ICD-9	Pages in ICD-10
1: Tabular List	773	1,231
2: Instruction Manual	included in Volume 1	160
3: Alphabetic Index (Volume 2 in *ICD-9*)[a]	659	750
Totals	1,432	2,141

All category codes in *ICD-10* start with an alphabetic character, including "I" and "O," which are ordinarily avoided in codes because of their confusion with the numerals "1" (one) and "0" (zero).

Many conditions were added, others were moved from one Chapter to another, and some categories were modified. One-to-one correspondence between the categories of *ICD-9* and those of *ICD-10* does not exist. Only a concordance (which also does not exist) would permit tracking a diagnosis from one version to the other.

a. In *ICD-9-CM*, Volume 3 was devoted to procedures.

The Plan to Change

The United States National Center for Health Statistics (NCHS) — responsible for disease classification — determined that, like *ICD-7*, *ICD-8*, and *ICD-9* before it, *ICD-10* would have to be modified for clinical use in the United States. As a result, a new clinical modification was created *(ICD-10-CM)*.

Background   **A look at the new *Clinical Modification* for diagnoses**

ICD-10-CM, the volume the United States government has produced for diseases, is a huge expansion over *ICD-9-CM*. In October 1998, *ICD-9-CM* contained 12,628 categories. *ICD-10-CM* in its Internet draft has about 60,000 categories.

The bulk of the growth seems to have been in the widespread adoption of "combination categories." Combination categories use early computer theory in direct opposition to the more modern relational database theory (see "Database 101," page 172). For example, today's theory would have one table giving the site of a disease (e.g., stomach) and a second table giving the condition (e.g., ulcer). Conditions and sites would only be linked dynamically when appropriate. A search for "stomach" problems could be carried out with a single look at that code.

In combination coding, each condition for which site is important has the site put right *into* the code for the condition. Thus a search for stomach problems requires a search of every code where the element "stomach" might have been included in the code itself. It's hard to overstate the complexity this introduces into the coding process as well as the retrieval process. For example, look at the following from *ICD-10-CM:*

"S02.974" is the code for "Open fracture of skull and facial bones, part unspecified with subarachnoid, subdural, and extradural hemorrhage with prolonged [greater than 24 hours] loss of consciousness, without return to pre-existing conscious level, or when an unconscious patient dies before regaining consciousness, regardless of the duration."

Also, the Health Care Financing Administration (HCFA), responsible for procedure classification, determined that the U.S. needed a new procedure coding system. Neither *ICD-10* nor *ICD-10-CM* contain codes for procedures. So HCFA created the *ICD-10 Procedure Coding System (ICD-10-PCS)*.

Background

The new codes for procedures

The procedure *coding* system commissioned by HCFA — *ICD-10 Procedure Coding System* — is exactly that. It is not a classification, as was found in Volume 3 of *ICD-9*, and generally in *CPT* and HCPCS; nor is it related to the classification, *ICD-10*.

ICD-10-PCS is an extremely complete but complex system which, like *SNDO* and *SNOMED*, requires the coupling of elements from several modules to form the code (with its nomenclature) for a procedure. There are 7 lists (modules), each with a potential of 34 alphanumeric entries (unlike *ICD-10*, the letters "I" and "O" have been omitted to avoid confusion).

Not all of the 52,000,000,000 possible combinations have been used, but some 200,640 codes are available for the male reproductive system, 482,000 for the female.

"Appendectomy" in the Alphabetic Index leads to the Tabular List, where one finds it possible to code 9 kinds of diagnostic partial appendectomies, nine kinds of therapeutic partial appendectomies, and nine kinds of complete appendectomies: 27 in all. Code "0D8JCZX," for example, means:

0	=	medical and surgical
D	=	gastrointestinal system
8	=	excision (partial removal)l
J	=	appendix
C	=	transorifice intraluminal endoscopic
Z	=	no device
X	=	diagnostic

> Presumably this is a valid code, because the *ICD-10-PCS* "Working Paper" states that "combinations of characters that do not constitute a valid procedure are not contained in the Tabular List."
>
> Despite the huge number of specific procedures which may be coded, *ICD-10-PCS* still must rely on wastebaskets such as "other device" to accommodate future inventions; e.g., a new procedure which uses tiny robots does not have a code.

Plans are underway to implement both *ICD-10-CM* and *ICD-10-PCS* in the near future.

Our Reimbursement System is Threatened

The federal government has been planning to introduce *ICD-10-CM* within the next several years, possibly as early as 2001. The effects of this on our reimbursement system could prove disastrous.

Billing in the United States is "prospective," in that prices are established for groups of patients ahead of time. The grouping for hospital inpatients is called Diagnosis Related Groups (DRGs), about 475 groups into which patients are fitted, primarily on the basis of their *ICD-9-CM* codes. All patients within a given DRG have, by definition, roughly the same resource consumption, so each patient episode falling within the DRG should be worth about the same payment. To develop the proper values for DRGs, the resource consumption is approximated by the hospital cost.

DRGs were originally defined from cases coded with *ICD-8*, at a time before hospital reimbursement was dependent upon the prospective payment system (PPS). When *ICD-9-CM* was introduced, series of cases coded under *ICD-8* were also coded under *ICD-9-CM*. This "dual" information, along with the accompanying cost information for each case, was provided to the researchers and the effects on the dollar values of each DRG were studied. Significant differences were found, and the DRGs got new definitions based on *ICD-9-CM* rather than *ICD-8*.

Only after the comparative cost study under both *ICD-8* and *ICD-9-CM* was completed, and the necessary adjustments made, were DRGs given the green light to govern payment for hospital care.

Now there has been a dramatic change in the situation. Hospitals are critically dependent on DRGs as major determinants of their incomes. Medicare, Medicaid, and most other payers are dependent on DRGs in planning their expenditures.

Yet no plans have been announced to carry out a study such as was done with the *ICD-8* to *ICD-9* changeover, that is, to collect the same data under both classifications and redefine DRGs in order to maintain fairness to both the payer and the provider.

This information is critically important prior to the introduction of any change. There should be study of statistically significant numbers of the same cases coded to both classifications, the financial impact measured, and the payment groups redefined as necessary before the nation is asked to shift. Needless to say, such a study would be both time consuming and very costly. It would probably delay the introduction of the new classification. But without such a study, financial chaos is almost a certainty.

An Alternative Plan

As this is being written in early 2000, it is understood that *ICD-10-CM* may be required in the billing system beginning in 2001. This does not leave enough time to develop a system for entity codes and code identification keys, develop an entity coding system, fine-tune it in actual clinical care, and carry out the critically important studies necessary to recalibrate the DRG and other prospective payment classifications. Yet it is clear that in the long run, an entity-coded front end in the medical record itself and in the electronic records derived from it — plus tagged codes — will give far better information for all purposes. And having these in place would also make the transition to *ICD-10*, and future classification changes, far simpler. How can we resolve this apparent impasse?

✓ An alternative path can be followed; we don't have to rush into a change.

In anticipation of changing to *ICD-10-CM*, the National Center for Health Statistics (NCHS) has had a "crosswalk" — a conversion table from *ICD-9-CM* to *ICD-10-CM* — prepared. [6] This is intended to assist in classifying cases to the new system — and it could provide the solution to the "time challenge."

The implementation of *ICD-10-CM* is spurred primarily to make it easier to put the United States national healthcare data into *ICD-10* for international exchange of information. The *ICD-9-CM* to *ICD-10-CM* crosswalk could, with minimal effort, be reworked to convert from *ICD-9-CM directly to ICD-10 itself.* The new crosswalk would be both simpler and more accurate — it's always easier to move data into larger categories than into smaller. *ICD-10* has only 13,000 (larger) categories, about the same number as *ICD-9-CM*, while *ICD-10-CM* has much smaller categories (about 60,000 of them).

Thus when information coded to *ICD-10* is required, as to meet the United States obligations to the World Health Organization, the new crosswalk could be used to easily convert the data from *ICD-9-CM* (in which it is already coded) directly to *ICD-10*. And this conversion can be done at the federal level — so the 500,000 or so coders across the nation needn't be concerned with it.

The crosswalk approach would allow us to simply continue with *ICD-9-CM* for all billing and other reporting purposes — while we get ready to add entity coding and code identification keys. The equilibrium of the payment system would not be disturbed. Furthermore, the nation can get all its statistics into *ICD-10* categories much sooner than if we had to wait to change the entire input across the healthcare system.

This alternative plan would require the following steps:

To Buy Time:

- Rework the existing NCHS crosswalk so that the conversion is from *ICD-9-CM* directly to *ICD-10*, where the data are needed for international statistical purposes.

---

6. For illustrative pages from the *ICD-9-CM to ICD-10-CM Conversion* table, see page 300.

- Continue using *ICD-9-CM* in billing and as input to the various groupers[7] now in use. No system change would be required. Coders are already experienced. The payment system is in equilibrium between payers and providers.

To Develop Entity Coding:

- Mount a project to create the basic entity coding tool — the master database of entity terms and codes. This would require close collaboration and "beta testing" in real life clinical settings.

- Simultaneously prepare the medical record systems to carry the entity coded data. Computer-assisted encoding programs should find adding entity codes relatively easy — they must already "recognize" many of the entities as they decide their category assignments. Vendors of electronic medical record systems should welcome the additional information their products would provide their customers.

- Implement entity coding as rapidly as the healthcare system finds it desirable.

To Identify Our Data:

- Establish standards, including identifying keys, for *all* healthcare codes.

- Designate or create master code lists, coordinating with the keys.

- Agree on standards for creation, usage, and registration of codes (after the model of other uniform code systems).

To Be Ready for the Future:

- Undertake a study of the whole health information system in the light of current information technology and the opportunities which will be made available with the corrections we propose in this book.

- Study the needs and how best to meet them.

---

7.   "Groupers" are software programs used for putting cases into payment groups, such as DRGs, using *ICD-9-CM* and accompanying data from medical records.

Advantages of this "Alternate Plan":

This course of action would have several advantages:

- The federal government would be able to handle its international and other needs for information presented in *ICD-10* categories much earlier than if it had to wait for the changeover to *ICD-10-CM* throughout the healthcare system.

- We could avoid many of the data quality problems inherent in the break-in period of a category coding system change, the time during which the entire health information system is trying to adjust itself.

- There would be no interruption in the reimbursement system for providers and payers.

In fact, the healthcare system might avoid the costs of implementing *ICD-10-CM* at the coder level entirely, because once entity coding has "incubated," and standard healthcare identification is a reality, we may decide to take a different route. For example, it might then be feasible to develop a classification specifically designed for reimbursement, and other "tailored" classifications for such purposes as facility planning, establishing public policy, and contributing to knowledge for evidence-based medicine.

A Great Opportunity

The coming of *ICD-10* is serving to focus attention on our health information system, at a time such attention is sorely needed. It is also providing a wonderful opportunity to enhance the system. A system with entity codes as well as category codes can better meet our needs, and save money.

The addition of entity coding will allow us to comply with one of the basic principles of information management:

✓ Keep data in its most discrete form.

From the discrete "building block" it can then be aggregated in any desired way. Entity coding keeps discrete information discrete. Category coding, although essential for its purpose, can never adhere to this rule, because, by its very nature, it aggregates data. Once aggregated, data can never be disaggregated.

Entity coding will permit the electronic medical record to have the flexibility needed to accommodate a vast range of information, allowing it to live up to its potential.

Tagging both entity and category codes (with "keys") will permit us to comply with two other basic principles:

✓ Never change the meanings of the codes.
Be sure you can tell what the codes mean.

Even if a classification changes the meanings of its codes, the keys will ensure that the "key + code" *combination* will never change meaning, because it has become unique. We will always be able to find out what the tagged code means.

If we take advantage of the opportunity offered at this time, there is much to look forward to:

- Classifications custom-tailored for reimbursement under various circumstances would become a welcome possibility.

- Changes in international demands and in clinical knowledge reflected in succeeding generations of *ICD* would never distort the information in medical records.

- In a reasonably short time, a substantial saving in information management cost could be achieved.

- We can rely on a much sounder base of health information.

Our medical records can get back to their fundamental business of helping in medical care, and our national knowledge of health and healthcare can become trustworthy.

Section 2: History & Background

Medical Records, Coding, and Healthcare Classification

2

Primer on Medical Records

THE MEDICAL RECORD[1] is the basic "record of original entry" (a useful term acquired from accounting) for healthcare information. A medical record is a file which is created by a healthcare provider, as an integral part of care, for each patient who visits that provider.[2] When the record pertains to both the individual's health and to healthcare as well, and is a continuous record over a long period of time, it is usually called a patient record rather than a medical record.

The fundamental purpose of the medical record is to aid in the patient's care, in two ways:

Memory The physician and other caregivers have fallible memories. Even when there was only the single physician involved, it was impossible to remember exactly what each patient's problems were, what was done, and the patient's course, without a written record.

Communication As more and more individuals became involved in the patient's care — nurses, consultants, and others — the record became vital for communication among them. The continually increasing complexity of today's care makes this function ever more important. This communication need extends, of course, from one time period to another in the patient's life.

---

1. This is also called the clinical record, chart, and perhaps other terms. "Medical record" is used throughout this book for consistency. Most of the record, today, is on paper. A term has recently been coined to describe paper documents as opposed to electronic ones — "treeware."

2. A person often has several medical records — one for each doctor visited, hospitalization, emergency room visit, etc. The unit of time covered in a segment of the record is typically an office visit or a hospitalization. Medical records for a given patient (within a hospital or office) are linked together over time in order to provide continuity, and kept physically at the provider's location. When the patient moves, copies of those records are usually sent to the new providers (at the patient's request).

Formation & Contents

Specifications for the medical record depend to some extent on the setting where it is kept, but there are usually certain minimum requirements. The broad statement of the Medical Record Standard of the Joint Commission on the Accreditation of Healthcare Organizations (JCAHO)[3] is that the hospital medical record must contain

> ... sufficient information to identify the patient, support the diagnosis, justify the treatment, document the course and results accurately, and facilitate continuity of care among healthcare providers.

The standard then states specifically that each record must have:

- The patient's name, address, date of birth, and the name of any legally authorized representative

- The patient's legal status, for patients receiving mental health services

- Emergency care provided to the patient prior to arrival, if any

- The record and findings of the patient's assessment

- A statement of the conclusions or impressions drawn from the medical history and physical examination

- The diagnosis or diagnostic impression

- The reason(s) for admission or treatment

- The goals of treatment and the treatment plans

- Evidence of known advance directives

- Evidence of informed consent for procedures and treatments for which informed consent is required by organizational policy

- Diagnostic and therapeutic orders, if any

- All diagnostic and therapeutic procedures and tests performed and the results

---

3.   JCAHO is an independent, nonprofit, voluntary organization sponsored by the American College of Physicians (ACP), the American College of Surgeons (ACS), the American Hospital Association (AHA), the American Medical Association (AMA), and other medical, dental, and health care organizations. Its main activity is the accreditation of health care facilities.

- All operative and other invasive procedures performed, using acceptable disease and operative terminology that includes etiology, as appropriate

- Progress notes made by the medical staff and other authorized individuals

- All reassessments, when necessary

- Clinical observations

- The response to the care provided

- Consultation reports

- Every medication ordered or prescribed for an inpatient

- Every dose of medication administered and any adverse drug reaction

- Every medication dispensed to or prescribed for an ambulatory patient or an inpatient on discharge

- All relevant diagnoses established during the course of care

- Any referrals and communications made to external or internal care providers and to community agencies

Specific additional items may be required for clinical investigations, various insurances, Medicare, a health maintenance organization, peer review organizations, and others.

How Information Gets Into the Record

In most clinical settings, the patient record itself is still kept manually, as a paper document. The information in it includes:

- findings and observations (history-taking, physical examination, laboratory, x-ray, and other techniques)

- assessment and diagnoses

- care and treatments rendered

- patient's course and responses to treatment

Traditionally, physicians and nurses (and others authorized to make entries) simply write down their contributions on paper.[4]

Handwriting has the obvious disadvantages that it is slow to do, the information is locked to the page where it is entered, and it is difficult to read (especially when written by physicians — in fact, handwriting is often stated to be the best form of security yet developed).

Under many circumstances, especially in hospitals and group practices, dictation and transcription have replaced handwriting as the main form of data entry. These offer speed, legibility, and the potential for manipulation by computer.

Unfortunately, that potential is still far from being realized. Although technology for automatic indexing of the content of the narratives simultaneous with its transcription is widely available, it has been slow to be adopted for medical records.[5] As a matter of fact, often the dictation is only in machine-readable form while it is in transit between the dictation and a piece of paper to be placed in the traditional record; a machine-readable version may not be saved at all. The dictated material is usually retrievable only in document form, even though it may have been committed to storage on a CD-ROM or other electronic storage medium. The use of the computer in this manner has merely been an improvement on microfilming.

Form

Medical record information presently exists in two forms:

The "Original" Medical Record

This is the clinical record which is created by the caregivers. We refer to it as the "original" record to distinguish it from others forms, such as summaries, abstracts, electronic submissions, which take their information from the original record.

---

4.   Each time something is added to the record, it must be "authenticated" to show it is authorized and accurate. This is typically done by the signature (or initials) of the person making the entry.

5.   There is software available to manage information so that it can be continually indexed and instantly searched for text. See "Indexing of Text," page 68.

The original medical record is traditionally kept in a file folder, with pages of notes, paper copies of test results, x-ray reports, etc., each affixed to the folder by a metal holder. In many hospitals and offices, pages are inserted as they come in, with the most recent on top among documents of the same type, i.e., laboratory reports in one section, X-ray reports in another, and so on. Other providers use the organization of the "Problem-Oriented Medical Record" (POMR), a system developed by Lawrence Weed, MD, which collects the data pertaining to each of the patient's "problems" together so that the reader can see not only what was done but why it was done.

Paper records — especially of hospitalizations — can easily become several inches thick (and there may be several records, one for each separate hospitalization, even if the illness is the same). Today, very few providers keep the entire original record in electronic format. However, as the record becomes more and more digital, space will be saved (both in the record and in the hospital or office) and the organization of the record will not matter much, since software will take the reader directly to the necessary information.

The Medical Record Abstract

Today the "abstract" of the record — a "subset" or condensed version of the original — is created primarily to bill for the care rendered. In some instances, special abstracts are created for data banks. Such abstracts contain specific items of information, typically that necessary to identify the patient and the caregiver (at least in code), the source of the document (hospital, physician's office), the purpose of the care, the treatment, and the outcome. Often, this information exists only in coded form, and may be totally digital, except when bills and reports are printed out. At that time, the computer prints out a stored statement which translates the codes into human words, often severely truncated.

Abstracts should really be called "extracts," because they provide only selected, rather than summarized, information. Abstracts are created by the administrative branch of the healthcare provider, and are generally stored in the provider's electronic database. The people extracting information are typically not clinicians. They are usually in the medical record and billing departments of the hospital, clinic, or physician's office.

Uses of Medical Record Information

Primary Use

The *primary* purpose of the medical record is to assist in the care of the patient. All other uses of medical record information must be considered secondary. The key implication of this statement is that medical record design, paper-based or electronic, must first make sure that it helps in the care of the patient. The medical record must not be constructed with administrative convenience first in mind, or as a derivative of administrative paper work. (See more about this on page 244.)

Informed Shared Decision Making

There is a growing movement in healthcare called "informed shared decision making" (ISDM). With ISDM, physician and patient collaborate in making healthcare decisions for the patient. Together they decide on diagnostic efforts to be made and treatments to be used. The traditionally authoritarian role of the physician changes to one of consultation and advice, and the passive role of the patient changes to an active one, with the patient bearing increased responsibility for his or her health. Adjustments are required by both physician and patient, as are new tools. The information in the medical record is vital to the success of ISDM.

Physicians have known for years that patients were more "compliant" with their diagnostic and treatment programs if they understood the rationales behind them. A major obstacle to patient understanding was the "knowledge asymmetry" between the patient and the physician. This barrier is breaking down rapidly as the result of two informatics events:

- The development of computer software and other tools which put reliable information into the patient's hands, information which is specific not only to the disease and treatment but also to the individual patient. Examples include:

- Problem Knowledge Couplers®[6]
- Shared Decision Making® (SDM™) programs[7]
- CHESS®[8]

- Patients have virtually unlimited access to biomedical information (good and bad) through the Internet. Often the patient has read more deeply than the physician on her particular problem and the diagnostic and therapeutic options.

The nonprofit Health Commons Institute (HCI)[9] has been formed to promote medical care that uses computer-based information tools to improve collaboration between patients and health care professionals. Emphasis is given to the use of computer-based clinical guidance (not guidelines) and decision support tools that can continuously inform them with the best biomedical knowledge tailored to the patient.

---

6. Problem Knowledge Couplers® are Windows® based point-of-care information tools for identifying patient problems and risk factors, eliciting and recording patient findings, and considering and refining diagnostic and management strategies. The Couplers® are a product of PKC Corporation, a clinical software company located in Burlington, Vermont, which builds "knowledge engineering tools" for the healthcare community. Their website is http://www.pkc.com.

7. Shared Decision-Making® (SDM™) tools are produced by Health Dialog, which provides services and educational materials based on the concept of Shared Decision-Making® as developed by the Foundation for Informed Medical Decision Making. For example, SDM™ video tapes and CD-ROMs are developed to assist patients in medical decision making by providing them with specific information about their condition. The tapes are provided on a complimentary basis to members of participating health plans. They've also developed web-based support tools, self-care handbooks, and an online knowledgebase. Health Dialog's website is at http://www.healthdialog.com.

8. CHESS® (Comprehensive Health Enhancement Support System) is a computer-based support system designed to remove or reduce barriers to the information and support needed by people facing health crises or concerns. It is a project of the CHESS Research Consortium at the University of Wisconsin, Madison. http://chess.chsra.wisc.edu/Chess.

9. Based in Falmouth, Maine. Its website is at http://www.maine.com/hci.

"Secondary" Uses

The information in the patient's medical record is often referred to for purposes beyond care. Such uses include those which are still related directly to the *unique patient* and the care that that patient received.

- Billing for services rendered, providing the information necessary for payment of the bill, and substantiating the bill should it be questioned.

- Quality review. Medical records individually, and patterns of the care revealed by aggregating their data appropriately, are the source information for quality review.

- Legal defense. In case of litigation, the medical record, as the record of original entry, is essential to show the care provided to the patient, its nature, its effects, and the rationale for its employment.

Other, broader uses exclude identification of patients, and the information in the record is aggregated with other care information to get a larger picture of patients and their healthcare services and needs.

For example, a physician or institution may use medical record information for:

- Administration
- Clinical research
- Determining educational needs
- Facilities planning
- Staffing planning

On a greater scale, society uses patient information for a number of purposes, including:

- Clinical research
- Benchmarking of practice (determining standards of care)
- Epidemiology
- International statistics
- Public policy
- Healthcare financing
- Actuarial analyses

Health Information Professionals

The Medical Record Department

Every hospital has a special department dedicated to processing, keeping, maintaining, retrieving information from, and safeguarding medical records.[10] In some ways it's like the vault of a bank — customarily in a protected area of the facility, with extra precautions to protect the paper and electronic storage media from harm, such as by fire, water, or other catastrophe.

The medical record department is a beehive of activity. Records are physically created, dictation is transcribed, cases are abstracted, information is obtained, and reports are made for medical staff, administration, and others.

The titles of medical record professionals keep changing to reflect the increasing complexity — and demands — of the health information field. The "medical record librarian" of the past is no more. These days, it takes a team of health information professionals, transcriptionists, and clerical workers to run the department and to meet the demands of its many "customers" — patients, physicians, insurance companies, government, and more.

---

10. Clinics, physicians' offices, and other healthcare facilities also have the equivalent of the hospital medical record department, even if on a much smaller scale.

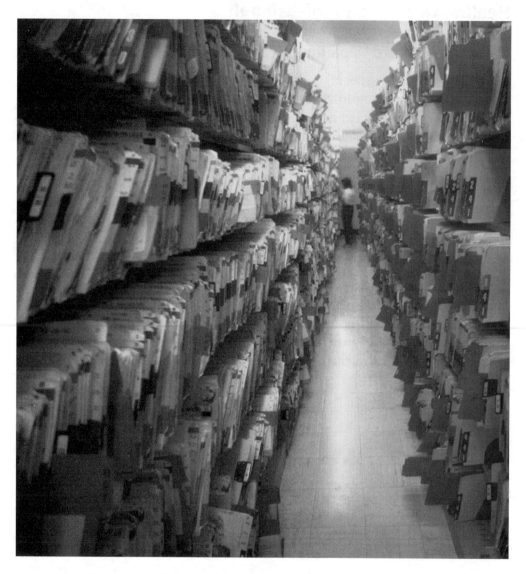

A traditional hospital medical record department. (Photo from Corel® Photo Studio.)

Health Information Administrator

The head of the medical record department is most often a "health information administrator" (HIA), but sometimes still called a "medical record administrator" (MRA).

The American Health Information Management Association (AHIMA)[11] describes the role of the health information administrator as

> ... providing reliable and valid information that drives the healthcare industry. They are specialists in administering information systems, managing medical records, and coding information for reimbursement and research. Health information management professionals are uniquely qualified to:

> - Ensure health information is complete and available to legitimate users

> - Code and classify data for reimbursement

> - Analyze information necessary for decision support

> - Protect patient privacy and provide information security

> - Enhance the quality and uses for data within healthcare

> - Administer health information computer systems

> - Comply with standards and regulations regarding health information

> - Prepare health data for accreditation surveys

> - Analyze clinical data for research and public policy

Registered Health Information Administrator (RHIA) A health information administrator who has been certified by AHIMA as meeting its standards in medical record science is called a "Registered Health Information Administrator" (RHIA).[12] An RHIA must have a baccalaureate degree in health information administration (HIA). AHIMA describes an RHIA as follows:

---

11. AHIMA (founded in 1928 as the AAMRL, American Association of Medical Record Librarians) is a national organization of registered record administrators and accredited record technicians with expertise in health information management, biostatistics, classification systems, and systems analysis. Definitions provided here are from AHIMA.

12. Prior to January 1, 2000, the title was "Registered Record Administrator" (RRA).

RHIAs are skilled in the collection, interpretation, and analysis of patient data. Additionally, they receive the training necessary to assume managerial positions related to these functions. RHIAs interact with all levels of an organization—clinical, financial, administrative— that employ patient data in decision making and every day operations.

In a recent membership survey, AHIMA found that more than half of the RHIA respondents were directors, managers, or consultants, with nearly 31 percent serving as health information management directors. Historically, most RHIAs have held the title of director of the health information management department of an acute care facility, but today other career opportunities abound. As patient records evolve toward computerization and as more entities such as third-party payers require health data, RHIAs benefit from a wide selection of roles in the industry. Information security and storage, data quality assurance, and advanced assistance to consumers with their health information are among the new domains.[13]

Health Information Technicians

The U.S. Department of Labor's *1998-99 Occupational Outlook Handbook*[14] projects "health information technician" (formerly "medical record technician") as "one of the 20 fastest growing occupations."

The "nature of the work" is described as follows:

Every time health care personnel treat a patient, they record what they observed, and how the patient was treated medically. This record includes information the patient provides concerning their symptoms and medical history, the results of examinations, reports of x-rays and laboratory tests, diagnoses, and treatment plans. Health information technicians organize and evaluate these records for completeness and accuracy.

When assembling patients' health information, technicians, who may also be called medical record technicians, first make sure the medical chart is complete. They ensure all forms are present and properly

---

13. From AHIMA's website, at http://www2.ahima.org/certification/index.html (12/31/ 99).

14. D.O.T. 079.362-014, -018. The number is from the *Dictionary of Occupational Titles* (D.O.T.), Fourth Edition, Revised 1991, U.S. Department of Labor. The D.O.T. is being replaced by O*NET, the Occupational Information Network, online at http://www.doleta.gov/programs/onet/.

identified and signed, and all necessary information is on a computer file. Sometimes, they talk to physicians or others to clarify diagnoses or get additional information.

Technicians assign a code to each diagnosis and procedure. They consult a classification manual and rely, also, on their knowledge of disease processes. Technicians then use a software program to assign the patient to one of several hundred "diagnosis-related groups," or DRG's. The DRG determines the amount the hospital will be reimbursed if the patient is covered by Medicare or other insurance programs using the DRG system. Technicians who specialize in coding are called health information coders, medical record coders, coder/abstractors, or coding specialists.

Technicians also use computer programs to tabulate and analyze data to help improve patient care or control costs, for use in legal actions, or in response to surveys. Tumor registrars compile and maintain records of patients who have cancer to provide information to physicians and for research studies.

Where they work:

Health information technicians held about 87,000 jobs in 1996. Less than one half of the jobs were in hospitals. Most of the rest were in nursing homes, medical group practices, clinics, and home health agencies. Insurance, accounting, and law firms that deal in health matters employ a small number of health information technicians to tabulate and analyze health information. Public health departments also hire technicians to supervise data collection from health care institutions and to assist in research.

Qualifications:

Health information technicians entering the field usually have an associate degree from a community or junior college. In addition to general education, coursework includes medical terminology, anatomy and physiology, legal aspects of health information, coding and abstraction of data, statistics, database management, quality assurance methods, and especially computer training. Applicants can improve their chances of admission into a program by taking biology, chemistry, health and computer courses in high school.

Technicians may also gain training through an Independent Study Program in Health Information Technology offered by the American Health Information Management Association (AHIMA). Hospitals sometimes advance promising health information clerks to jobs as health information technicians, although this practice may be less common in the future. Advancement generally requires 2-4 years of job experience and completion of the hospital's in-house training program.

Most employers prefer to hire Accredited Record Technicians (ART), who must pass a written examination offered by AHIMA. To take the examination, a person must graduate from a 2-year associate degree program accredited by the Commission on Accreditation of Allied Health Education Programs (CAAHEP) of the American Medical Association, or from the Independent Study Program in Health Information Technology that requires 30 semester hours of academic credit in prescribed areas. Technicians trained in non-CAAHEP accredited programs, or on the job, are not eligible to take the examination. In 1997, CAAHEP accredited 157 programs for health information technicians.

Employment Outlook:

Job prospects for formally trained technicians should be very good. Employment of health information technicians is expected to grow much faster than the average for all occupations through the year 2006, due to rapid growth in the number of medical tests, treatments, and procedures which will be increasingly scrutinized by third-party payers, regulators, courts, and consumers.

Hospitals will continue to employ the most health information technicians, but growth will not be as fast as in other areas. Increasing demand for detailed records in offices and clinics of physicians should result in fast employment growth, especially in large group practices. Rapid growth is also expected in nursing homes and home health agencies.

Registered Health Information Technician (RHIT) A health information technician who passes a credential examination and meets other requirements of AHIMA becomes a "Registered Health Information Technician (RHIT).[15]

Certified Coding Specialist (CCS) Another speciality within health information is the "coding specialist." AHIMA describes certified coding specialists as professionals:

> skilled in classifying medical data from patient records, generally in the hospital setting. These coding practitioners review patients' records and assign numeric codes for each diagnosis and procedure. To perform this task, they must possess expertise in the ICD-9-CM coding

---

15. Prior to January 1, 2000, the title was "Accredited Record Technician" (ART).

system and the surgery section within the CPT coding system. In addition, the CCS is knowledgeable of medical terminology, disease processes, and pharmacology.

Hospitals or medical providers report coded data to insurance companies or the government, in the case of Medicare and Medicaid recipients, for reimbursement of their expenses. Researchers and public health officials also use coded medical data to monitor patterns and explore new interventions. Coding accuracy is thus highly important to healthcare organizations because of its impact on revenues and describing health outcomes.

Certified Coding Specialist—Physician-based (CCS-P) A CCS-P is a coding specialist with "expertise in physician-based settings such as physician offices, group practices, multi-specialty clinics, or specialty centers."

Medical Transcriptionist

A vital member of the information team is the "medical transcriptionist" — the person who must listen to and transcribe dictated clinical reports. The *1998-99 Occupational Outlook Handbook* describes the work:

> Using a transcribing machine with headset and foot pedal, medical transcriptionists listen to recordings by physicians and other healthcare professionals dictating a variety of medical reports such as emergency room visits, diagnostic imaging studies, operations, chart reviews, and final summaries. To understand and accurately transcribe dictated reports into a format that is clear and comprehensible for the reader, the medical transcriptionist must understand the language of medicine, anatomy and physiology, diagnostic procedures, and treatment, and must be able to translate medical jargon and abbreviations into their expanded forms. Editing as necessary for grammar and clarity, the medical transcriptionist transcribes the dictated reports and returns them in either printed or electronic form to the dictator for review and signature, or correction. These reports eventually become a part of the patient's permanent file.

The Medical Transcriptionist Certification Program (MTCP) is the credentialing program of the American Association for Medical Transcription (AAMT). MTCP offers a voluntary two-part certification exam to individuals who wish to become certified medical transcriptionists (CMTs).

A number of vendors offer "outsourcing" for medical transcription services, so that hospitals can send dictation elsewhere for transcription.

Clerical Support Staff

Clerical support needs in a medical record department are substantial. For one thing, an enormous amount of photocopying now takes place in the medical record department — insurance companies often request paper copies of the entire record to verify a claim, and copies are still sent in paper format to consulting physicians, attorneys, and others with need for the patient's files. The medical record department must assure that such copies go out only with proper authorization. Original records are checked out by physicians, for review or completion; it is the medical record administrator's responsibility to keep track of these records, making sure that all records are completed and returned to the department.[16]

The Electronic Medical Record (EMR)

A strong effort has been mounted, in both the public and the private sectors, to replace the manually-kept, paper medical record with an electronic version. Technology offers great promise in improving medical care. Already, some electronic record systems can collect patient information from multiple sites, such as several hospitals and physicians' offices. The computer can present this information at the touch of a finger, with legibility and helpful dispay techniques. Time series of laboratory values, for example, can be shown graphically, abnormal values can be color-coded — features not possible with paper-based records. Patient education can be both triggered and provided within the sophisticated systems. Patient and physician reminder notices can be generated automatically. Medical care can be made much more efficient and less error-prone.

Despite its many real advantages, though, adoption of the electronic record has been slow, largely because it has required changes in the habits of physicians and other caregivers, and because the input methods have slowed down the care process (at least initially). Physicians have been loath to devote learning time. Time saved later in care — the promise of "delayed gratification" — has not been enough to overcome these

---

16. A big advantage of the electronic medical record is that it doesn't physically leave the medical record department, and in fact can be accessed by several people at once. And if insurance companies are willing to forego their paper copies, a lot of trees will be saved.

problems. Several techniques have been adopted in an effort to overcome these roadblocks, among them keeping the electronic record looking and feeling like the familiar paper-based record (and in so doing, failing to take advantage of many of the computer's capabilities) and providing simplified data entry.

What is an Electronic Medical Record?

"Electronic medical record" (EMR) does not have a specific definition, but is used loosely today to describe any medical record kept in digital form (on a computer), with constant instantaneous access via a computer terminal. The term "computer-based patient record" (CPR), while sometimes used synonomously with EMR, has become more distinctly defined.[17] In general, the term "CPR" should be reserved for the "ultimate" form of digital record which is the long-range goal (see the discussion below). For the range of "intermediate steps," which represent the state of computerization today, we shall use the designation "EMR" in this book.[18]

The official impetus for the development of electronic medical records was a study carried out by the Institute of Medicine (IOM) beginning in 1989 and completed in 1990.[19] The study report specifically recommended that:

---

17. And of course CPR, perhaps more commonly, also stands for "cardiopulmonary resuscitation."

18. *See* Andrews, William and Richard Dick. "On the Road to the CPR: XIX." *Healthcare Informatics*, May 1996, 50-XIX. This article defines the *electronic medical record (EMR)* as "an electronic, machine-readable version of much of the patient data typically found in today's PPR [paper-based patient record]. It contains structured and unstructured patient data obtained from both disparate, computerized ancillary systems and document imaging systems ... The PPR is the legal patient record." It then states that the *computer-based patient record (CPR)* is "a representation of all of the data found in the PPR in a coded and structured, machine-readable form. It incorporates a messaging standard for common representation of all pertinent patient data ... The CPR is rapidly becoming the legal patient record."

19. The Study was reported in *The Computer-based Patient Record: An Essential Technology for Health Care*, by Richard Dick, Study Director, and Elaine Steen, Study Officer, published by the National Academy Press, Washington, DC, 1991. A revised edition of the study (1997) contains not only the original volume in its entirety, but a new preface which discusses changes in the health care scene in the intervening six years, and also two new chapters: (1) a progress report on CPR development in the United States and (2) a corresponding chapter on the scene in Europe.

1. The computer-based patient record (CPR) become the standard for medical and all other records related to patient care.

2. The public and private sectors together form a Computer-based Patient Record Institute (CPRI) to "promote and facilitate development, implementation, and dissemination of the CPR."[20]

3. Research, research and development, and demonstrations should be carried out with federal, foundation, and vendor support.

4. CPRI should promulgate uniform national standards for data and security.

5. CPRI should review federal and state laws and make efforts to remove any statutory barriers to the CPR.

6. The costs of CPR systems should be shared by the users.

7. Educational institutions should enhance educational programs in computers, CPRs, and CPR systems.

The IOM report presented twelve "Gold Standard" attributes for the computer-based patient record (CPR):[21]

1. Offers a problem list

2. Has ability to measure health status and functional levels

3. Can document clinical reasoning and rationale

4. Is a longitudinal CPR and has timely linkages with other patient records

5. Guaranteed confidentiality, privacy, and audit trails

---

20. CPRI was in fact organized, in 1991, by a coalition of about 35 interested groups, which included the American Medical Association (AMA), the American Health Information Management Association (AHIMA), and the US Chamber of Commerce. Membership is for corporations only (there were approximately fifty corporate members in 1995); there are no individual memberships, although individuals may obtain the newsletter and participate in certain activities and work groups. Additional and updated information is available on CPRI's Internet home page, http://www.CPRI.org.

21. Dick, Richard, and William F. Andrew. "Explosive Growth in CPRs: Evaluation Criteria Needed." *Healthcare Informatics* (1995): 110-114.

6. Offers continuous access for authorized users

7. Supports simultaneous multiple user views into the CPR

8. Supports timely access to local and remote information resources

9. Facilitates clinical problem solving

10. Supports direct data entry by physicians

11. Supports practitioners in measuring or managing costs and improving quality

12. Has flexibility to support existing or evolving needs of clinical specialties

Another writer, Peter Waegemann of the Medical Records Institute, identifies more stages along the continuum from the paper-based to the computer-based patient record, using a slightly different terminology.[22] His stages (paraphrased) are:

Level 1: Automated Medical Records. In general, we are at this stage, with medical records in paper format, although as much as 50% of the information in them is created by computers.

Level 2: Computerized Medical Record System. This appears to be Level 1 with the addition of *scanned images* to the system (ultrasound images, for example).

Level 3: Electronic Medical Records. This is a step up, with the requirement that the system be institution-wide, and that it contain such elements as integration with practice management systems, "expert software" such as "clinical reminders," and programs for patient education.

Level 4: Electronic Patient Record Systems. The key distinction here is the definition of a patient record as having a wider scope of information than a medical record, having additional information about the person, going beyond the walls of the institution.

Level 5: The Electronic Health Record. This includes "a network of provider and non-provider settings with the patient at the center. The information is not based only on healthcare; it is based on a person's health and wellness." (Presumably the label CPR would be reserved for this stage.)

---

22. Waegemann, C. Peter. "The Five Levels of Electronic Health Records," *M.D. Computing*, Vol 13, No. 3, 1996.

Much progress has been made toward the goal of a "complete" CPR. Unfortunately, well over two hundred products (at last count) claiming this designation (CPR[23]) are currently offered and are being employed, but none of them fulfill all of the requirements. There is not yet consensus on standards for content, formats, security, etc. (see page 247 for more about health information standards). Meanwhile, vendors and investigators are going forward with a variety of approaches, including central storage of the medical record information with local access via the Internet — the "online medical record."

The potential inherent in EMR technology cannot be denied, but both implementation and adoption are progressing more slowly than technically possible. Some things are clear in the current scene: despite official pronouncements, the nomenclature and definitions are still in a state of flux, and the transition from the paper-based record to a totally computerized record will not happen in a single step by a specified date.

---

23. Or, confusingly, "electronic medical record" (EMR) or "electronic health record" (EHR) or "online medical record" (OMR), none of which have precise definitions or standards.

Electronic Record Systems Today

In general, the emerging electronic medical records do not substantially change the format of the traditional medical record. The record on the computer screen looks a lot like a paper record; it is essentially a replica of the paper record. There are folders with tabs on which the mouse can be clicked. The sequence of content is easily understood. The implicit assumption in the system design is that "changes can be made over time as needed."[24]

Electronic Input

In many hospital and medical information systems, information created in digital form throughout the institution is transferred to the medical record department and deposited in the medical record. For example, the admission process in a hospital initiates a good deal of the demographic portion of the medical record, while at the same time setting up the accounting records, sending notifications to various hospital departments, and so on. Some laboratory reports are automatically transmitted to the medical record, as well as to the nurses' station and to the physicians' offices. Writing prescriptions is frequently done on a computer, and thus the medical record entry and the prescription are created simultaneously. These documents and reports may be both in electronic form and also printed out as hard copy.

Images

Other portions of the record are harder to handle digitally. They include:

- Text, such as an X-ray report

- Graphic materials, such as an electrocardiogram tracing, a radiographic image, or a photograph

- Holographic documents, such as a handwritten note, or a required signature (when an electronic signature is not permitted or possible)

---

24. But will they be made? The more the users adapt to the system, the harder will be changes in the future, even though they may be necessary if the electronic potential is to be achieved.

The current trend is to have such documents digitized. This is done by optically "scanning" the document, using a device that looks like a small photocopier, and then storing it as a digital image.[25] Digitizing is an improvement over microfilming, in that the digital information is easier both to store and to retrieve.[26]

The "Paperless" Record

A commonly stated goal is the achievement of a "paperless" medical record. Those concerned about helplessness when all the information is in the computer are comforted to know that paper copies of the images, as well as the other contents of the EMR, are readily available on demand. In fact, most people agree that the EMR has, as a result of this demand, resulted in the use of more paper than before the EMR was introduced. Reasons for paper reproduction include the physician's and others' familiarity with the use of paper documents, quick local retrieval which is not dependent on a computer terminal, and general lack of confidence that the computer record will really be there when it is needed. Paper copies are also used for transmittal of information to others, as in the case of requests for consultations outside the electronic system.

"Paperless" means different things to different people.

The physician imagines it to work just like the paper record, but without paper, and to solve one paper-record problem which bothers him. That problem is that whatever he dictates for the paper record is not available for him to read for at least a day or two, until it has been transcribed. To get around this he also must make handwritten notes. In his mind, the magic of the computer should solve this problem. The computer should also substitute for his handwritten notes.

---

25. Vendors of the digitizing processes have adopted the word "imaging" instead of "digitizing," thereby creating confusion with the term "imaging" as used for years by radiologists for radiographic, ultrasound, and other diagnostic processes which produce images. Both disciplines now are obliged to use adjectives, e.g., "archival or document imaging" for the "scanning" process and "diagnostic imaging" for x-rays, etc.

26. The fundamental difference between microfilm and scanned images is that the former is still *analog*, while the latter is *digital*, which is inherently more maneuverable by computer.

Of course, he understands that the computer can later retrieve information by an electronic search. And he thinks that it will be easy to search for specific terms, e.g., diagnoses themselves (not their "*ICD codes*"). For this to become a reality, the information must be in searchable form.

The current vendors of electronic medical records, on the other hand, interpret paperless to mean that no paper records need be consulted. Thus, a medical record is "paperless" if it can be viewed entirely without reference to paper, even though its content may not be electronically retrievable. For example, a picture of the patient can appear on the screen, even a motion picture, but the content, meaning, can't be teased out with the computer.

Under either definition, we have not yet reached the paperless stage.

Accessing Digital Information

Presently, the physician's narrative in the medical record is almost always created by dictation. The dictation is then transcribed by medical record department personnel using a wordprocessing application, which may be part of a proprietary institutional information system, a dedicated word processor, or a personal computer. The transcription is then printed on paper and inserted into the medical record. In some instances, the electronic wordprocessing files themselves are kept as part of the medical record. Such files are amenable to being searched by the "find" features of the wordprocessing system. However, this is a laborious process, since one must repeat the search for each file in the medical record, or expend the effort to find out which particular file is most likely to contain what one is looking for.

Indexing of Text

We should design a medical record system in which the transcribed text, already in digital format, is indexed automatically by an indexing "engine" and then stored in a single infobase.[27] This single infobase would include all of this patient's medical record. This is important because one should be able to search through the entire medical record with a single search, if desired. The next step would be to group all of a provider's medical records into a single infobase, allowing instant information access across all patients with a single search. If this technology (available today) were used in medical records, all could be quickly searched for any information item at any time. For example, one could readily find all patients given a certain drug who also exhibited confusion as a transient finding, even though "confusion" might not have been recorded as a final diagnosis.

Even non-transcribed narrative (for example, handwritten or typed notes and reports) could be converted to digital format for indexing purposes. Such documents could be scanned optically and digitized with the use of optical character recognition (OCR) technology. Also, as voice recognition technology (VRT) matures, the caregiver may dictate into the medical record directly, bypassing the transcription process altogether. Video clips, with or without sound, may also be digitized. Once in electronic format, the information can be added to the patient's "infobase."

---

27. The term "infobase" was coined by, and has been used in relationship to a commercial software product called Folio Views®. This program, in widespread (but not always well-known) use for about the last decade, is built on an interesting technology mix that includes elements of a word processor, a database, text compression, and a variety of tools to organize, navigate, and publish large amounts of complex information.
    While the basic structure of an infobase is "record" oriented, and while it also supports "fields", the infobase is extremely 'free-form' compared to typical databases (hence the name). Virtually any kind of information can be stored in a single infobase, and no two records need have a similar structure, unless desired. Also, from the very beginning (long before the world wide web), infobases included hypertext capabilities to make their contents more useful.

Indexing of Image Content

The actual images of x-rays, ultrasounds, and other visual medical reports have long been excluded from the medical record. While the interpretation of the information, such as the radiologist's report, was inserted into the record, the original information was kept elsewhere — in the x-ray department or, eventually, in "dead storage" (off-site, and often difficult to access), or even destroyed (accidently or on purpose). Now, more and more, this information is being preserved by scanning it or otherwise converting it to an electronic (digital) image format. This allows compact storage and rapid retrieval of the total document, for example, a picture of the x-ray image for the specified patient, or a copy of the patient's electrocardiogram. "Telemedicine" is encouraging this digitizing of images.[28] Increasingly, it is possible to transmit them over the Internet in order to obtain consultation and advice on patient care.

Images must be indexed in some manner as to their content, in addition to their "ownership" (i.e., the patient to whom they belonged), if they are to have advantages over and above easy storage and quick retrieval — that is, if they are to be accessed to add information to our body of healthcare knowledge. However, very few documents stored as images today are provided with content indexing. Sometimes "exception indexing" on the basis of the content, such as "unusual chest abnormality" or "case for Grand Rounds," is done manually as an extra step, but this approach is rare.

Designing the EMR for Patient Care

See "Optimizing the Electronic Medical Record," page 237, for more about the electronic medical record, including problems, solutions, and maximizing the EMR as a tool for patient care.

---

28. Telemedicine is medical care provided through telecommunication when the patient and the caregiver are at separate physical locations, or when the patient and the primary caregiver are at one location, but a specialist or other consultant is at the distant location. It involves application of interactive audio-visual technology in patient care and education of physicians and other health care personnel, as well as the more traditional access to medical and related records. Sometimes called "telementoring".

3

Expression of Clinical Concepts

ONE THING complicating the attainment of a streamlined information system is the language used in healthcare: *there is no standardized language.* Words used by physicians, nurses, other healthcare professionals, patients, and their families and friends, vary greatly from place to place, and from person to person. The words used to express symptoms, diagnoses, and so forth are influenced by the geographical and political region, the schooling of the writer, the "world" language used (e.g., Spanish, Hmong), and local practices and customs. To fully understand the complexities of a health information system, one must be acquainted with matters of healthcare language.

Background

"Labels" in healthcare

Kerr L. White, former chairman of the United States National Committee on Vital and Health Statistics (NCVHS), in commenting on the thousands of different "labels" available to assign to health problems, stated:

"For our diverse manifestations of ill health and related suffering there are lay and colloquial terms, symptoms, complaints and problems, functional and feeling states, handicaps and disabilities, accidents, injuries and poisonings, fetal deaths and "voodoo" deaths, and finally diseases."[a]

a. From Lamberts and Wood, *Historical Introduction to ICPC, International Classification of Primary Care*, Oxford University Press, 1987, Chapter 1.

Types of Language

There are several "subsets" of language, shown in the illustration on the following page. While related, these subsets have important distinctions. Each will be discussed in greater detail below.

Figure 3.1 Expression of Clinical Concepts: Definition of Terms

"Natural" Language
All of the words *actually*
used by real people –
providers & patients

    Vocabulary
    All of the words *used* ——————— **Controlled Vocabulary**
    within a specific field   Those terms which
    or group   *a system* is permitted
        to accept

        Terminology   **Taxonomy**
        All of the words which ———— A terminology
        have a *special meaning* arranged per a
        within a field   particular *relationship*

           Nomenclature   **Standardized Nomenclature**
           A list of terms   A single nomenclature
           officially approved ————— *accepted and used* by
           for use within a field all in the field

                    Modular Language
                    Terms comprised
                    of *components* from
                    several universes

                    Preferred Terms
                    A list of *defined terms*
                    with medical criteria for
                    use of each term

                    Biomedical Concepts
                    A description and name
                    of each *concept* in a field,
                    arrived at by consensus

Illustration showing the sometimes subtle distinctions in the ways we "group" language.

Natural Language

"Natural" Language
All of the words *actually used* by real people – providers & patients

Language is a universe of expressions used to communicate ideas. "Natural language" as used here refers to the spoken or written words actually used by people in healthcare — by both those treating and those being treated. They will draw these words from their native language (e.g., English, Spanish, Estonian), the common language (e.g., English in most U.S. hospitals), their learning, their culture, their experiences, and their beliefs.

Natural language is how people express themselves, every day, as a natural part of who they are. When healthcare professionals record information in the medical record (whether directly in writing or by dictation), they will use their natural language to the extent possible. This is how they have learned to express themselves. Health professionals will use, in addition to everyday language, special language learned in studying healthcare. Patients will use their own natural language, which may include a vast vocabulary, or be very limited in ways to express their feelings and symptoms. They will not necessarily "speak the same language" as the caregiver.

Two assumptions must be made:

- It is probably *impossible* to stop people from expressing themselves in their own, personal, natural language. The failed efforts to control language in medicine are discussed later in this chapter.

- It is probably *undesirable* to deny the use of natural language. Language can be very rich, and expression of ideas can be very difficult. Any filter used will cause some information to be lost.

Vocabulary

"Natural" Language
All of the words *actually*
used by real people –
providers & patients

Vocabulary
All of the words *used*
within a specific field
or group

A vocabulary is a set of words used (or available for use) by an individual or group, or within a particular type of work or field of knowledge. Teenagers have their own (constantly changing) vocabulary, as do dockworkers, singers, and gardeners.

The contents of a medical record draws from a broad vocabulary, including all of the kinds of information carried in the system, from laboratory values to narrative text. Designing the electronic medical record to accept "objective" data — blood pressure, temperature, pulse rate — is relatively easy.

The tough part is the vocabulary used in the narrative contents of the paper-based record, especially that for the patient's problems, observations made, diagnoses recorded, and procedures performed — that is, the information normally expressed in natural language.

In fact, a special problem with health information is that, since some essential information is provided by the patient (who is typically not a healthcare professional and thus unlikely to be familiar with the healthcare vocabulary), the "vocabulary" of healthcare must necessarily expand to the entire sphere of natural language. There is a real hazard of the caregiver translating the patient's words into something the patient didn't intend. The patient's words should be preserved as faithfully as the physician's.[1]

Terminology

Vocabulary
All of the words *used*
within a specific field
or group

Terminology
All of the words which
have a *special meaning*
within a field

"Terminology" is the set of all the words (or groups of words — "phrases") which have a special meaning within a given field of knowledge. The words and phrases are called "terms."

Some terms will be exclusive to the field; for example, one is not likely to encounter "otorhinolaryngology" outside of the medical world. On the other hand, common words may take on special meaning when used within a specific field. For example, "typing" commonly refers to a way of putting words on paper; in blood banks, it means determining certain characteristics of a blood sample. "Risk" to many people has to do with taking a chance — but a financial expert sees "risk" as a special kind of chance, that of losing money. An insurance adjuster will see "risk" as the odds of having to pay an insured for a loss (a hospital "risk management" department tries to minimize this type of risk). A physician will see the likelihood to a patient of disease, injury, or death —

---

1. Interestingly, the physicians using the *International Classification of Primary Care (ICPC)* do translate the patient's problems into the *ICPC* category codes, but the conscientious doctors use the phrases, the problems as expressed in the *ICPC* classification, to negotiate with the patient and achieve better understanding of each other when they come to agreement. They also preserve the patients' words in the medical record. See page 473.

a person with high blood pressure, for example, is "at risk" for stroke or heart disease.

Terminology includes not only "proper" language, but also acronyms, eponyms, initialisms, abbreviations, and local jargon. Terminology varies regionally, and even varies within the same healthcare institution. It involves terminology from all of the disciplines which record information in the medical record — nursing, medicine, physical therapy, radiology, etc. Because of all these characteristics, healthcare terminology is an uncontrolled (and uncontrollable) set of terms. The set must include any term which is actually used, even if only locally and only for a few individuals, and whether everyone likes it or not.

Terminology	Taxonomy
All of the words which _____	**Taxonomy**
have a *special meaning*	A terminology
within a field	arranged per a
	particular *relationship*

A "taxonomy" is a terminology arranged according to the logical relationships of the terms with respect to a particular viewpoint, e.g., diagnoses would have different taxonomies — e.g., relationships —from the point of view of their etiology (cause) than their physiological manifestations (symptoms, for example).

Nomenclature

Terminology
All of the words which
have a *special meaning*
within a field

Nomenclature
A list of terms
officially approved
for use within a field

A "nomenclature" is a subset of the terminology for a given domain, discipline, or universe. It consists of names for the terms (or groups of terms) in a terminology. Each "name" is called a "nomen" (from the Latin for name). A nomenclature is created not by chance or usage, but by an official body or publisher of some kind which is seeking to organize (and/or standardize) the terminology.

A nomenclature is like a *classification*[2] of the contents of a terminology — every term in a terminology must find its home under one of the "nomens "[3] of the nomenclature. The nomenclature cannot ignore any of the terms in use as though they did not exist. In most classifications, this problem is handled by "categories" labeled "other." That solution won't work in a nomenclature, since a meaningless nomen would be created.

A nomenclature is a much more stable set of terms than the terminology, but it can change from time to time. There can be a number of nomenclatures within a given terminology, even if only one nomenclature is allowed in an individual setting for a given universe (such as diagnoses or procedures). There can also be two or more lists of words and phrases, advertised as nomenclatures, competing for the same universe. For example, today both *SNOMED*[4] and Medcin[5] are advertised (and sold) as nomenclatures for clinical medicine. Perhaps the closest to an "official" nomenclature in the United States is that used in the Unified Medical Language System (UMLS) of the United States National Library of Medicine[6] to express biomedical concepts.

Uniformity in Clinical Language

Biomedical progress often is enhanced by the fact that various investigators and research centers use their own terminology, reflecting subtle differences in concepts.

---

2. "Classification" is discussed more fully beginning on page 133.

3. A "nomen" is one of the pigeonholes of a nomenclature. In a classification, the pigeonhole is called a "rubric."

4. See "Systematized Nomenclature of Human and Veterinary Medicine (SNOMED International)," page 85. For more information about *SNOMED*, see page 429 in the appendices.

5. For more about Medcin, see page 497.

6. For more about UMLS, see page 425.

However, the variances in language usage, discussed above, make clear documentation of clinical information — and understanding of that information — seem almost impossible. So for years, many have sought to control the way that healthcare professionals use clinical language.

Controlled Vocabulary

Vocabulary	Controlled Vocabulary
All of the words *used*	Those terms which
within a specific field	*a system* is permitted
or group	to accept

Writers on the subject of the electronic medical record refer frequently to the desirability of (or the necessity for) a "controlled vocabulary," by which is meant a list of all the words and terms which the computer system would be permitted to accept; no other terms would be allowed.

One cannot argue with the simplicity which a controlled vocabulary would introduce into the handling of the information. Once it was established, all system design and computer programming could proceed smoothly, with no surprises.

But a controlled vocabulary appears to be an impossible goal, at least for the healthcare system as a whole. There are major problems in compiling it, maintaining it, and enforcing its use.

Compiling

The first problem with a controlled vocabulary is its construction or, better stated, its compilation. Presumably, it would have a term for everything which the medical record should contain. But, as experience shows, it would start out biased by who its authors were and what they thought the record should contain.

For example, for one such compilation on the market, the authors are all medical specialists — and at that, not all medical specialties are represented (e.g., family practice was not included). The rich nursing diagnostic terminologies are not included, nor are complementary medicine terms accommodated. In addition, no provision has been made for the inevitable use of local initialisms, abbreviations, and acronyms.

Picture the enormity of constructing the list. The nomenclature *SNOMED* (discussed below, page 85, and in the appendices, page 429) was the brain child of one man, a pathologist, who developed the first list just for pathology. Then he gathered individuals and groups as followers, and the list of SNOMED's contents gradually grew over decades. It sought to become the nomenclature for medicine. Today it embraces both human and veterinary medicine — plus occupations, chemicals and physical agents, and more. It will never be finished.

The Unified Medical Language System (UMLS) of the National Library of Medicine is an ongoing effort to corral and define all of the biomedical concepts in order that the various terminologies and nomenclatures can have a common link for their various synonyms and expressions. One of the reasons it was launched was that "the same concepts are expressed in different ways in different machine-readable sources and by different people." The purpose of UMLS is to make it possible to find textual, visual, and other materials in the Library's collection, no matter how the subject matter (concept) is expressed. By 1999 it had drawn its input from about 50 "source" vocabularies. Developing and refining UMLS, too, remains a continuing process.

Maintaining

Once a controlled vocabulary is established, there is a constant demand for its maintenance, improvement, adjustment, and expansion. It must be ready to respond instantly to

- New things
- New thinking

Both *SNOMED* and UMLS are ponderous and costly. The bigger they become, the slower they are to respond to demands for new terms and to changes in biomedical thinking. Yet healthcare is an ongoing system which cannot stop or even slow down — patients must be cared for and the business of healthcare must be paid for. Neither process can wait days or months or years for the answers to questions as to language (or codes) to be used.

For example, *Coding Clinic* for *ICD-9-CM* for 1st Quarter 1998 contains an inquiry as to how to code "Gulf War syndrome," a term in use since 1992. A long discussion is provided about the lack of agreement in medicine that such a condition exists. The reader is advised to code to "late effects of war" plus to whatever symptoms are presented (an inquiry in November 1999 obtained the same answer). Yet, obviously, the term "Gulf War syndrome" (sometimes called "Persian Gulf illness") is being encountered in medical records. Without its recognition in the vocabulary and coding system, our knowledge base is being deprived of a valuable tool for further study of the condition, and perhaps the patient is being deprived of the information in the medical record, as well. In fact, the ultimate determination of whether or not the syndrome exists, and if so, what it is, might well be made much sooner and more accurately if suspected cases were immediately recognized by the coding system.

Enforcing

There seems to be an assumption that the only places the controlled vocabulary would have an impact on the healthcare system would be at the input to and the output from the electronic system. It is as though the electronic system's demands would automatically and painlessly control the daily usage of language. Or that the language in the record need not particularly relate to that in the electronic system. But people can't be expected to change their patterns of expression to conform to the machine's demands, especially in the healthcare setting. And the people involved include the patient and other caregivers in addition to the physician.

- Individuals are loath to abandon their favorite modes of expression — after all, others understand what they mean now.

- Individuals with different geographic, ethnic, educational, and social backgrounds bring ingrained patterns of speech and expression which are virtually impossible to dislodge, "y'all."

The problems of enforcing the common language from one institution to another, and from one geographic region to another, are greater by an order or more of magnitude. So the third problem with a controlled vocabulary is — controlling people. No one has yet been able to do this successfully and consistently, in any context.

Standardizing the Meanings of Terms

Nomenclature	Standardized Nomenclature
A list of terms *officially approved* for use within a field	A single nomenclature *accepted and used* by all in the field

More important than "controlling" language, however, is to know the meanings of terms used — the meanings of terms must be discoverable. In the context of coding information, the "thing" (whatever the original information is) to be coded must be defined. The meanings of the entries in medical records should be clear and unambiguous.

Acronyms and abbreviations are an especially difficult (and somewhat terrifying) means of medical expression. Neil Davis has published a volume, now in its 9th Edition, entitled *Medical Abbreviations: 14,000 Conveniences at the Expense of Communications and Safety.*[7] Just one entry suffices to prove the point of the title:

"CS" is used to mean:

cardioplegia solution	congenital syphilis
cat scratch	conjunctiva-sclera
cervical spine	consciousness
cesarean section	conscious sedation
chest strap	consultation
cholesterol stone	consultation service
cigarette smoker	coronary sinus
clinical stage	corticosteroids(s)
close supervision	Cushing's syndrome
conditionally susceptible	cycloserine

---

7.   Neil M. Davis Associates, Huntingdon, PA, 1999.

And, as the title says, there are 13,999 more such examples.[8]

Davis also supplies an example of what a physician might actually write in a typical medical record:

> 64 YO WDWNWM BIBA admitted
> to CPETU c/o PND & DOE. TBNA in
> ER last wk for CP relieved by NTG.
> Prev Adm for PTCA 1986, NSRP
> 1992, & LC 1996. Dr Wynn CTSP by
> SMR.

And this sample doesn't even include the physician's handwriting ...

In the case of diagnoses and procedures, the goal is that the language used must describe the "clinical concepts." Further, these "things," themselves, must be accepted as concepts by those in the particular field. However, it is rare that there is complete consensus, even within a field, as to what each concept means.[9]

Be that as it may, the concepts must be defined, and their expression (it is argued) must be standardized. A number of attempts have been made to achieve such standardization, and in some fields, such as chemistry, standardization has been well worked out and is in use. Let's examine the situation in medicine.

---

8. Recognizing the pervasiveness and the importance of the "shorthand" problem, the Joint Commission on the Accreditation of Healthcare Organizations (JCAHO) has required each hospital to create, maintain, and enforce the use of a list of the abbreviations, acronyms, and initialisms permitted in the institution.

9. See "The Concept of AD/HD," page 266.

The desire to standardize medical language and its usage has been the stimulus for a number of vigorous efforts over the years.[10] Two paths have been followed in the efforts to achieve a uniform, healthcare-wide, nomenclature. Some have attempted to link the nomenclature to coding, some have not. The two paths have been:

- modular languages
- preferred terms

Modular Languages

Standardized Nomenclature
A single nomenclature
accepted and used by
all in the field

Modular Language
Terms comprised
of *components* from
several universes

Modular languages use components which are taken from different universes or axes and then linked together.[11] The following provides an excellent example:

> After years of hacking through etymological thickets at the U.S. Public Health Service, a 63-year-old official named Philip Broughton hit upon a sure-fire method for converting frustration into fulfillment (jargon-wise). Euphemistically called the Systematic Buzz Phrase Projector,

---

10. The term "standardized language" is often misused with reference to one of the "classifications," such as the series of International Classifications (*ICDs*). However, none of these volumes has ever been offered as standardized language or nomenclature, although they are frequently and erroneously referred to as such. They have always been labeled "classifications." Copies of the Introductions to *ICD-6* and *ICD-9* are included in the appendix for those curious about the actual intentions of the World Health Organization in their publication, and the methods followed in their creation; see page 364. A complete discussion of classifications begins on page 133.

11. For more about universes and axes, see page 133.

Broughton's system employs a lexicon of 30 carefully chosen "buzzwords".

The procedure is simple. Think of any three-digit number, then select the corresponding buzzword from each column. For instance, number 257 produces "systematized logistical projection," a phrase that can be dropped into virtually any report with that ring of decisive, knowledgeable authority. "No one will have the remotest idea of what you're talking about," says Broughton, "but the important thing is that they're not about to admit it."[12]

Figure 3.2 Broughton's Systematic Buzz-Phrase Projector

Column A	Column B	Column C
0 Integrated	0 Management	0 Options
1 Total	1 Organizational	1 Flexibility
2 Systematized	2 Monitored	2 Capability
3 Parallel	3 Reciprocal	3 Mobility
4 Functional	4 Digital	4 Programming
5 Responsive	5 Logistical	5 Concept
6 Optional	6 Transitional	6 Time-phase
7 Synchronized	7 Incremental	7 Projection
8 Compatible	8 Third-generation	8 Hardware
9 Balanced	9 Policy	9 Contingency

"Systematic Buzz Phrase Projector" created by Philip Broughton. From *Style, an Anti-Textbook*, by Richard A. Lanham, Yale University Press, 1974.

Modular languages to express clinical concepts are slightly more complex. One module might consist of anatomical sites, in standard terms, with codes. All possible "injuries," also expressed in standard terms, might form another module. Thus, a fractured arm would be represented by a standard term for "arm" plus a standard term for "fracture." Use of modular languages is a transformation process,

---

12. From *Style, an Anti-Textbook*, by Richard A. Lanham, Yale University Press, 1974.

resulting in transformation coding (see "Modular Language Coding," page 127). Three modular languages have been prominent, and a fourth is on the horizon:

- *Standard Nomenclature of Diseases and Operations (SNDO)*

- *Index for Radiological Diagnoses (IRD)*

- *Systematized Nomenclature of Human and Veterinary Medicine (SNOMED International)*

- *ICD-10 Procedure Coding System (ICD-10-PCS)*

Standard Nomenclature of Diseases and Operations (SNDO)

The American Medical Association published the first edition of its *Standard Nomenclature of Diseases and Operations (SNDO)* in 1933. While in use for many years, this attempt to standardize medical language, nomenclature, and coding eventually failed, and the last edition was published in 1961. For more about *SNDO*, see "Coding Problems with SNDO," page 114, "The Early Years Using SNDO," page 151, "Procedure Classifications for Hospital Use," page 176, and the appendices, page 407.

Index for Radiological Diagnoses (IRD)

The American College of Radiology published the first edition of its *Index for Radiological Diagnoses (IRD)* in 1955. The fourth edition appeared in 1992. This system is in use in a number of radiology departments. It is discussed more fully in the appendices on page 483.

Systematized Nomenclature of Human and Veterinary Medicine (SNOMED International)

The College of American Pathologists has sustained the modular language concept since the publication, in 1965, of the *Systematized Nomenclature of Pathology (SNOP)*. The current generation is the *Systematized Nomenclature of Human and Veterinary Medicine (SNOMED International)* (sometimes referred to as *SNOMED III* or just *SNOMED*), which was published in 1993.[13]

---

13. For more background on *SNOMED*, see page 429.

SNOMED III is designed to accommodate diagnoses, procedures, and other items of biomedical information. At this writing, it is being referred to by some as the prime candidate for a standardized nomenclature for medicine in the development of the electronic medical record (EMR) (see page 60). In fact, vendors of EMR systems today typically state that they are "using "*SNOMED*"." Advocates for *SNOMED* seem to base their contention on the fact that *SNOMED III* has the longest list of "defined terms" — just under 157,000. However, the 157,000 terms are the total found in eleven "modules," the most extensive of which is the "D" module, "Diseases/Diagnoses," with roughly 41,500 terms. EMR vendors are apparently using only the "D" module, which effectively limits the real breadth of *SNOMED* to 41,500 terms. From this total must be subtracted the 3,400 terms with the suffix "V", which indicates that they are purely veterinary terms. This leaves about 38,100 human diagnostic terms. And at that, a lot of the D codes must be for "other" if *SNOMED* is to accommodate all the diagnoses there are. The necessity for many "other" terms in the D module makes it impossible for this to be a true nomenclature (see page 76).

A "definined term" under *SNOMED*, however, does not by itself describe a concept. Its "rules of use" require that terms be taken from each appropriate module and linked together. For each diagnostic concept, one must use at least the following formula:

> 1 entry from Topography ("T" module) (12,000 terms)
>
> +   1 entry from Morphology (M) (5,000 terms)
>
> +   1 entry "cause," i.e., from Living Organisms (L) (24,000 terms) or Chemicals, Drugs, and Biological Products (CC) (14,000 terms) or Physical Agents (P) (1,400 terms)
>
> +   1 entry from Function (F) (16,000 terms)
>
> _____
>
> =   1 diagnosis (concept)

The user is given free rein to "mix and match" from the modules at will. It is clear that in terms of number of possible concepts that *SNOMED III* could handle, the mathematics is multiplication, not addition. So, using the smallest cause list, P, for a condition caused by a physical agent, the number of possible diagnoses is

$$12,000 \times 5,000 \times 1,400 \times 16,000 = 1,344,000,000$$

If each module has every possible subconcept, e.g., if every anatomical site is in the topography ("T") module, every morphology is in the "M" module, and every cause is in one of the cause modules, then the system can indeed accommodate every possible diagnostic concept, and for each there would be a unique code—provided all coders used the same logic in creating the assembly of modular codes.

If the use of *SNOMED* in the EMR means only use of the Diseases/ Diagnoses (D) module, "use of *SNOMED*" becomes a preferred term transformation for those conditions for which it has provided terms (see below), rather than one of modular language for the specific diagnosis. The degree to which the D module list of terms would satisfy the daily demands of clinical medicine in all of its specialties, along with the demands of other caregivers, including the statements of the patients' problems and the usage of alternative medicine, has not been examined.

ICD-10 Procedure Coding System (ICD-10-PCS)

This is the new modular system developed for the Health Care Financing Administration (HCFA) for *coding* procedures; it is discussed in detail later (see "ICD-10-PCS — A New Coding System," page 191).

Preferred Terms

Standardized Nomenclature
A single nomenclature
accepted and used by
all in the field

> Modular Language
> Terms comprised
> of *components* from
> several universes
>
> **Preferred Terms**
> A list of *defined terms*
> with medical criteria for
> use of each term

There have been several major movements to express clinical concepts in "preferred terms." In each of these, the terms are given and their concepts defined, giving medical criteria which should be met for the use of each term. These include:

- Current Medical Terminology
- Obstetric-Gynecologic Terminology
- International Nomenclature of Diseases
- Diagnostic and Statistical Manual of Mental Disorders (DSM)

Current Medical Terminology (CMT-CMIT)

The American Medical Association took up the preferred term approach following its abandonment of *SNDO* (1961), and in 1963 published the first in its "Current Medical Terminology" series, which dealt with diagnoses only, not with procedures.[14]

---

14. The American Medical Association's *Current Procedural Terminology (CPT)* (1966–), while at a glance a similar volume, is quite different (page 183). *CPT* was created not as a system of terminology (despite its name), but as a vehicle for the reporting of services provided — i.e., for billing.

The foreword to *Current Medical Information and Terminology (CMIT)*, the fourth and final edition in the series (1971), described it as "essentially a distillate of medical knowledge" — a sort of mini-*Merck Manual*.[15] Each preferred term (concept) was followed by as many of the following items of information, in skeletal fashion, as were relevant:

> additional terms (AT)
>
> etiology (ET)
>
> symptoms (SM)
>
> signs (SG)
>
> complications (CM)
>
> laboratory data (LB)
>
> pathology (PA)
>
> x-rays (XR)

Its foreword further stated that *CMIT* contained 3,262 preferred terms and about 5,500 additional terms for diseases, i.e., eponyms and synonyms. The fourth edition was considerably bulkier than earlier editions, with the inclusion of French, German, and Spanish Cross Reference Sections for the terms themselves, a "KWIC" (Keyword in Context) Index[16] of about 70 pages, and an alphabetic index for each of 10 body systems. There was also a section of abbreviations and a small glossary.

One noteworthy feature of the *CMT-CMIT* series was the use of "random numbers" which were apparently "accession numbers" for the

---

15. The *Merck Manual* is a widely-used reference on diagnosis and treatment of disease, published by Merck, Sharpe, and Dohme.

16. A KWIC index was an early method of automatic indexing by computer. In one form, the computer took a series of perhaps seven keywords, usually the title of the document, and "rotated" the series of words so that each word in turn was the first in the string. Thus one seven-word title would have seven permutations. All the strings resulting from the process were then alphabetized on the first word in the permuted string. In *CMIT* the KWIC index was described as "essentially an [alphabetic] arrangement of etiologies and signs that appear in the main body [of the volume]," and thus an early attempt to provide an electronically produced aid to the physician in his or her decisions.

preferred terms.[17] Presumably these numbers were unique, i.e., the same number would never be used for a different term. No information is given as to how these numbers were used, except that the *CMT* authors called them "reference and filing numbers" for information pertaining to the diagnosis so numbered.[18]

The authors of *CMT* believed that it would be possible to get physicians to standardize their language and use only "preferred terms," presumably by the influence of these books.[19] The chief method employed to exert the necessary influence was to give the criteria only for the use of the preferred terms. Synonyms which had been identified were indexed with "see [preferred term]." At the preferred term entry, the synonyms were shown as "additional terms," e.g., "hiccup" was the preferred term, "clonic spasm" and "singultus" the synonyms. With this fourth edition, 1971, AMA abandoned this effort. Not surprisingly, its dream of "one concept, one term" has never been realized, at least in everyday usage.

Obstetric-Gynecologic Terminology

The American College of Obstetricians and Gynecologists created an authoritative list of preferred terms and their definitions in its *Obstetric-Gynecologic Terminology* (1972). It made no effort to provide codes for the terms it defined, or to indicate where they would fit into *ICD* or any other classification. A second edition never appeared.

International Nomenclature of Diseases (IND)

In 1977, the International Conference for the Ninth Revision of the *International Classification of Diseases* recommended that the "possibility of preparing an International Nomenclature of Diseases, as

---

17. Accession numbers are numbers assigned to things in the order they are acquired, or in the order in which they are listed, with no significance other then identification of the item.

18. For preferred terms the code numbers from both *SNDO* and *ICD* were given, and this convention was continued through the third edition (1966). It was abandoned in the fourth edition. That edition, however, added code numbers for one of ten body systems to each of the accession numbers. See "Code or classification?," page 117.

19. Personal communication from Burgess Gordon, MD, author of *Current Medical Terminology*, 1963, the first volume in the series.

an improvement to the Tenth Revision of the International Classification of Diseases" be investigated.[20]

Work toward establishing an "International Nomenclature of Diseases" (IND) had been initiated in 1970 by the Council for International Organizations of Medical Sciences (CIOMS). In 1975, the World Health Organization (WHO) joined CIOMS in the project. The project published its tenth (and last) volume in 1992; further publication was suspended due to lack of funds. The first four volumes are attributed to CIOMS alone, the final six jointly to CIOMS and WHO.

Subsequently, WHO has published 5 more volumes described as having "diagnostic definitions." All 15 volumes are listed:

IND (International Nomenclature of Diseases): Diseases of the Lower Respiratory Tract, Volume III (CIOMS 1979)

IND: Infectious Diseases, Volume II, Part 2: Mycoses (CIOMS 1982)

IND: Infectious Diseases, Volume II, Part 3: Viral diseases (CIOMS 1983)

IND: Infectious Diseases, Volune II, Part 1: Bacterial Diseases (CIOMS 1985)

IND: Infectious Diseases, Volume II, Part 4: Parasitic Diseases (CIOMS/WHO 1987)

IND: Cardiac and Vascular Diseases, Volume V (CIOMS/WHO 1989)

IND: Diseases of the Digestive System, Volume IV (CIOMS/WHO 1990)

IND: Metabolic, Nutritional and Endocrine Disorders, Volume VI (CIOMS/WHO 1991)

IND: Diseases of the Kidney, the Lower Urinary Tract, and the Male Genital System, Volume VII (CIOMS/WHO 1992)

IND: Diseases of the Female Genital System, Volume VIII (CIOMS/WHO 1992)

The ICD-10 Classification of Mental and Behavioral Disorders: Clinical Descriptions and Diagnostic Guidelines (1992)

The ICD-10 Classification of Mental and Behavioral Disorders: Diagnostic Criteria for Research (1993)

---

20. For more about the recommendations of the Conference, see the Introduction to *ICD-9* on page 385 in the appendices. The specific recommendation for the *International Nomenclature of Diseases* is on page 400.

Lexicon of Alcohol and Drug Terms (1994)

Lexicon of Psychiatric and Mental Health Terms (1994)

Lexicon of Cross-cultural Terms in Mental Health (1997)

The intention of the IND was to provide a single "recommended" name for each "morbid entity." The names were to be, as much as possible, specific (apply to only one disease), unambiguous, self-descriptive, simple, and based on cause. Each name carried with it a brief definition and list of synonyms, if any.

CIOMS/WHO described *Metabolic, Nutritional and Endocrine Disorders* as follows:

> A dictionary of over 750 metabolic, nutritional, and endocrine disorders, each entered under a single recommended name, concisely defined, and accompanied by a comprehensive list of synonyms. Diseases are defined on the basis of their cause or pathogenesis, an approach which posed particular problems in view of the many newly detected metabolic disorders whose underlying biochemical or genetic defect remains to be elucidated ...

Diagnostic and Statistical Manual of Mental Disorders (DSM)

Although the *Diagnostic and Statistical Manual of Mental Disorders* (*DSM*) has been listed here because of its influence on the preferred use of language, its prime purpose over the 42 years between the 1st and 4th editions (1952-1994) has been to record the evolution of the biomedical concepts the field of mental illness. It is discussed in some detail beginning on page 94.

Identifying Biomedical Concepts

Standardized Nomenclature
A single nomenclature
accepted and used by
all in the field

Modular Language
Terms comprised
of *components* from
several universes

Preferred Terms
A list of *defined terms*
with medical criteria for
use of each term

Biomedical Concepts
A description and name
of each *concept* in a field,
arrived at by consensus

It seems clear that the efforts to standardize language which have relied on transforming the terms commonly used in medical communication, written and oral, into modular expressions have not succeeded in changing professional usage in a trial period of over 60 years (*SNDO* was first published in 1932). It is hard to see how continued effort along this line is worth pursuing for the purpose of changing the language in daily use.

Nor have the attempts at forcing conformity in the usage of terms, that is, controlling usage so that only preferred terms are employed, proven successful.

The alternative, which seems far more attractive as a way to standardize the usage of terms, is to continue along the educational path to identify biomedical concepts. This path involves mobilizing each profession to set up an ongoing process of study of its concepts and come to a consensus on describing and naming them. It also requires determining where the terminology actually in use fits into the defined concepts.

At least three endeavors are under way or already in use:

- Diagnostic and Statistical Manual of Mental Disorders (DSM)

- Read Clinical Classification System (now National Health Service Codes)

- Unified Medical Language System (UMLS)

Diagnostic and Statistical Manual of Mental Disorders (DSM)

The American Psychiatric Association entered the field of defining the terms in its universe in 1952 with its *Diagnostic and Statistical Manual of Mental Disorders (DSM)*, now in its fourth edition, *DSM-IV* (1994). Each edition has become more and more precise and explanatory as to the meanings of the diagnoses used in psychiatry, because this is its purpose. It has also, of course, reflected the changes in psychiatric thinking and definition of concepts over the years.[21] Literally thousands of American and hundreds of international participants were involved in its construction and in its field trials. It has remained a work addressed at clarifying psychiatric thinking as well as terminology.

The volume does contain *ICD-9-CM* codes, but they are given simply for the convenience of psychiatrists when they must record and report their diagnoses by placing them in the *ICD* categories.[22] However, the classification *(ICD)* has not been permitted to influence the medical thought. APA makes no representation that the *ICD-9-CM* codes are equivalent to the actual psychiatric diagnoses. Those who decode psychiatric data from *ICD-9-CM* will often be misled as to the actual diagnoses, just as others are who draw the same inferences when decoding from *ICD-9-CM* in other fields of medicine.

---

21. See the example on page 266 of the changes in the definition of Attention Deficit/ Hyperactivity Disorder (AD/HD) from 1979 to 1994.

22. In view of the US decision to create a clinical modification of *ICD-10*, *ICD-10-CM*, the *DSM-IV* reference table will be made obsolete because of the differences between *ICD-10-CM* and the parent volume.

DSM-IV is the first United States volume to provide users with similar assistance for *ICD-10*, the new edition of *ICD*.[23] A table in *DSM-IV* gives, for each of the diagnoses, the appropriate *ICD-10* category. The table below illustrates the relationship of the concepts to their classification in both *ICD-9-CM* and *ICD-10*. Note the much closer correspondence with *ICD-10*, the result of close collaboration between the American Psychiatric Association and the World Health Organization in the creation of *ICD-10*.

Figure 3.3 DSM-IV / ICD-10 Table

DSM-IV	ICD-9-CM		ICD-10	
Term	Code	Category Label	Code	Category Label
Pain disorder associated with psychological factors and a general medical condition	307.89	Other psychalgia	F45.4	Pain disorder
Pain disorder associated with psychological factors	307.80	Psychogenic pain, site unspecified	F45.4	Pain disorder
Adjustment disorder with depressed mood	309.0	Brief depressive reaction	F43.20	Adjustment disorder with depressed mood
Adjustment disorder with anxiety	309.24	Adjustment reaction with anxious mood	F43.28	Adjustment disorder with anxiety

---

23. Additional publications have appeared to assist in the use of *DSM-IV*. One, published by the American Psychiatric Association itself, is entitled *DSM-IV Guidebook*. Another, published by the American Health Information Management Association, entitled *DSM-IV to ICD-9-CM Crosswalk*, contains instructions as to what to do when the wordings of concepts in *DSM-IV* and *ICD-9-CM* are different or the *ICD-9-CM* conventions require additional information, e.g., when *ICD-9-CM* requires an "E" (external cause) code and a specific drug to be stated.

Figure 3.3 DSM-IV / ICD-10 Table *(continued)*

Circadian rhythm sleep disorder	307.45	Phase-shift disruption of 24-hour sleep-wake cycle	F51.2	Circadian rhythm sleep disorder not due to a substance or known physiological condition
Hallucinogen intoxication	292.89	Other specified drug-induced mental disorder	F16.00	Hallucinogen intoxication
Hallucinogen persisting perception disorder	292.89	Other specified drug-induced mental disorder	F16.70	Hallucinogen persisting perception disorder

Table developed from DSM-IV.

It should be emphasized that the evolution of the *DSM* series is a demonstration of the evolution of thinking, knowledge, and conceptualization in the field of psychiatry. Similar changes in concepts are natural developments in all fields; they are not peculiar to the biomedical fields.

Read Clinical Classification System (NHS Codes)

The United Kingdom National Health Service has adopted concept coding which was developed as the "Read Clinical Classification System."[24] Previously referred to as the "Read Codes," they are now called the "NHS Codes."

At the NHS Centre for Coding and Classification, directed by Dr. Read, careful study is given to each term encountered and a decision is made as to whether the term expresses a new concept or is some alternative form of a recorded concept. If it is an alternative, that is noted, and the system codes the alternative term to the concept code. Mapping tables are provided which place the concept codes into the rubrics of the classifications with which data are to be reported in Great Britain. This

---

24. The system is described in detail in the appendices; see "NHS Codes (Read Codes)," page 459.

includes mapping to *ICD-9-CM* and *ICD-10*. Other mapping tables can readily be developed.[25]

Unified Medical Language System (UMLS)

The Unified Medical Language System (UMLS) of the United States National Library of Medicine is designed to (1) identify biomedical concepts and (2) determine into which concepts the various terms encountered in healthcare fit. The purpose of UMLS is to provide a bridge between inquiries (using whatever language) and information (both printed and images) in order to link the inquirer to the archives of the library. See page 425 for more about UMLS.

Admittedly, identifying concepts is a lengthy process requiring much effort and much patience. *DSM-I* was published in 1952, and there is no indication that the task is finished. There will be new knowledge, new thinking, and new formulation of the concepts. It is likely that new generations of *DSM* will appear periodically, as they have in the past. Family practice in Great Britain has, with the Read Codes (now called the NHS Codes) also started on the task in a determined, careful, and sustained fashion. The UMLS project is a vast and continuing undertaking.

Language Can't — and Shouldn't — Be Controlled

Clinical disciplines will continue to define new concepts and redefine old concepts, and to organize and often provide codes for the terms in their universes. This is a natural part of the growth of our knowledge and understanding. But no matter how sophisticated the terminology and nomenclature become, nothing ever will — or should — get physicians and others in healthcare to always communicate and record information in preferred terms, or specifically defined concepts, or standard nomenclature.

People will always use their own words — their natural language. Even if professionals were to be trained to adhere to standard terminology, they would want to add more information than that terminology can express. And laypeople (which patients sometimes are) will hardly ever

---

25. Note, however, that to be accurate in classifying *cases*, mapping tables must take into account more than just the diagnosis; see "Entity Code Classifying," page 320.

use clinical terms. No one wants to be — and probably no one can or should be — restricted in their means to express themselves (as a matter of fact, we said something about this in our national Constitution).

This is really a basic fact of human behavior, and we might as well face it. But we can't let this facet of behavior allow essential information to escape the electronic health information system. We must be able to capture the actual expressions of the people involved — the natural language of providers and patients. To do this, each individual term, whether a defined concept, standard nomen, preferred term, or none of these, must be somehow recorded (and coded, to permit digital manipulation) as it is expressed. The system can then access exactly what was stated, and changes in knowledge and language can be accommodated without distortion. To be sure, this is no easy task; it presents a real challenge in system design.

4

Retrieval of Medical Record Information

WITHIN THE HOSPITAL or physician's office, retrieving information about an individual patient in order to provide patient care has, until recently, been a simple matter, depending only on the filing system used and the care with which it is managed. The record is looked up by the patient's name or number, starting with a "Patient Index" (alphabetic listing by patient name). Special tracers have to be employed when the record is removed from the file for consultants or processing, but these are relatively small problems, with local solutions.

Before the 1950s, medical records in hospitals began to be called upon for uses in addition to direct patient care (and billing). The records were:

- the source of information for the hospital's "professional activity" statistics
- counted and analyzed to review each physician's use of the hospital
- used to document a surgeon's experience when seeking credentials such as board certification
- brought together in "series" of cases in preparation of scientific papers
- assembled in groups for review of the quality of care

These uses of medical record information led to the development of four more standard indexes of the records, in addition to the Patient Index:

- Diagnosis Index (patient records listed by diagnosis)
- Operation Index (patient records listed by operation)
- Physician Index (patient records by admitting physician)
- Surgeon Index (patient records by operating surgeon)

To be accredited, a hospital was required to keep all five indexes.[1] In establishing these indexes, hospitals typically used Kardex visible files, with the records referenced under the codes for their diagnoses and operations, using the *Standard Nomenclature of Diseases and Operations (SNDO)*.[2] Compiling statistical information from these medical records was, in almost all hospitals, a hand-sorting, clerical task.

Access to Information

Until about 1950, there was only one way to find out about anything that was in a patient's medical record: go to the hospital (or office or clinic) with the necessary authorization, have the medical record librarian locate the record for you, and read it.[3] This was not so bad for one patient. If you wanted to study a group of patients, it could become tedious. If you wanted to compare patients among more than one hospital, it started becoming costly as well as time-consuming. And when the numbers of patients became of even modest size, it became impossible.

---

1.   "Accreditation" is the process of (1) evaluation of an institution or education program to determine whether it meets the standards set up by an accrediting body, and (2) if the institution or program meets the standards, granting recognition of the fact. Accreditation is a process performed by a non-governmental agency at the request of the institution or education program. Hospitals (and today, other healthcare institutions) are accredited by the Joint Commission on Accreditation of Healthcare Organizations (JCAHO) in the United States and by the Canadian Council on Health Facilities Accreditation (CCHFA) in Canada.

2.   See "Standard Nomenclature of Diseases & Operations," page 407, for more information.

3.   The term "medical record librarian" was later replaced by "medical record administrator," then by "health information administrator." For more about health information professionals, see page 53.

Example	Retrieving case information in 1953
	The senior author spent three weeks in 1953 with a physician colleague visiting 15 general hospitals within a 100 mile radius in order to compile information on several series of cases: 1,647 appendectomies, 1,109 diabetic admissions, and 2,269 pneumonia admissions. The studies required the laborious reading of 5,025 medical records. The data extracted from each medical record were placed in a punch card and the analyses were developed with tabulating machines, an early such application. This was a very expensive study.[a]

a.   Eisele, C. Wesley, Vergil N. Slee, Robert G. Hoffmann. "Can the Practice of Internal Medicine be Evaluated?" *Annals of Internal Medicine*, 44, No. 1 (1956): 144-61.

In the middle of the last century, two major developments drove the system to find more efficient ways to retrieve patient information:

- The appearance of health insurance
- The evaluation of the quality of clinical care

Healthcare Insurance

When healthcare insurance came along, hospitals had to prepare a bill for each individual patient's care and submit it to the insurance company.[4] The care had to be described and justified in ways that could be understood by the insurance companies. Bills previously prepared for individual patients to pay had been under far fewer constraints, and did not have to be standardized among hospitals.

As a practical matter, bills to insurance companies were, from the very first, coded documents. The coding primarily pertained to the physician's and surgeon's identities, and to diagnostic and surgical information, but it was also applied to such information as the patient's origin and other items wherever coding led to more compact and "specific" information.

It was interesting that, in general, the demand of the insurance company was only that enough diagnostic and surgical information be provided so

---

4.   The insurance company was the original "third party payer." Before that, only two parties were involved in payment — the provider and the patient. Thus the insurer was called the "third party."

that the claim could be granted or denied. For example, a question was asked as to whether the problem was a mental illness or alcoholism (these were simple coded "yes or no" categories). Knowing that these conditions were not covered, providers began to "game" the system: the physician typically reported an "approved" — meaning not denied — primary category in such cases, such as "pneumonia," in order to be paid and, if the mental problem or alcoholism was mentioned at all, it was "incidental," i.e., shown as a secondary diagnosis.

Evaluation of Care

There was a growing movement to evaluate the quality of clinical care, both in hospitals and in office practice. Paul Lembcke's "Medical Evaluation Study" was one step (see below). The medical audit, introduced by C. Wesley Eisele, MD, was another step,[5] as was a project of the American College of Surgeons (ACS) to pursue a methodology for evaluating the quality of care for all patients in the hospital.[6]

These pioneers in evaluating care recognized the need for statistical bases to undergird the review of individual cases.[7] Patterns of care, which could only be developed by aggregating information from individual patients, were more important than occasional misadventures in individual instances. Patterns lent themselves to educational interventions, and improving care was the goal rather than punishing physicians or others for isolated incidents. Multihospital statistical comparisons were essential to provide, in many cases, the baselines (now called "benchmarks") — what one hospital or clinical department or physician could achieve, so could others. The goal was to let physicians learn from their own and others' experiences in caring for patients.

---

5.   Eisele, C. Wesley, Vergil N. Slee, Robert G. Hoffmann. "Can the Practice of Internal Medicine be Evaluated?" *Annals of Internal Medicine*, 44, No. 1 (1956): 144-61.

6.   The latter project was called "The Evaluation of the Quality of Patient Care." Surgical patients were already being reviewed by the hospital's Tissue Committee, pioneered by the American College of Surgeons. Both Eisele's work and the ACS project were supported by the W. K. Kellogg Foundation.

7.   An audit trail from the statistics to the individual cases which contributed to them was, of course, an essential, but often overlooked, element of an adequate information system.

Hospital Discharge Abstract Systems

Stimulated by the desire of a few forward-looking hospitals to "compare notes" on clinical experiences, data management technology emerging in the middle of the 20th century began taking on the job of processing patient information. To permit this, a way had to be found for information in individual patient records to be handled by machine. This led to the appearance of hospital discharge abstract systems.

In the early 1950s, the Rochester (NY) Regional Hospital Council set up a system for its hospitals so that they could compare statistics on their clinical activities. A few years later, in Michigan, the senior author, under a grant from the W. K. Kellogg Foundation to the Southwestern Michigan Hospital Council (SMHC), installed an adaptation of the Rochester system for the Council's hospitals. The program in Michigan was called the Professional Activity Study (PAS).[8]

The Rochester program, as well as the first attempt in the fifteen or so participating hospitals in the Southwestern Michigan Hospital Council, required the hospitals to send to the hospital council headquarters copies of statistical reports of their activities. At the headquarters, comparison tabulations were made across the hospitals, showing such basic information as average lengths of stay for adults and newborns, percentages of patients operated on, percentages falling into the medical, surgical, and obstetric services, death rates for each service, and so on.

It was soon clear that *more than half of the statistics from the hospitals were unreliable, not because of carelessness or lack of interest, but because the underlying data were not handled uniformly in the hospitals:*

- Some hospitals, despite the rule stating that "the day of admission is a day, the day of discharge is not," counted both days within the length of stay.

---

8. The Rochester program, instituted by Paul Lembcke, MD, was called the "Medical Evaluation Study." This name was quickly replaced in Michigan by the more neutral term, "Professional Activity Study," because not only was there resistance by physicians to the term "evaluation," but also there was little or no evidence at that time that such an approach could evaluate the quality of care.

- The "cause of admission" was taken from the face sheet of the medical record in one hospital as the first diagnosis written by the physician; in another hospital, the medical record librarian searched among the list of diagnoses for the one which, in her or his opinion, was the "most important;" while in a third hospital, a real attempt was made to select the diagnosis which answered the question, "why was the patient hospitalized?" The reason for hospitalization had to be known, because the statistics called for tabulations indicating the clinical service on which the patient was treated.[9]

- What was a patient on the surgical service in one hospital might be a gynecological patient in another.

Because of these insurmountable problems in obtaining standardized information from each hospital, an alternative was proposed: that the system be changed to one in which uniform clinical information about each individual hospital patient was collected, and the statistics be uniformly prepared by tabulating machines.

To gather uniform information about patients, a "punch card" needed to be created to carry a summary of each patient's hospitalization. A punch card was an early device used for database management. Instead of an electronic record, each record was placed on a punch card, made of heavy paper.

---

9.   A "clinical service" is a division of the medical staff according to clinical specialty, such as surgery, internal medicine, obstetrics and gynecology, pediatrics, neurology, and the like. In some hospitals, clinical services are called departments; for example, the surgical service may mean the same thing as the surgical department. In other instances, a service may be a subdivision of a department; for example, the orthopedics service may be part of the larger department of surgery.

Figure 4.1 Hospital Discharge Abstract Punch Card

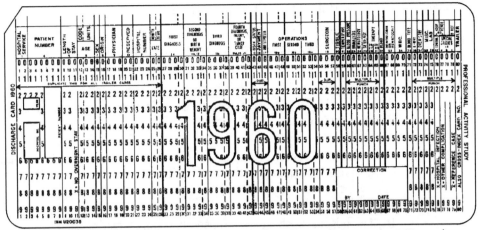

The "Discharge Card" used by the Professional Activitity Study in 1960. PAS used a standard IBM 80-column keypunch card, customized to receive the required information. Into this single card was punched an entire case abstract.

A keypunch machine was used to punch holes in the card corresponding to the information required. Mechanical tabulating, statistical, and printing machines then "read" the punched holes to analyze and print out the data.

After patient information was keyed into the punch cards, the statistical reports would be compiled at a central point. Not only would the use of punch card methodology permit the previously compiled reports to become more uniform, it would also provide the ability to handle information about patients in a variety of ways, giving new insights into physician and hospital practices.

When the idea was proposed, the task of providing the information for the punch cards appeared to put a significant burden on the hospital. However, it was pointed out that the hospital medical record department was already required by custom and accreditation to carry out several information processing tasks. First, as discussed above, hospitals had to keep patient, diagnosis, operation, physician, and surgeon indexes to remain accredited. In addition, hospitals regularly compiled statistics which were termed "Professional Activity Statistics" by Malcolm MacEachern, the prime authority on hospital administration.[10]

---

10. See, for example, MacEachern, Malcolm T. *Hospital Organization and Management*. Chicago 1935: Physicians' Record Co.

Background

The powerful – but limited – punch card

Punch cards were first used in 1801 by a French weaver, Joseph Jacquard, who devised them to control the pattern of cloth woven on his special looms.

In the mid-nineteenth century, Charles Babbage, assisted by Ada Lovelace, devised a calculating machine controlled by information on punch cards. This is considered the "birth" of the computer.

In the late 19th century, Herman Hollerith invented the Hollerith machine – which used the punch card –for tabulating the 1890 census. Thus, the card was often called a "Hollerith card."

The first hospital abstract system used IBM punch cards. Each card had 80 columns with 12 possible punches in each column, thus 960 holes could be punched in each card. But all were not available to carry different items of information. A 5-digit patient number occupied 5 columns and took 60 holes out of use, and so on.

In view of the physical limitations imposed by a "single-punch card" system, the abstract designers were reluctant to use up an entire punch card column for a single "yes" or "no" (binary) entry, when logic insisted this could be expressed at a single position (hole) in the card – "yes" could be expressed by a hole; the absence of the hole could mean "no." Under this theory, one column could contain 12 items of information.

Special innovative modifications were made to the card punch machines by PAS in order to permit "multiple punching" to achieve this end. This at least doubled the capacity of the single punch card.

These were all tasks which could easily be delegated to tabulating machines. To test the feasibility of this, the Professional Activity Study obtained another grant from the W. K. Kellogg Foundation. The School of Public Health of the University of Michigan[11] offered statistical

---

11. Notably Clarence Velz, Chairman of the Department of Biostatistics, and Fay Hemphill, Associate Professor and the key statistician in the evaluation of the Salk poliomyelitis vaccine.

consultation, tabulating facilities, and office space, and system design began. This was the birth of PAS, the prototype "hospital discharge abstract system." PAS was started and run originally by the Southwestern Michigan Hospital Council. The nonprofit Commission on Professional and Hospital Activities (CPHA)[12] was then founded, in 1956, with its first mission to make PAS available nationally.[13]

Designing the Abstract

The primary question was, what should go into the abstract? The cards had limited physical space, and technical considerations at that time mandated that there be only one punch card per hospital "discharge," so there were constraints on the amount of data collected. In addition, the data was collected from only one source, the medical record. Data input was done in the medical record department, by hand: the medical record librarian studied the actual record and filled out a single-page case abstract form.[14] Sharing of accounting and other information, from other departments, was difficult; in those days it required a change in hospital procedure to even obtain the expected source of payment, e.g., Blue Cross, commercial insurance, self-pay. This put constraints on the type of information collected.

---

12. CPHA's founding sponsors were the American College of Physicians, the American College of Surgeons, the American Hospital Association, the American Medical Association, and the Southwestern Michigan Hospital Council.

13. After the Professional Activity Study (PAS) was established, the Commission on Professional and Hospital Activities (CPHA) pioneered in evaluation of care by developing a special system called the Medical Audit Program (MAP). MAP took information derived from PAS and displayed statistics relevant to the quality of care for a number of conditions and procedures, along with audit trails to the individual cases involved.

14. The form on which this information was collected became known as a "discharge abstract" because it was completed after the patient was discharged from the hospital (a "discharge" is a single period of hospitalization) and it contained a coded summary ("abstract") of the hospitalization. See the illustration on page 112.

Key Elements of Information

The designers had to carefully consider what information about each patient should be placed on the abstract in preparation for its entry onto the punch card (for an example of some of the possibilities, see the list on page 142). Obviously, there had to be the information which was needed to create the statistics and indexes the hospital had been maintaining manually. This determined the initial array of items, which today would be called the "basic data set." Other items were selected on the basis of their likely value in better understanding the clinical activities in the hospitals. Several classes of information were considered, and key elements were selected:

Administrative information The identification of the patient and the patient's medical record, as well as dates of admission and discharge, were essential, as was the outcome of the hospitalization. (There are three "possible" outcomes of hospitalization: discharged alive, died, or transferred. These outcomes are not the same as the patient's outcome, which might be "return to work," for example.)

Demographic information The patient's age on admission and sex were obviously necessary basic items. To economize in punch card usage, the age was carried in a 2-digit "value" field with a third digit indicating hours, days, weeks, months, years, and "over 100." (With today's technology, of course, one would have recorded the date and time of birth and the computer would have calculated the age.) Other demographic information, such as marital status, residence, and educational attainment, which appealed to some of the planners, was seen by hospitals and their physicians as of little or no value to them, and so was not included.

Physicians The physician(s) caring for the patient were needed, including, of course, the surgeon(s), if any.

Cause of admission Clearly, one needed to know why the patient was admitted to the hospital. The reason was usually expressed as a medical diagnosis, although it was often very vague. Hospital study of the patient was often necessary to clarify the situation, and often the discharge diagnosis was quite different from the admitting diagnosis. So the system called for the "final diagnosis causing (explaining) admission"; this was commonly called the patient's "primary diagnosis." Often, the medical record librarian had to make a judgment, using the record, as to what *was* the "primary diagnosis."

Other diagnoses Other diagnoses, especially those which were known to be important in understanding the management of the patient (such as diabetes and heart disease), were also wanted. These were called "secondary diagnoses." Punch card capacity limited the number of diagnoses permitted, and the length of the codes determined the number of punch card columns required for each. The shorter the codes, the better.

Operations These were not only a major kind of intervention, but they were also, of course, needed for creation of the surgeon's index. Statistical reports often tabulated "major" and "minor" operations. This distinction was abandoned when the only definition which surgeons could agree on was, "a major operation is one that I perform or that is performed on me." Here also, code length and punch card capacity were critical determinants.

Investigative procedures These included laboratory and X-ray work, along with other procedures, such as the then-common "basal metabolism test." These had to be accommodated by simple "done" or "not done" entries which would give some estimate of diagnostic effort expended and, in some instances, the credibility of the resulting diagnoses, e.g., there would be some doubt about a diagnosis of diabetes in a hospital record without a blood sugar determination recorded.

Treatment There was interest in what else was done in the hospital to treat the condition, in addition to, or in the absence of, surgery. This included such therapy as blood transfusions and the use of other blood products, radiation, and the use of certain classes of drugs, such as antibiotics. Again, the system had to be content with "used" or "not used" except in the case of blood transfusions, in which the number of units given was recorded as 1 through 8, and "9 or more."

Payment The only information here was the source of expected payment — self-pay, Blue Cross, commercial insurance, or other. This was included because of the allegation that third parties were being exploited — that the physician and hospital, knowing that a third party would pay, would be less frugal.

There was insufficient interest in dollar amounts to persuade the hospital to establish the new procedures required to give the charges to the medical record department, and for the record librarian to go to the extra work to include them. (Of course, hospital cost accounting had not progressed to even an approximation of costs rather than charges.)

Optional data Opportunity was provided for the hospital to submit limited amounts of other coded information of local interest, such as a finer breakdown by race than the standard one at that time. One hospital in Hawaii, for example, wanted to keep track of something like 30 different ethnic groups.

Limitations

Physical limitations did not provide the only constraints on the information to be abstracted. Several other factors influenced the design of the abstract:

Clerical data input The abstracting of the medical records — including coding of diagnoses — was a "clerical task," meaning, in this context, one performed not by the physicians, but by medical record personnel who transferred information from the original record to the case abstract. Not all medical record personnel were equally trained or qualified for this task.

Objectivity The abstracter needed to be able to simply pick up the data exactly as recorded in the medical record, without making judgments about it or drawing conclusions from it, i.e., without interpreting it. This represents a basic principle of data gathering: the information should be as objective as possible. For example, a standard question used at that time for statistics was, "did the pathology diagnosis agree with the preoperative diagnosis?" This question, while apparently objective, often could not be answered even by a physician because of variations in the language used, and so was never included in the case abstract.

Standardization A basic core of information on each discharge had to be required. Thus the system had to pick up exactly the same items of information about every patient. Otherwise, standard tabulations and valid comparisons would be impossible. (Additional information, unique to an individual hospital, could be added.)

Case Summary Code Sheet

Based on these considerations, the first "case abstract" — a single-page "Case Summary Code Sheet" — was drawn up and provided to the fifteen small Michigan hospitals which had earlier been sending to the hospital council copies of their standardized monthly statistical reports as specified by the council's project.

Following is an illustration of the first code sheet, which used SNDO. Note the length of the diagnosis and operation codes, and how many columns they required, thus greatly limiting the number which could be accommodated.

Figure 4.2 Case Summary Code Sheet (full page)

SOUTHWESTERN MICHIGAN HOSPITAL COUNCIL
PROFESSIONAL ACTIVITY STUDY
CASE SUMMARY CODE SHEET
BATCH ______ PAGE ______

REPORTING HOSPITAL (CODED) 1. ☐

DATE OF DISCHARGE 2. ☐☐ ☐

PHYSICIAN — Code Number Assigned by Hospital 3. ☐☐

ADMISSION NUMBER — THIS ADMISSION
UNIT NUMBER 4. ☐☐☐☐☐☐

1. In-Patient, 1st Admission
2. In-Patient, 2nd thru 4th Adm.
3. In-Patient, 5th thru 9th Adm.
4. In-Patient, over 9th Adm.
5. Out-Patient, 1st Visit
6. Out-Patient, Other Visits
7. Out-Patient, 1st Visit for Follow-up Rx
8. Out-Patient, Other Visits for Follow-up Rx
9. Newborn remaining after Mother

5. ☐ PATIENT STATUS

LENGTH OF STAY, DAYS — Day of admission is a day, day of discharge is not.
6. ☐☐☐

AGE ON ADMISSION
Units:
1. Newborn.
2. Year (year or over)
3. Months (over 27 days, under 1 yr.)
4. Days (27 days or less).
5. Years plus 100.

7. Unit ☐ Age ☐☐

1. Male
2. Female
Incomplete Chart —
3. 7 Days or Less
4. Over 7 Days
5. Incomplete Chart — Data Not in

8. ☐ SEX

1. White
2. Non-White
3. Not Recorded

9. ☐ RACE

1. Admitting Diagnosis Same as Discharge Diagnosis
2. Admitted for X-Rays
3. Admitted for Observation and Diagnosis
4. Admitted without Stated Diagnosis
5. Emergency Admission without Doctor's Exam
6. Admitting Diagnosis Different from Discharge Diag.
7. Admitted with Symptoms Listed Only

10. ☐ ADMITTING DIAGNOSIS

Enter Total Number of Different Disease States, NOT Manifestations
11. ☐ NUMBER OF DISCHARGE DIAGNOSES

PRIMARY DIAGNOSIS* 12a. ☐☐☐☐–☐☐☐☐•☐

SECONDARY DIAGNOSIS* 12b. ☐☐☐☐–☐☐☐☐•☐

Enter Total Number During Hospitalization
13. ☐ COMPLICATIONS

1. Tissue Confirmed Pre-Op Diagnosis
2. Tissue Did Not Confirm

PRIMARY OPERATION* 14. ☐☐☐–☐☐☐

15. ☐ TISSUE

SECONDARY OPERATION* 16. ☐☐☐–☐☐☐

Enter Total Number During Hospitalization
17. ☐ CONSULTATIONS

A–
1. Out-Patient
2. Recovered
3. Improved
4. Not Improved
5. Not Treated
6. In for Diagnosis
7. Trfd. to Other Hosp.
8. Discharged Against Medical Advice
9. Died

B–
1. Discharged Alive
2. Died Over 48 Hrs.–Autopsy
3. Died Over 48 Hrs.–No Autopsy
4. Died Under 48 Hrs.–Autopsy
5. Died Under 48 Hrs.–No Autopsy
6. D. O. A.–Autopsy
7. D. O. A.–No Autopsy
8. Stillborn–Autopsy
9. Stillborn–No Autopsy

18. A ☐ B ☐ DISCHARGE STATUS

A–
1. Chest
2. For Fractures
3. Extremeties (other than fractures)
4. Gastro-Intestinal
5. Gall Bladder
6. G-I Plus G. B.
7. Uro-Genital
8. Any Combination 1 to 7
9. Repeat Exams for Re-evaluation
X. All Others

B– Total Number of X-Ray Exams

19. A ☐ X-RAY STUDIES B ☐☐

Enter Total Number During Hospitalization
20. ☐ Number of Operations

1. Gross Exam Only
2. Papanicolaou
3. Microscopic Exam
4. Microscopic plus Special Stain
5. Frozen Section plus Routine Microscopic
6. Alcohol
7. Chem. Studies–Sedatives, Poisons
8. Toxins plus Tissues

21. ☐ Tissues/Toxicology

1. Routine - s Microscopic
2. Routine - c Microscopic
3. Routine plus Fat
4. Routine plus Blood
5. Routine plus PSP, DIL, Conc.
6. Routine plus Repeat Sugars
7. Routine plus Bile and/or Urobilinogen
8. Routine plus 17 Keto Steroids
9. Routine plus Other Special Studies
X. Routine plus 2 or More Special Studies

22. ☐ URINALYSIS

1. Bleeding and/or Coag. Time
2. Hemoglobin (RBC not done)
3. RBC (with or without HGB)
4. Hematocrit
5. WBC
6. CBC Including Differential
7. CBC plus Sed. Rate (or sed. rate only)
8. CBC plus Hematocrit
9. CBC plus Other Special Tests
X. Bone Marrow (CBC implied)

23. ☐ HEMATOLOGY

1. Sugar
2. Nitrogen Derivatives
3. Total Proteins -c or -s A/G Ratio
4. Prothrombin Time
5. Cholesteral -c or -s Esters
6. Liver Function Tests
7. Electrolytes
8. Amylase, Vitamins, Others
9. Tests from 2 Groups Above
X. Tests from 3 or More Groups Above

24. ☐ CHEMISTRY

25.

1. Kahn
2. Kahn plus Rh if Not Transfused
3. Special Human Antibodies
4. Bacterial Agglutination
5. Heterophile
6. Quantitative Kahn
7. Kahn plus 2 or More from Above

26. ☐ SEROLOGY

1. EKG
2. EKG–2 or More Exams
3. EKG with Special Leads
4. BMR
5. BMR–2 or More Exams
6. BMR–Special Circumstances
7. EKG plus BMR
8. Electroencephalogram

27. ☐ EKG—BMR

1. Gastric or Vomitus for Blood
2. Stool for Blood
3. Stool Fat
4. Stool–OVA plus Parasites
5. Stool–Bile and/or Pigments
6. Gastric–Fractional as for HCl
7. Sputum–Other Than Bacteria
8. Both Gastric and Stool

28. ☐ Gastric-Stool

1. Direct Smear Only
2. Smear and Culture
3. Sub-Cultures for Identification
4. Anti-Biotic Sensitivity
5. Animal Inoculation
6. Sent Away for Study
7. Blood Culture
8. Skin Tests for Allergy
9. Skin Tests and Bacterial Studies

29. ☐ Bacteriology

1. Cell Count Only
2. Pandy or Other Protein
3. Routine inc. Count, Sugar, Protein
4. Routine Smear
5. Kahn and/or Colloidal Gold
6. Others

30. ☐ SPINAL FLUID

TOTAL NUMBER OF LAB PROCEDURES
31. ☐☐

A– Enter Number Whole Blood Transfusions 500 ml. Each or Less

B–REACTIONS
1. None Recorded
2. Subjective
3. Allergic -c Rash
4. Pyogenic
5. Mistake in Type plus X-Match
6. Due to Frequent or Many

32. A ☐☐ BLOOD B ☐

1. Private
2. Commercial Insurance
3. Workmens Comp.
4. Blue Cross
5. Local Welfare
6. Veterans
7. Crippled Children
8. Charities
9. Other

33. ☐ PAYMENT

REMARKS: ______

FOR SPECIAL STUDIES
34. ☐☐

*CODED BY STANDARD NOMENCLATURE

Form No. SWMHC-100—4-53

Reproduction of the Case Summary Code Sheet, Professional Activity Study, 1953.

Figure 4.3 Case Summary Code Sheet (close-up)

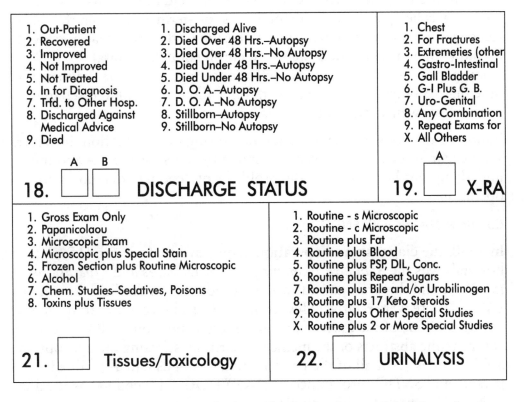

1. Out-Patient
2. Recovered
3. Improved
4. Not Improved
5. Not Treated
6. In for Diagnosis
7. Trfd. to Other Hosp.
8. Discharged Against Medical Advice
9. Died

1. Discharged Alive
2. Died Over 48 Hrs.–Autopsy
3. Died Over 48 Hrs.–No Autopsy
4. Died Under 48 Hrs.–Autopsy
5. Died Under 48 Hrs.–No Autopsy
6. D. O. A.–Autopsy
7. D. O. A.–No Autopsy
8. Stillborn–Autopsy
9. Stillborn–No Autopsy

1. Chest
2. For Fractures
3. Extremeties (other
4. Gastro-Intestinal
5. Gall Bladder
6. G-I Plus G. B.
7. Uro-Genital
8. Any Combination
9. Repeat Exams for
X. All Others

A B

18. ☐☐ **DISCHARGE STATUS**

A

19. ☐ **X-RA**

1. Gross Exam Only
2. Papanicolaou
3. Microscopic Exam
4. Microscopic plus Special Stain
5. Frozen Section plus Routine Microscopic
6. Alcohol
7. Chem. Studies–Sedatives, Poisons
8. Toxins plus Tissues

1. Routine - s Microscopic
2. Routine - c Microscopic
3. Routine plus Fat
4. Routine plus Blood
5. Routine plus PSP, DIL, Conc.
6. Routine plus Repeat Sugars
7. Routine plus Bile and/or Urobilinogen
8. Routine plus 17 Keto Steroids
9. Routine plus Other Special Studies
X. Routine plus 2 or More Special Studies

21. ☐ **Tissues/Toxicology**

22. ☐ **URINALYSIS**

Detail from the Case Summary Code Sheet, showing how some of the information was abstracted from the medical record. Each box could accept only one digit.

Using the System

The Michigan program was a success from the start, creating the first multihospital discharge abstract system. The initial distrust of the machines, which had resulted in the maintenance of the old manual systems in parallel with the new, quickly disappeared. Hospitals became "hooked" on the manifest advantages of computerization (machine tabulation), both for their internal uses, and because of the challenge provided by the interhospital comparisons. Meticulous input in the form of carefully prepared abstracts from each medical record was quickly perceived to pay off as the new statistics and indexes replaced the old. Without exception, the pilot participants dropped their old manual methods of indexing and statistical tabulating.

The hospitals were then, of course, dependent on the new external hospital discharge abstract system. The work had been "outsourced." Since it was being provided only under a short-term grant from the W. K. Kellogg Foundation, an emergency extension of the grant was approved to allow time to refine the system and enroll enough hospital participation to make the project self-supporting. It may be of interest to note that solvency was achieved with only about 1,000,000 discharges per year, at twenty-five cents per discharge.

Improved methods of retrieving and processing of information, however, soon began to uncover problems. Among the most serious — and those underlying this book — were the problems of "coding" diagnoses and operations.

Coding Problems with SNDO

In 1950, the diagnosis and operation coding system in use in U.S. hospitals was the *Standard Nomenclature of Diseases and Operations (SNDO)*, and this was, naturally, the one adopted in the first version of PAS.[15] There were relatively few trained medical record librarians in the 1950s, and one of the most important of their functions in PAS was to complete the abstracts of the medical records by selecting the appropriate *SNDO* codes. Not all of the participating hospitals had a qualified person, and *SNDO* (pronounced "SNOWDOUGH") coding, as it came to be called, proved quite a challenge.

✓ Coding problems which were formerly concealed within each individual hospital were now put on display as data comparisons across hospitals began and as increasing use was made of the diagnosis and operation indexes.

Odd information often turned out simply to reflect faulty coding. Further, the nature of *SNDO* made it impossible even to know whether or not a valid code had been used. There was no list of "legal" codes against which the recorded codes could be compared, and thus be used to control the quality of information (nor could there ever be such a list).[16]

---

15. SNDO is discussed further in the appendices; see page 407.

16. For more about valid codes, see page 131.

Incomplete Series of Cases

Equally as critical as the accuracy of the codes was the virtual impossibility with *SNDO* of retrieving a satisfactorily complete series of cases. The basic reason for this was that *SNDO* permitted the same condition to be given a variety of valid codes by different coders, and the existence of all these variations could never be detected. Thus a person attempting to retrieve all patients with "diabetes mellitus," for example, was unlikely to know how to look for patients who had been given different codes for the same condition by another coder (or even by the same coder at another time).

Changing to ICD

The solution to the diagnosis and operation coding problem at that time was to change to using the codes of the *International Statistical Classification* (commonly called "*ICD*") categories into which the *SNDO* codes would fall.[17] The *ICD* code was found adjacent to the *SNDO* code in the Fourth Edition of *SNDO*. This edition of *SNDO* also had an Appendix which was entitled, "List of 3-Digit and 4-Digit Categories of the International Statistical Classification [6th Revision] with Standard [i.e., "*SNDO*"] Numbers Included in Each International Category."

This change was greatly facilitated by the assistance of two enterprising medical record librarians — Loyola Voelker, CRL, of the United States Public Health Service Hospital in Baltimore, and Dorothy Kurtz, CRL, of the Columbia-Presbyterian Medical Center in New York — who had modified the 6th Revision of the *International Classification* to meet the data needs of their own hospitals. Their modifications, generally providing increased detail, were provided to the Professional Activity Study, and later formed the basis of the modifications and subdivisions used in all United States hospitals (and still in use today).[18] This was a

17. See "Classifications & Classifying," page 133 for more information on *ICD*.

18. These modifications are contained in the "Clinical Modification" of the *International Classification of Diseases*. The current edition is *International Classification of Diseases, Ninth Edition, Clinical Modification (ICD-9-CM)*. More about *ICD-9-CM* is contained on page 354.

much better solution to the "retrieval of series of cases" problem, and offered advantages in the coding step and in data processing as well.[19]

With abandonment of SNDO, which had a 6-digit modular operation coding system, a replacement was required. CPHA,[20] at the request of the federal government, developed a 3-digit operation classsification (later expanded to 4-digits) which was published by the government in Publication 719, *International Classification of Diseases, Adapted for Indexing of Hospital Records and Operation Classification.* PHS 719 is the nucleus of the operation classification found in Volume 3 of *ICD-9-CM*.

Though each succeeding volume of *ICD* has provided some improvement for assisting in retrieval of clinical information — primarily by permitting greater detail, i.e., having more categories — many of the early coding and classifying problems still remain with *ICD*:

- Its codes are for categories of diagnoses, rather than for individual diagnoses.

- The contents of many of the categories change with each generation of the classification, so that there often is no continuity from one revision to the next (even in the rare instance where categories in succeeding generations have the same numbers and labels).

- Many of the code numbers for categories (labels) also change; even if the category itself contains the same diagnoses, its contents will have different number. So diagnosis AAA in one generation may become diagnosis BBB in the next.

- Dual codes are still, in some instances, provided for the same condition in the *ICD* volumes from WHO (World Health Organization) (see "Dual Coding," page 139).

These problems are discussed in greater detail in later chapters.

---

19. Not the least of the advantages was that the *International* codes were shorter and thus they permitted more diagnoses to be entered into the punch card.

20. Commission on Professional and Hospital Activities, which ran PAS (Professional Activity Study).

5

Codes & Coding

In our electronic health information system today, a great deal of patient data is carried in coded form — that is, instead of all the original medical record information (from handwritten notes to dictated x-ray reports), what we give the computer to work with most of the time is coded material. For each patient, a whole lot of strings of characters (alphanumeric codes) tell that person's story.

Background

Code or classification?

One of the root causes of the problems in our health information system is the failure to understand (and appreciate) the differences between "code" and "classification." The words are often used interchangeably. But their meanings and functions are so entirely different, it is essential to distinguish between them.

Basically, *codes are identifiers*, and *classifications are organizers*. When we use both codes and classifications in the plural, as we have just done, this is simple enough because we are comparing "things" to "things". When used in the singular, however, a "classification" can be either a "thing" or an "activity."

As a "thing," a classification is an organizer, a set of pigeonholes into which to place other things. A code is a "thing" substituted for something else.

As an activity, classification means the same as "classifying" — the *process* of placing things *into* the categories of another "thing" (which happens to be also called a classification). *Coding* is the process of substituting the code for the original thing.

The definitions of these words — particularly the dual meaning of "classification" — have led to a great deal of confusion in the health information world.

Further, once a thing has been assigned to its category in a classification, that same thing is often *also assigned a code* to indicate where it has been classified. In fact, in healthcare *classifying and coding are almost always done at the same time*, which makes them look even more like one and the same thing.

Because of these vagaries of our language, we need to be sensitive to the problems they raise. It's not possible to discuss a single classification and not use the word classification in the singular. But when we mean the process of classification, we do have an option, and we try in this book to use either the single word "classifying" or the phrase "classification process." We may slip somewhere, though, so please try to think about which usage is intended whenever you encounter the word "classification" — in this book, and everywhere else, as well.

(Classifications and classifying are covered in detail in the next chapter; see page 133.)

The Code: An Information "Identifier"

A code is something substituted for something else — an individual item (of information, for example). There are several reasons for using a code:

- To obscure meaning. Examples include secret codes used in espionage, or in hospitals to protect the privacy of the physician or patient.

- To shorten information and facilitate its handling, especially by electronic means. For example, the use of product codes in mail order catalogs.

- To increase precision in communication. The single word Mayday is an internationally recognized code used to signal distress. In the sometimes jumbled world of radio-telephone communications, this single word can have no other meaning.

All three purposes can be served by coding health information.

The type of code used in an information system is customarily (but not necessarily) a numeric or alphanumeric string of characters, substituted for a term expressed in natural language (such as English). Some examples of commonly used codes are shown below.

Figure 5.1 Commonly Used Codes

Kind of Code	What It Represents	Example of Code
Social security number	Identity of a specific, unique individual	355-34-3222
Emergency information	A specific kind of emergency, to notify those who must take immediate action	Code Blue
Telephone number	Electronic pathway to a specific telephone	651-699-0666
URL (Uniform Resource Locator)	Electronic pathway to a specific page (file) on the World Wide Web (WWW)	http://www.tringa.com/ hccc.htm
Catalog number	A specific item of merchandise	HQ47588
Healthcare classification code	A specific category within a specific classification	473.1
Entity code	A specific, unique item — code is assigned to the smallest available relevant item of information	ISBN 0-9615255-2-5

Every code can in theory be decoded, meaning that it can be "translated back" into the original thing for which it was substituted. For example, in a mail order catalog, a code may look like this:

HQ47588 = "women's low cut blue jeans"

And the following comes from the diagnosis classification system currently used in U.S. hospitals, *ICD-9-CM,*[1]

508.9 = "Respiratory conditions due to unspecified external agent"

---

1.   *The International Classification of Diseases, 9th Revision, Clinical Modification.*

✓ We refer to the actual characters that make up the code in the examples above — "HQ47588" and "473.1" — as the code "value." We refer to the original information that it represents as the "equivalent."

It should be noted that codes are sometimes displayed with additional formatting characters to make them easier to be read by humans (e.g., the hyphens in phone numbers). Depending on the rules established for the use of the particular code involved, those characters may or may not be part of the code's value (see the box below).

Background

Codes: format vs. content

Frequently, codes are displayed in certain formats, typically to make them easier to be comprehended by humans. This sometimes leads to confusion about what the "real" value of the code is.

A diagnosis code's value might be "510.0" — requiring 5 characters (since in this example the decimal and its position are deemed significant). It would not be accurate to simply describe this as a "4-digit" code.

The value for a Social Security Number (SSN) code might be "333-44-6789". In this example, if the hyphens are significant, it is an "11-character" code. If they are not significant (used only for "formatting"), the SNN code might safely be called a "9-digit" code.

Other common codes which employ these "formatting characters" include telephone, ISBN, and credit card numbers. If the only purpose for the presence of these characters is to make the codes easier for humans to read and use, they aren't really part of the code's value. You don't dial the parentheses or hyphens when making a phone call. Computers don't need to store these characters in their databases either — they are simply inserted by the computer software whenever the code is displayed or printed for human consumption.

How Classifications Get Their Codes

Designing an effective classification is not an easy task. The creators of healthcare classifications are most concerned with organizing the items (e.g., diagnoses) in groups, according to their thinking, to serve the purposes of the classification. Once the schema is laid out, the categories are usually numbered to make it easy to put them in sequence. The designers leave "lots of room" between one group of categories and the next, always with the hope that there will be places for new things as needed. These numbers end up being used as "codes," since they are "equivalent to" the labels of the categories. This method of assigning codes has the helpful added feature that similar items can be "grouped" by their code numbers, and also sorted easily.

So, many healthcare classification codes — *ICD*, for example — really started out as "sequence numbers" used for ordering and sorting the classification. The assignment of codes was not intended to give any particular meaning to the codes themselves, except insofar as their placement indicated a relationship to other diseases/diagnoses with adjacent numbers.

✓ Thus while the classification itself is a scientifically designed schema, the coding system has not been planned and thought out in a similar way.

Shortcomings of "Sequence" Codes

There's a very big drawback to the "sequence" method of assigning codes: when new terms overflow the "lots of room" between existing categories, or new thinking reclassifies items, the only options for assigning codes to them are to:

- move items from one category to another to match the thinking, or
- add more categories if needed

Most critically, when the new categories outnumber the vacant spaces, there is no option but to *change the numbers*, so that the classification layout (sorting in the proper order) can be accommodated.

Perhaps the best illustration of this growth is in the field of genetics. In *ICD-9*, written in 1975 and published in 1978, 186 genetics categories ("pigeonholes") were provided, and nine of them were for chromosomal abnormalities. In *ICD-10* (written in 1989 and published in 1992, prior even to the vast explosion in knowledge in this field), the category number had grown to 709 categories, with 77 allocated for chromosomal abnormalities. No one predicted this growth in knowledge in 1975.

Chapter XVII in *ICD-10*, the "Q-codes" chapter where genetics disorders are found, allows space for only 23 more chromosomal abnormality groups. When the inevitable need to exceed this appears, major changes in the schema will be required, e.g., adding to the numbers of digits in the 3-character code and making it 4 or more digits, or rearranging other sections of the chapter so that the chromosomal abnormalities could start before code Q90. To do this, it might be necessary to rearrange and therefore renumber the chapters on either side of "Q" so it could start earlier or extend into the territory now occupied by "R."

Ideally, a code would never change its meaning, so that it could always be decoded to one and only one thing. To do this, the code cannot also serve as the device for sorting the items in the universe into a logical sequence. Developers of classifications should divorce the sorting mechanism from the codes which represent the meanings of the items. Up until recently, this has been an unwieldy, and perhaps impossible, task, because printed books were used and had to be revised and reissued with changes.

Today, such a "divorce" has become not only possible, but essential in a world of exploding technology and information. The classification's categories and their contents can be maintained in a database and updated as often as airline schedules, if necessary. Sorting can then be done instantly by the computer, which is instructed where to put each new code. Printed versions of the classification, when needed, can be produced from the database at a moment's notice.

Coding Processes

The process of assigning a code to an item (or group of items) of information is called "coding." Several processes are used for coding. Note that the *outcomes* of the "coding" processes vary greatly:

- some codes will describe the thing coded — *"what it is"*

- other codes will describe the category in which the thing belongs — *"where it goes"*
- still other coding processes result in telling how (somebody else thinks) the thing should be expressed — *"how to say it"*

Yet each process is commonly referred to as "coding." The three processes are distinct, as follows:

"What it is" — Entity coding This is the simple process of replacing the original term — a disease, for example — with its own, unique code. Entity coding, by itself, does not involve any classification schema or classifying of information. It simply identifies each piece.

"Where it goes" — Category coding This is the process of giving the original term the code belonging to the *category* into which the term should be placed, in the classification being used.

"How to say it" — Transformation coding This is a process of changing clinical terminology into a kind of "standardized language," usually accompanied by codes. There are two kinds of transformation coding:

- Modular language coding

This is the process of transforming a term (or a group of items or terms) into a structured set of coded components.

- Concept coding

This is the process of using only a single "preferred term" for a biomedical concept as defined by experts, instead of any synonyms which might have been used. The synonyms are discarded during the coding process. In fact, this is a kind of classifying process, as all synonyms are classified to the same preferred term for the concept.

Entity Coding

Entity coding is the "purest" form of coding. It of itself does not involve any classifying. There is a one-to-one relationship between entity and code, and the code is permanent.

Data maintained in entity code form can forever be retrieved unambiguously (decoded) when necessary, and it can be precisely and correctly classified from the coded state into any groupings desired, for any purpose.

Entity coding, and its application to health information management, is discussed in greater detail later; see page 277.

Category Coding

Category coding is the process most widely used in the United States today for coding clinical information.[2] In this system, patients ("cases") are assigned the code number for the classification category ("pigeonhole") into which they presumably fit. The code the patient receives does not represent that patient's diagnosis; rather, the code stands in for the *category* into which that patient fits.

The loss of specificity caused by category coding is illustrated in the table below, which shows how diagnoses coded into the system are eventually identified when retrieved. The first column gives the original diagnosis, as stated by the physician in the medical record, the second shows the code assigned in the medical records department, the third shows how the code would be translated. Note how specificity is lost, if not the actual diagnosis itself.

Figure 5.2 Diagnoses as Distorted by Coding to ICD-9-CM

Diagnosis in the Medical Record	ICD-9-CM Code Assigned	Decoded "Diagnosis"

Cold agglutinin disease	283.0	AUTOIMMUNE HEMOLYTIC ANEMIAS
		(which includes:
		    Autoimmune hemolytic disease
		      (cold type) (warm type)
		    Chronic cold hemagglutinin disease
		    Cold agglutinin disease or hemoglobinuria
		    Hemolytic anemia:
		      cold type (secondary) (symptomatic)
		      drug-induced
		      warm type (secondary) (symptomatic)
		and excludes:
		    Evans' syndrome (287.3)
		    hemolytic disease of newborn (773.0-773.5))

---

2.   For more about category coding, see "How We Code Today: Category Coding," page 205.

Figure 5.2 Diagnoses as Distorted by Coding to ICD-9-CM *(continued)*

Diagnosis in the Medical Record	ICD-9-CM Code Assigned	Decoded "Diagnosis"

Empyema of the gallbladder	575.0	ACUTE CHOLECYSTITIS
		
		(which includes:
		  Abscess of gallbladder without mention of calculus
		  Angiocholecystitis without mention of calculus
		  Cholecystitis without mention of calculus:
		    emphysematous (acute)
		    gangrenous
		    suppurative
		  Empyema of gallbladder without mention of calculus
		  Gangrene of gallbladder without mention of calculus
		and excludes:
		  that with:
		    acute and chronic cholecystitis (575.12)
		    choledocholithiasis (574.3)
		    choledocholithiasis and cholelithiasis (574.6)
		    cholelithiasis (574.0))

Pseudomonas meningitis	320.82	MENINGITIS DT GR-NEG NEC[a]
		
		(which includes:
		  Aerobacter aerogenes
		  Escherichia coli [E. coli]
		  Friedlander bacillus
		  Klebsiella pneumoniae
		  Proteus morganii
		  Pseudomonas
		and excludes:
		  gram-negative anaerobes (320.81))

Figure 5.2 Diagnoses as Distorted by Coding to ICD-9-CM *(continued)*

Diagnosis in the Medical Record	ICD-9-CM Code Assigned	Decoded "Diagnosis"

Hyperkeratosis	701.1	KERATODERMA, ACQUIRED
		
		(which includes:
		  Acquired:
		    ichthyosis
		    keratoderma palmaris et plantaris
		  Elastosis perforans serpiginosa
		  Hyperkeratosis:
		    NOS
		    follicularis in cutem penetrans
		    palmoplantaris climacterica
		  Keratoderma:
		    climactericum
		    tylodes, progressive
		  Keratosis (blennorrhagica)
		and excludes:
		  Darier's disease [keratosis follicularis]
		    (congenital) (757.39)
		  keratosis:
		    arsenical (692.4)
		    gonococcal (098.81))

a. This is the computer truncation of "meningitis due to gram-negative bacteria, not elsewhere classified." Such truncation is used in most computer printouts of codes, forced by the limited space allowed.

Only if a category has been designed to contain *only one diagnosis* will decoding return the name of that specific diagnosis. This would be strictly accidental, because categories are constructed to contain groups of items, and by far the majority of them do contain groups, not single entities.[3] And even if a "single-diagnosis" category was maintained as

---

3. *ICD-9-CM* has over 100 categories which each contain more than 100 individual diagnoses. Thus over 10,000 discrete diagnostic terms are being replaced by 100 group labels. Similar losses occur with the coding of procedures and treatments. Diagnosis Related Groups (DRGs) are a special class of category coding in that the "terms" placed in the DRG categories are themselves the categories of *ICD-9-CM* (see "Diagnosis Related Groups," page 421).

such from one generation of the classification to another, it would quite likely have another code because of rearrangement of the classification.

Transformation Coding

Some types of "coding" processes actually serve to transform clinical terminology into "accepted" terms or phrases. The purpose of such coding is not to classify as such, but to create a standardized terminology for a specific discipline (for more about this subject, see "Standardizing the Meanings of Terms," page 81). There are two main kinds of such transformation processes: Modular Language Coding and Concept Coding.

Modular Language Coding

Transforming information into a modular language[4] is typified by "coding" with the *Standard Nomenclature of Diseases and Operations (SNDO)*, which was used for many years in the United States health information system. Here the ordinary diagnostic term or procedure was transformed into a "standard nomenclature" when the coder replaced the diagnostic term with codes representing:

a. the part of the body affected (topography),

b. the cause of the aberration or condition encountered (etiology),

c. the manifestation, when appropriate, and

d. (sometimes) other information.

A procedure was expressed by starting with:

a. the involved part of the body (topography), and adding

b. a code from a very simple classification of operations.

For example, the coder could look up "diabetes mellitus" in the alphabetic index to *SNDO*. There the reference was to a page in the "Standard Nomenclature of Diseases" section of the book. In the designated section, there were a number of options given. Some were for

---

4. Modular languages create terms by taking components from different universes or axes and linking them together. See "Modular Languages," page 83.

diabetes in conjunction with other diseases or manifestations. One of these could be chosen, or the coder could create a code representing (1) a condition of the pancreas, (2) caused by something, and (3) perhaps manifested by, e.g., glycosuria. Each of these three segments had its own code number, and their appearance in the prescribed sequence was the total "term" (and its code) to be given to the disease — the disease name was transformed before coding.

Decoding this string of segment codes transformed the diagnostic term into an often unrecognizable concatenation of words. For example, even if the coder used the simplest code for diabetes mellitus, 871-785, decoding it literally yielded (871) "pancreas, insular tissue" + (785) "insular tissue, decreased function" — clearly a transformation of the original terminology — and that string of words could hardly be called the "standard nomenclature" for diabetes mellitus.[5]

A similar transformation process is the foundation of the College of American Pathologists *Systematized Nomenclature of Human and Veterinary Medicine (SNOMED International* or *SNOMED III)*, and of the American College of Radiology's *Index for Radiological Diagnoses (IRD).*[6]

For example, using *SNOMED II*, here's how "pulmonary tuberculosis" would be coded:

> T-28000 + M-44060 + E-2001 + F-03003

This decodes to:

> Lung + granuloma + M. tuberculosis + Fever

With *SNOMED III*:

> T-28000 + M-44060 + L-21801 + F-03003

Which decodes to:

> Lung + Miliary granuloma + Mycobacterium tuberculosis hominis
> + Increased body temperature

---

5. Coding with SNDO is treated in some detail in the appendices; see page 407.

6. *SNOMED* and *IRD* are discussed more fully in the appendices; see page 429 and page 483.

SNOMED also has a module entitled "Diseases/Diagnoses" which can be used instead of the modular construction. "Pulmonary tuberculosis" using this method (the method employed in electronic medical record systems which accommodate SNOMED) produces the following coding:

SNOMED II:

D-0188 = Tuberculosis

SNOMED III:

DE-14800 = Tuberculosis, NOS (not otherwise specified), or

DE-14813 = Tuberculosis of the lung with cavitation, or

DE-14814 = Tuberculosis of lung with involvement of bronchus.

This change between *SNOMED II* and *SNOMED III* may have been one of clarification of the concept or a change in the concept itself. In any case, the strings of code numbers which depicted pulmonary tuberculosis under the two transformations were radically different. The decoder would have to know whether *SNOMED II* or *SNOMED III* was involved, and the clue provided — "D-" vs "DE-" — is a subtle one indeed.

SNOMED is a highly complex, structured transformation method, and decoding the product of the transformation cannot retrieve the natural language input from which the structured code was derived. Sometimes even the concept is distorted. Because of this, the codes do not reflect precisely what was in the records of original entry.

Concept Coding

The second kind of transformation is used in "concept coding." This primarily consists of using all the synonyms or other alternative terms for a given concept as "input" to a system which then "reports out" the "preferred term," i.e., the concept for which the synonyms, at a given point in time, are considered to have the same meaning.

In a general dictionary, vertigo has as its synonyms dizziness, lightheadedness, giddiness, instability, and wooziness (colloquial). While these terms may be used alternatively in ordinary conversation, such usage probably would not satisfy various medical specialists, among whom they might have different definitions. So even the decisions as to which terms are synonyms and which are not is a task for experts.

The rules for transforming a clinical or biomedical term to a modular language classification do not appear to have been written; the process is virtually an art. The *Diagnostic and Statistical Manual of Mental Disorders (DSM)* of the American Psychiatric Association describes concepts, and approaches concept coding in its correlation with *ICD-10*; see page 94.

Concept coding is also used in the Read Clinical Classification System in Great Britain (NHS Codes) and in the Unified Medical Language System (UMLS) of the National Library of Medicine.[7]

Identifying the Type of Coding

The best way to find out whether the process in question is entity coding, category coding, modular language coding, or concept coding is to decode — look up the code to see what it means.[8] And to be sure about it, one needs to have at hand the natural language which was the original input.

Only if it is *entity coding* of a clinical term will decoding retrieve the exact natural language term which was coded, instead of a category or transformed term. If decoding doesn't retrieve that term, but rather brings out the label of a group or category, the process is *category coding*. If the retrieved string of words is an array of modular components which describe an entity, or if it is the label given a concept or is a preferred term, the process used was one of *transformation* (i.e., either *modular language* or *concept coding*).

Maintaining Data Integrity

While, as we have seen, there are a number of benefits to coding information, there is also the risk of assigning the wrong code, either by a mistake in judgment or by simple clerical error. The same computer-

---

7. For more detail on these, see the appendices, "NHS Codes (Read Codes)," page 459 and "Unified Medical Language System," page 425.

8. The decoding, itself, can be very difficult — see the discussion on page 291.

based electronic health information system that uses the codes can also be designed to minimize the risk of coding errors occurring in the first place.

Validity

A computer can easily be made to check the validity of the data which comes into it. It does this by applying "validation rules." Data which don't comply with the rules are called "invalid," and are rejected by the system. This greatly improves the accuracy in an information system. Of course, "valid" data may still be inaccurate or even wrong, but eliminating the possibility of invalid ("obviously wrong") errors goes a great way to improve the quality of the data overall.

Well-designed data entry systems can achieve very high accuracy rates. In some manual-entry systems, for instance, everything is keyed in a second time, a process called "key verification" — any discrepancy reveals an error. Systems employing barcode scanners make use of an extra "check digit" encoded in the barcode symbol itself.[9] This extra digit allows the scanner software to mathematically determine if the code just scanned in is valid. This concept allows barcode data entry to have as few as one error for every three million entries — as opposed to the 30,000 errors a human would normally make doing the same task manually.

Some validation rules are built into almost every modern database program. For example, a numeric field is not permitted to receive alphabetic characters. This prevents the common error of someone using a lowercase "L" ("l") rather than the digit "1". Another consistent rule is that a numerical field for months cannot have a number higher than 12.

Impossibility

Another way the accuracy of data can be improved is to have the software check for certain combinations of data items — many combinations are improbable or impossible. For example, any patient data linking a male with an obstetrical or gynecological diagnosis or procedure code is "illegal." Similarly, a procedure for newborns could

---

9. See an example of this in the ISBN barcode symbol on the back of this book; see also "The ISBN Code Example," page 307.

not be "legally" performed on someone over six months old. Impossible or illegal code combinations can be written into the rules as invalid.

A specific classification may have its own set of rules, tailor-made for that classification. For these, someone familiar with the classification and its conventions compiles a list of "legal" terms and codes. The list is called "valid codes" or "valid values." First of all, any such list will include all of the codes in the classification itself — any code which is not included somewhere in the classification is, of course, not valid. The computer sends such codes back for correction. In a classification where modules are combined (e.g., *SNOMED*), valid codes would be limited to biomedically possible combinations. Compilation and maintenance of such a list would require a truly monumental effort, as the number of possible combinations would be astronomical.

A little known fact about *SNDO*, which was used in U.S. hospitals until the 1950s, was that virtually any combination of numbers of the correct configuration was, so far as the computer was concerned, a legal code in *SNDO* — yet it could easily be absolute clinical nonsense (the same problem is presented by *SNOMED*). *ICD*, on the other hand, had a finite, auditable list of valid codes, and any invalid code could be blocked from entry (and thus sent back for correction) by programming of the computer.[10] Thus when hospitals moved from *SNDO* to the *International Classification*, a quantum improvement in data quality was the immediate result of the switch.

---

10. One problem with the new coding system being developed for procedures, *ICD-10-PCS*, is that there is not yet a list of valid values, and it may be impossible ever to create such a list. See "ICD-10-PCS — A New Coding System," page 191.

6

Classifications & Classifying

A CLASSIFICATION is a set of categories into which all the things in a given universe are to be placed, along one or more axes. "Classification" as used here must be distinguished from *nomenclature*, which refers to approved terms used in a particular field or science, and *terminology*, which refers to the terms actually used in the field, whether "approved" or not.[1]

The concept of a "universe" is as simple as it sounds: it could be all known diseases, all recognized healthcare procedures, or all the items in your attic. "Axes," the other key concept in defining a classification, is just a bit more complex.

Axes An "axis" is an attribute or "property" that all items in the classification's universe share. (The plural of axis is "axes".) Think of an axis in a classification as the term that completes the phrase "organized by ... " (size, color, weight ...).

Items in a universe often have more than one attribute by which they can be described (organized). Diseases, for instance can be organized by which parts of the body they affect (topography), or by their cause (etiology). Healthcare procedures may be organized by whether they are surgical or not, inpatient or outpatient, or even whether they are covered under Medicare or not. An axis for the universe of items in your attic is whether they are yours or whether they were left there when your kids moved out. In the context of classifications, an axis is simply an organizing framework for arranging the contents of a universe.

Real world classifications often require more than one axis to be useful. While the "white pages" of a telephone directory needs only a single axis (last name, in alphabetical order), the "yellow pages" typically uses two

---

1. And from "taxonomy," which is a kind of terminology. For more about these distinctions, see "Expression of Clinical Concepts," page 71.

or more axes. The primary axis is the type of product or service provided, and the secondary axis is the name of the vendor. Directories in larger urban areas sometimes use a third axis which organizes vendors by their location. Such classifications are called "compound" (see page 136).

The Classification: An Information "Organizer"

The categories of the classification can be seen as a set of "pigeonholes" into which all of the things you want to organize can be put. The selection of categories and the way *they* are organized is referred to as the "schema" of the classification.

✓ The classification schema is a plan of organizing information in the way most helpful *to those who designed the schema*.

Below is a small segment of a larger classification. Each line is one category, with indentation indicating that the indented items are subsets (subcategories) of the less indented, broader, category:

> Pneumothorax
>> Spontaneous tension pneumothorax
>> Iatrogenic pneumothorax
>> Other spontaneous pneumothorax
>> Paradoxical thorax[2]

As we saw in the previous chapter, codes are often assigned to each category (and subcategory) to make the classification easier to work with (see "How Classifications Get Their Codes," page 121). This is the case, for example, in the *International Classification of Diseases, 9th Revision, Clinical Modification (ICD-9-CM)*, used by United States hospitals today. The decimal subdivisions serve the same purpose as the indentations shown above:

---

2.   A "condition in which the pleural membrane presents a singular appearance" — this fictitious diagnosis was invented by Souther F. Tompkins, MD, a classmate of the senior author.

512   Pneumothorax
  512.0   Spontaneous tension pneumothorax
  512.1   Iatrogenic pneumothorax
  512.8   Other spontaneous pneumothorax
  512.X   Paradoxical thorax

In this example, the code value itself ("512" etc.) comes simply from the *sequence* in the classification where nosologists believe, at a given time in biomedical thought, the category belongs.[3] Each code value for the category in *ICD-9-CM* comes from its use in *sorting* the information to place it in the order prescribed periodically by the World Health Organization.[4]

Because of the proximity of the "code" (numeric value) to the "category" (the name of the disease), the code is often mistaken for the category, and the code system is mistaken for the classification schema. However, the codes in *ICD-9-CM* have no meaning in themselves; they are only "labels" for the category names.[5]

Attributes of a Classification

A classification has certain basic properties:

Defined universe. Each classification deals with a defined universe, i.e., a set of items which have something in common. For some purposes, a universe may be dissected into subsets of items; these subsets are also, in themselves, universes. For example, a telephone directory may be set up to list all telephone subscribers in a given area. In this directory, universe = all subscribers. Or the subscribers in the same area may be divided into

---

3.   A nosologist is a specialist in the classification of diseases.

4.   And by the United States Coordinating and Maintenance Committee for *ICD-9-CM*. This official committee is made up of federal employees who meet periodically and consider changes in the categories, new subcategories, and their content. Its recommendations, after approval by the National Center for Health Statistics (NCHS) (for diagnoses) and the Health Care Financing Administration (HCFA) (for procedures), are made official by publication in the *Federal Register* and disseminated in a publication, *Coding Clinic for ICD-9-CM*, published quarterly by the American Hospital Association's Central Office on *ICD-9-CM*.

5.   For more detail on sequence coding, see page 121.

two universes, residential and business, and placed in two directories. Thus, universe of directory 1 = all residential subscribers, and universe of directory 2 = all business subscribers.

Purpose. Each classification is devised to meet some need, i.e., it has a specific purpose. The purpose determines not only the universe to be classified, but also the schema (design and organization) of the classification.

Groups of items. A classification groups the items in its universe, and uses as few groups (categories) as are consistent with its purpose. The joking statement that persons who design classifications are either "groupers" or "splitters" reflects the differences in the purposes for which the classifications are developed.

Logical schema. Each classification organizes the groups in its universe logically according to a schema (design and organization) which is created in response to its purpose. In general, the simpler and more consistent the schema of the classification, the more useful the classification. The schema is expressed by the axis or axes used in forming the classification.

Accommodates all items. A classification must accommodate its entire universe, i.e., it has to have a pigeonhole for every member of its universe, even if one of the pigeonholes has to be labeled "other" (such pigeonholes are usually called "wastebasket categories"). As a corollary, a classification cannot accommodate items which do not belong to its universe. As a matter of fact, the first step in using a classification is to classify the items presented for classifying as either belonging "in" or "out."

Simple vs. Compound Classifications

Simple Classifications

When a classification deals with a single universe, distributed along a single axis, it is called a simple classification. For example, one attribute of a shoe is sex. Another is size. Each of these universes has its own simple classification along an appropriate axis. Sex is male or female. Size is numerical. Granted that stocking purely by sex or size would not make much sense, these descriptions illustrate simple classifications.

In medicine, there are a number of universes, such as body systems, causes of disorders, physiological disturbances, and anatomic sites. Parts of the body could be "found along" an anatomic or topographic axis. All causes of disease could be arranged along an "etiologic" (cause) axis. One classification of diseases could have a single axis, such as the probable fatality of the diseases themselves, progressing from trivial to lethal. Another classification of diseases could have a different single axis, such as the parts of the body affected. The skeleton could be classified on an axis of sizes of the bones, from small to large.

As a matter of fact, for each of the attributes used in classifications in healthcare, there are several simple, comprehensive classifications. Etiological classifications have been worked out for such major subdivisions as neoplasms, infections, genetic abnormalities, trauma, and the like. Anatomic (topographic) classifications have been worked out on axes such as head, upper extremities, torso, lower extremities, and so on. "System" classifications are built around the circulatory system, nervous system, respiratory system, endocrine system, reproductive system, and the rest. Each of these simple classifications is drawn on in developing the more complex classifications used in healthcare to describe patients.

The various modules of the *Systematized Nomenclature of Human and Veterinary Medicine (SNOMED)* are actually a series of such classifications.[6] For example, the Topography module classifies anatomy by system and by region and provides classifications of cellular and subcellular structures and the products of conception and embryonic structures. The Morphology module classifies according to disease processes: traumatic, congenital, inflammatory, degenerative, growth, and neoplastic. For neoplasms, *SNOMED* uses the *International Classification of Diseases for Oncology (ICD-O)* from the World Health Organization. *ICD-O* has its own topographic classification plus a morphologic classification which is modified by a supplementary code showing the behavior of the particular neoplasm.

---

6. For more about *SNOMED*, see "Systematized Nomenclature of Human and Veterinary Medicine (SNOMED International)," page 85 and the appendices, page 429.

Compound Classifications

A classification may deal with more than one axis at a time, and in fact most do. Such classifications are called compound — they take into consideration more than one attribute. Compound classifications often include axes within axes.

The shoe store must, in real life, use a compound classification in its stock room. The axes of sex, size, color, style, manufacturer, and others, such as season, are all used in arranging the shelving for the single universe of shoes.

As described earlier, in medicine there are a number of universes, thus a medical classification is likely to be compound, and to have primary and secondary (or more) axes. For example, the primary axis for diagnoses could be anatomical, the secondary etiologic — in which case for each body site, the causes of the disease would be categorized. Then the diseases might be alphabetically arranged within each cause. Some diseases might have multiple causes, of course, and the schema becomes more complicated than ever. Designing a compound classification is not a simple task.

Variable Multiaxial Classifications

The *International Classification of Diseases (ICD)* has been called a "variable multiaxial" classification, so constructed because of its need to try to satisfy so many constituencies. For example, early in the volume there is a chapter concerning infectious diseases. A later one covers respiratory diseases. It is likely that the user will not want to count the same condition (or patient) more than once. Where, then, to place pneumonia? It is both an infectious disease and a respiratory disease.

This, and myriad similar conditions which cross one or more boundaries between chapters of the classification, are at the root of the many problems facing a person trying to classify a case. They are responsible also for the amount of instructional materials for the use of *ICD*, both within *ICD* itself and in "coding aids" published by others. They are also responsible for the numbers of "inclusion," "exclusion," and other instructional notes found accompanying more than half of the categories in some chapters of the Tabular List (for examples of some of these, see "Walking Through: Coding "Polyneuropathy" with ICD-9-CM," page 206).

Dual Coding

The preference in the United States for classifying a given case only once was a prime motivator for the creation of *ICD-9-CM* — to get rid of the "dual coding" feature of *ICD-9* (and still in the new *ICD-10*). This is usually referred to as the "dagger (†) and asterisk (*)" feature.

Dual coding applies to some, but not all, of the diagnostic statements. It is used when the statement contains " ... information about both an underlying generalized disease and a manifestation in a particular organ or site which is a clinical problem in its own right." Where it is used, the dagger (†) marks the underlying disease, and the asterisk (*) marks an optional additional code for the manifestation. Discussion of this usage is found in Volume 2 of *ICD-10* along with all the instructions for use of the classification. A dagger code, for example, is:

A30.0† Meningococcal meningitis [use also code] (G01*)

The asterisk code is:

G01* = Meningitis in bacterial diseases classified elsewhere

Objections to the "dagger and asterisk" feature were that the user could not be depended on to use both codes consistently, as directed in the instructions. Both would always have to be searched, and there would be no assurance as to whether cases were being counted once or twice. Elimination of the dual coding was one argument which led to the clinical modification of *ICD-9* in the United States, so that this confusion simply could not occur.

Patient Information for Classifications

The classifications developed for use in today's healthcare have many different purposes, including:

- billing for care
- compiling mortality statistics
- compiling morbidity statistics
- comparing the health of our nation with that of other nations
- studying the effects of drugs and other treatments — providing information for evidence-based medicine

- controlling and improving the quality of care

- developing our healthcare policies

- epidemiological research, such as studying AIDS and other contagious diseases

- planning our facilities

- developing our local and national healthcare budgets

✓ For responding to each of these demands, the universe in healthcare is *patients*, not just diagnoses or procedures.

Each patient[7] — or "case" — who comes into contact with the healthcare system must be "classified" in one or more ways. Often, this is done on the basis of their diseases or of procedures performed on them. The various healthcare classifications in use are not, though their titles seem to imply, classifications of diagnoses or operations per se, but rather of *persons*.

Patient Data Sets

For each person, there exists a patient data set[8] made up of multiple universes of information, many of which are recorded in medical records. A subset of the items in the medical record is kept today in "derivative" records, such as record abstracts and patient bills. These derivative records are, almost without exception, electronic, and the electronic records are the source for virtually all of our information about healthcare. Increasingly, the derivative records are also the sole source of information on individual patients — not just patient groups.

---

7.   A patient is a person who has established a contractual relationship with a health care provider for that provider to care for that person. A patient may or may not be ill or injured. A patient who is ill or injured, or who otherwise presents a health problem, is often referred to as a "case."

8.   A data set is a group of items of information, usually in the context of an electronic database. The data set will be made up of "fields" which describe the type of information in each piece of data — for example, name, address, phone. The pieces of data are then specific within each field: name = Jane, address = 423 Fifth Street, phone = 222-5555. The data set is this collection of information.

When one asks questions about people, only rarely is there use for data from a single axis of information about them; seldom does a simple classification suffice. Sometimes a question pertains only to the sex distribution of a population, or to its age distribution. But usually such questions are asked without careful thought, and immediately are followed by a request for more information, such as the age distribution of each sex, or vice versa — the sex distribution of each age.

In a hospital, it may be useful to know the proportion of patients handled by each of the clinical services, but an immediately following question is likely to be, "what diagnoses or problems did each service see?" or "what procedures were performed on the patients?" or "what was the age distribution of these patients?" In a proper information system, such compound queries, requiring compound classifications, should be available on an "ad hoc" basis. In this way, anyone needing information can ask their own specific questions of the data, and receive immediate answers.

Patient Attribute Universes

It is not possible to list all the attributes which could be used in one or another classification of persons or patients, i.e., attributes which might be taken into account, under some circumstances, in describing an individual and that individual's experiences with regard to health or healthcare. There are some attributes which would be useful for retrieval of information about a given individual, while others would be primarily useful for placing the individual in a category for some specific purpose. A number of attributes come readily to mind, however, since they are already incorporated in many of the data systems used in healthcare today (and more data items are being added regularly).

Following is a list of commonly used patient attributes. The Uniform Hospital Discharge Data Set (UHDDS)[9], initiated for Medicare billing and subsequently adopted by other payers, could be considered the absolute minimum list of these attributes. UHDDS items are **bolded**. (Items relating solely to administration, charges, billing, and insurance are excluded from this list.)

---

9.   *UB-92 HCFA-1450.* U. S. Health Care Financing Administration (HCFA).

Figure 6.1 Patient Attributes

Individual identification
  Patient name
  Address
  Social Security number
  Date of admission (or visit)
  Medical record number
  Date of birth (DOB)
  Age (in variable detail: smallest
     units in infancy – minutes,
     hours, days, months; largest
     in adulthood – years)
Sex
Marital status
Race/Ethnicity
Past medical history
Family medical history
Physical attributes
  Height
  Weight
Genomic information
Problems of the individual
  Chronic
  Acute
  Social
  Mental
Investigations employed
  Physical
  Laboratory
  Imaging
  Others
Diagnoses
  Admitting diagnosis
  Principal diagnosis
  Other diagnoses

Treatments received
  Procedures (surgery, etc.)
  Physical therapy
  Radiation
Drugs
External factors
  Environment
  Occupation
Trauma
Physical fitness
Activities of daily living (ADL)
  capability (a series of attributes)
Preventive measures
  Vaccinations
  Education
Life style
  Nutrition
  Exercise
  Relevant habits
Provider (care system used)
  Office
  Clinic
  Hospital/clinical service
  Hospice
  HMO
  Others (listed)
Caregivers (who are also the
     sources of information)
  Patient
  Physicians
  Nurses
  Home health aides
  Others (listed)

Example of patient attributes which might be used in a database. The bolded items comprise the Uniform Hospital Discharge Data Set (UHDDS).

The list is virtually endless. And, as we see below, for each of the universes listed there are usually a number of additional axes which may be relevant under some circumstances:

Laboratory procedures May be classified by the specimen tested, or the technology used in their analyses, or the branch of science to which they pertain, e.g., bacteriology or chemistry, or the kind of laboratory in which they are performed, e.g., clinical or forensic, and so on.

Imaging diagnostic procedures May be classified by the technology, e.g., X-ray, ultrasound, MRI, or by the part of the body examined, or by the type of abnormality discovered, and so forth.

Surgical procedures May be categorized by the kind of surgeon doing them e.g., orthopedist or neurosurgeon, or by the kind of procedure, e.g., incision, repair, removal, or by the part of the body, and more.

Utilizing a Data Set

The demand on patient data for any useful classification will require taking into account more than one (often many) of the attributes of each individual patient.

✓ It is the job of a *classification* to declare, first, what patient attributes are required for that particular classification.

The classification must then specify how attributes are to be compounded — how each patient's data with regard to each attribute will be used in conjunction with some or all of the other attributes. Finally, the classification writes the rules for placing the patient in one of its classes (a category of the classification), i.e., creates an algorithm for the process.

Because of the versatility of a data set, there is no need to arrange attribute lists in any logical order. The computer can do the arranging "on the fly," according to the information needed and questions asked of it. From a computer standpoint, each attribute is a *field* in a patient database, where each patient is a separate *record*.

The *classification* provides the questions to be asked of the data, the rules for retrieval, and a blueprint for displaying the data once retrieved.

The Process of Classifying

Classifying, meaning "to put things into categories," is a process requiring care, knowledge, judgment, experience, and decision making. It includes three steps:

- Step 1: Determine the identity of the item to be classified.

    - This requires detailed *knowledge about the items.*

- Step 2: Decide whether or not the item belongs to the universe in question (if it doesn't belong, it gets "classified out" — a decision must be made to reject it).

    - This step requires knowledge of the *boundaries of the universe.*

- Step 3: If it does belong, allocate it to the correct category ("pigeonhole") of the classification being used.

    - This requires knowledge of the *organizing principles of the classification* and the *rules for its use.*

✓ Even if the classifier allocates the item to the code representing the category, the process is still classification, not coding. The item has not merely been assigned a code — it has been assigned to a category in a classification.

The reasons for using codes to represent the categories of a classification is discussed at "How Classifications Get Their Codes," page 121.

Example: Classifying Cars The process of classifying occurs millions of times a day. In the automobile industry, the number of classifications which may be constructed is virtually endless. There can be classifications based on size, numbers of doors, weight, purpose (trucks or passenger vehicles), manufacturer, and so on and so on.

Let's say a sales associate is asked to put all cars on outdoor display by color.

For Step 1, the associate will go to where the stock is kept, and determine for each vehicle whether it is a car or not.

For Step 2, the associate will bring out all the cars and leave all of the trucks, RVs, and SUVs where they were.

For Step 3, the associate needs adequate color vision and knowledge of the language used (often a cute term, like "sunset") to describe the colors. No other information about the cars, such as horsepower or body style, is needed.

The associate must also know, though, how the "color" classification schema works. Are the automobiles simply to be grouped as red, green, and "other?" Or does the grouping schema require a finer breakdown? How many shades of red must be distinguished? What are the rules for handling two-tone paint? Does metallic paint go in the same group as the color without the metallic sheen? A list of rules to answer these questions would be immensely helpful — but even with such a list, the classifier still needs to learn, understand, and apply the rules.

Classifying Healthcare Data

Most day-to-day classifying is probably taken for granted and done without much thought. Sometimes this happens with healthcare information. Most people dealing "at arm's length" with medical data, for example, think that what must be done with the data is to "code" it — simply look up each item in a list and find its code number there. Indeed, this process does not appear to be *classifying*, at all. But not only *is* it classifying, it is classifying information in the most complex and serious way. And it takes a much larger storehouse of information, skills, and experience than that needed to shelve shoes.

First of all, *what*, in our health information system today, is actually to be "coded"? It appears that we're coding just the diagnostic term(s), and any procedures performed, which have been recorded in the medical record — but it's not that simple.

In fact, the task in the health information system is to place the *case*, of which diagnosis and procedure are merely attributes, in its proper category.

A *case* is a patient *and* his or her medical problem. A *problem* is a disease, injury, or any other condition or situation which brings an individual into contact with the healthcare system.[10] Certain conditions, such as alcoholism, are not admitted by all to be "diseases," but they do bring individuals to healthcare, as do ill-defined symptoms, behavioral problems, the need for well-person examinations, and the like. Chapter XXI of *ICD-10* — *Factors influencing health status and contact with health services (Z00-Z99)* — lists, among others, the following "conditions":

> loss of love relationship (code number Z61)
>
> removal from home (Z61)
>
> failed exams in school (Z55)
>
> stressful work schedule (Z56)
>
> extreme poverty (Z59.5)

"Coding" a case under our present system isn't simple at all. For one thing, attributes of the patient other than the diagnosis per se almost always influence the placement of the case in a category. This is true because most healthcare classifications are complex — they have multiple axes (sets of attributes) involved in grouping and arranging the items in their universes.

In considering diagnoses, the *category coder* (who is really a *classifier*) must not only be able to recognize medical words (even when misspelled), but also must understand the meaning of most of them. And the classifications used for grouping them have far more rules (called "conventions"), exceptions, and modifiers, than the simple illustration, above, of automobile color. Examples throughout this book should make clear the complexity of the issue, whether the classification is *ICD-9-CM* or one of the other classifications used in the past.[11]

In classifying procedures, similar situations are encountered with *Current Procedural Terminology (CPT)* and the *Health Care Financing*

---

10. For each encounter between an individual and a healthcare provider, there must be some reason (if only for payment purposes) for that visit; each reason gets a code number (or at least the "most important" ones do).

11. See "How We Code Today: Category Coding," page 205.

Administration's Common Procedure Coding System (HCPCS) (see more about these on page 175.

In fact, there are a number of classifications used in U.S. healthcare today:

- *International Classification of Diseases, 9th Edition, Clinical Modification (ICD-9-CM)* (for diseases and, in the hospital, procedures)[12]

- *Physicians' Current Procedural Terminology (CPT)* (for physician procedures)

- *Health Care Financing Administration's Common Procedure Coding System* (HCPCS)

  - Level 1: *CPT*[13]

  - Level 2: National Codes

  - Level 3: Local Codes

- Diagnosis Related Groups (DRGs)[14]

- Ambulatory Care Groups (ACGs)

The proliferation — and complexity — of these systems shows the impossibility of a single classification meeting all of the needs in healthcare.

---

12. Discussion of *ICD* begins on page 155; for *ICD-9-CM*, see page 162.

13. *CPT* is described on page 183. For HCPCS, see page 188.

14. DRGs and ACGs are described further on page 163. There is also an appendix on DRGs; see page 421.

7

Diagnosis Classifications

THE PROCESS OF USING a disease or diagnosis classification to code clinical healthcare information has been an evolutionary one. Prior to about the 1930s, classifications in health care had been of diseases, injuries, and causes of death — these classifications were used for mortality and morbidity statistics.[1]

Since the 1930s, when coding and classifying came into widespread use in clinical[2] healthcare, two major diagnosis/disease classifications have been involved. Hospitals initially used the American Medical Association's *Standard Nomenclature of Diseases and Operations (SNDO)*.[3] Then hospitals, as well as other elements of the healthcare system, began using one generation after another of the *International Classification of Diseases (ICD)*, a product of the World Health

---

1. The history of these uses, going back to about the early 18th century, is well covered in the Introductions to the International Classifications *ICD-6* and *ICD-9* (these are reproduced in the appendices; see page 364). In this book, "coding" refers to *clinical* coding unless otherwise specified.

2. "Clinical" refers to direct contact with or information from patients and to the course of illness; "things" medical about a patient. Thus personal (bedside) contact with the patient is clinical contact, a laboratory which examines blood and other specimens from patients is a clinical laboratory, the patient's medical record is a clinical record, research involving patients is clinical research, a nurse taking care of patients is a clinical nurse.

3. Plunkett, R.J., and A. C. Hayden, editors. *Standard Nomenclature of Diseases and Operations*. 4th Ed. 1952. Amer Med Assn, Chicago. See "Retrieval of Medical Record Information," page 99, and the appendices, page 407, for more on *SNDO*.

Organization.[4] It is still the primary classification in use in the United States.

As over time more and more uses were found for clinical information, existing classifications were simply adopted and adapted to meet current needs. Once set in motion, coding simply grew, like cities grow, without a comprehensive plan.

✓ There has never been a "stopping place" at which planners in healthcare (that is, everyone with an interest) could examine what was happening and what was needed, and lay out a system accordingly.

The result has been, inevitably, a less than ideal system. One of the key figures in the development of health statistics in the United States in the 1970s and 1980s commented,

> The International Classification of Diseases (ICD) grew in size, as a consequence of unbalanced pressure from diverse sub-specialist groups, and in rigidity, through control of successive revisions by vital statisticians and epidemiologists who were increasingly removed from the realities of clinical practice and especially from the vast uncharted realm of primary care. In the absence of any organizing principles, the ICD became an unstructured amalgam of chapters based variously on anatomy, clinical manifestations, changing views of "causation," clinical specialties, and age groups. In trying to accommodate everyone, it pleased few.[5]

By examining the history of development of clinical coding, we can gather clues for making it better.

---

4.   The initial title of this classification was the *The International List of Causes of Death*. The name was later changed to *The International Classification of Diseases, Injuries, and Causes of Death*, resulting in the acronym "ICD." The forthcoming 10th revision has a new name — *The International Statistical Classification of Diseases and Related Health Problems* — but the shorthand use of "ICD" is likely to remain.

5.   Kerr L. White, *Historical Introduction to ICPC, International Classification of Primary Care*, Oxford University Press, 1987. Dr. White served as chairman of the United States National Committee on Vital and Health Statistics (NCVHS).

The Early Years Using SNDO

Prior to the mid-1950s, hospitals coded their diagnoses to the *Standard Nomenclature of Diseases and Operations (SNDO)*. "Snowdough" (as it was called by the medical record professionals) presented problems. Its codes were long and awkward, requiring that the diagnosis be translated into descriptions along two (and sometimes three) axes in the classification.

Every condition needed identification as to:

1. Axis 1, its topography (portion of the body affected), and

2. Axis 2, its etiology (cause of the disorder); many also required recording of

3. Axis 3, its manifestations (found in a "supplementary code").

Topography could require up to five or six digits, as could etiology, and manifestations several more. Digits were not only decimal, but also "x" and "y" (since punch cards had twelve rows, representing "0 through 9" and also "x" and "y"). Decimal points were also used, and their location was, of course, significant.

Additional suggestions for classifying were made in the *SNDO* text. For example, "mental deficiency" was accompanied by a note to include intelligence quotient (IQ) when available (although where to place it in the code, and how to tell that the numerical IQ was not a code itself, were not specified). Of course, before the use of punch cards and tabulating machines for indexing, more detail, including the physician's actual terminology, would often be simply written on the index card.

SNDO in fact offered a one-page list of "non-diagnostic terms for the hospital record"! Examples:

> alcoholic intoxication (simple drunkenness)
> boarder
> pregnant, not
> Wassermann reaction, positive
> experiment only

... and the famous "y00-y00" code, pronounced "YOYO" (like the toy), which was literally interpreted "diagnosis deferred." This was the ultimate "wastebasket code." This led, of course, to stating that a given patient had "YOYO's disease."

Not only was the coding process time consuming, but it required a great deal of knowledge. *SNDO* was a thick volume. The first thing in the book was the schema, giving two orderly lists, one the anatomic sites, and the other the etiologies envisioned. Then a much larger section listed diseases, where site and etiology were joined, and a code giving "topography-etiology," in that order, represented a given diagnosis. Often, of course, the manifestations, found elsewhere, were also essential.

Near the back of the book was an alphabetic list of diagnoses, which gave the user not the code itself, but simply the page number where the diagnosis would be found in its proper anatomic-etiologic sequence. The page number was occasionally used by accident as the code number, a practice sometimes undetected for years — after all, the medical record librarian was asked to find the series of cases with a given diagnosis. They might as well be filed under the page number as anywhere.

In general, there were two paths which could be followed in coding. One could either try to look up the term in the alphabetic index (but only a few of the thousands of possible terms were found there) and find the corresponding code, or one could simply construct the code from component parts. Diabetes could be constructed from the anatomic site, the pancreas, plus the etiology (a bit stickier). Whether or not a manifestation code was required was another conundrum. Then the resulting "compound" code had to be written down in such a manner that the reader could tell which number represented which axis, since codes for different axes looked the same.

Inspection of patients' codes assigned using *SNDO* revealed that a good many must have been put together this way, because the end products were sometimes weird and wonderful. A "fracture of the skin," for example, was entirely codable.

Who Should Code?

Initially it was thought that, in view of the amount of medical knowledge required and the complexity of the "coding" decisions to be made, the person doing the coding should be the physician. No non-physician, it seemed, could cope with such a challenge. Yet of all the tasks assigned to the physician of any rank, from intern to department chairman, none was more irritating to the physician — more "beneath his or her station" — than coding (unless, of course, the physician had a personal incentive for coding, such as a research project in which the data were of great importance).

Not surprisingly, coding by physicians was awful. Late at night, confronted by a stack of medical records to be coded, the intern learned how to do it as quickly and easily as possible. A common procedure was to simply put down codes which were "in the ball park" (in that they pertained to the general part of the body involved), and be sure to use codes that were in the book, since they were far less likely to be challenged by the medical record librarian.

✓ In view of the terrible results from physician coding, there soon emerged a basic rule in healthcare data management: never let physicians code. After all, who wants both useless data and physicians in rebellion?[6]

So the response of the system was to develop the coding skill of the allied health professional already responsible for medical records — the medical record librarian (MRL).[7] An essential part of the in-school and continuing education in medical records management became the mastery of *SNDO* and, later, of the succeeding classifications employed. Coding became an arcane art of the medical record professional — and physicians were delighted that this was so.

---

6.   Today, in view of the importance of the codes in the payment system, more physicians are taking an interest in this issue.

7.   Now called "health information administrator" (HIA) and other titles. See "Health Information Professionals," page 53.

✓ Today, however, much of the coding burden has fallen back on the physician, at least in the office. This is due to pressure from the reimbursement system (in particular, HCFA) to code accurately to (1) get reimbursed for services, and (2) avoid charges of Medicare fraud or abuse.[8]

So physicians increasingly must spend time to learn the system — not from nosologists, so that classification is accurate and clinically valuable — but from specialized "coding consultants," to ensure payment of claims.

SNDO's Failure

SNDO was widely used until the mid-50s, when it was finally abandoned, not only because of the work entailed in coding with it but, more importantly, when used for retrieval of medical records, relevant cases were often not found. Cases were retrieved by reference to the hospital's disease or procedure index, which were maintained by the code numbers.

The chief user of series of cases was the physician who wanted the series for clinical studies, and needed all the cases which might be relevant. It was better for her or him to retrieve some cases not wanted (and simply send their records back to the file) than to miss cases that should be in the study. With *SNDO* it was virtually impossible to think of all the codes which might have been coded into the group of cases which a physician might want, and *SNDO* provided no grouping mechanism built along the lines of a physician's interest. For example, patients with diabetes mellitus might have been found under any of the more than thirty codes listed in the book for that diagnosis. Here are a few examples of ways diabetes mellitus might have been coded:

> Diseases of the Insular Tissue
>> 870-785, Diabetes mellitus
>> 870-953.6, Sclerosis of insular tissue due to
>>> unknown cause, With diabetes mellitus

---

8. See "The Impact on Physician — and Patient," page 232.

Diseases of the Skin, Subcutaneous Areolar Tissue, and Superficial Mucous Membranes

    114-785, Xanthoma diabeticorum

Diseases of the Nervous System, Generally

    906-785, Encephalomyelopathy due to diabetes

Or the coder might have created equally logical, but unlisted and unrecorded, combinations of site and etiology.

Some medical record librarians solved this problem by coding at first to both the *SNDO* codes and the *International Classification of Diseases (ICD)* categories. Retrieval of cases was then done by using the appropriate *ICD* category.[9]

The International Classification of Diseases

It didn't take long for the record librarians to say, "if this is how we're going to find series of cases anyhow, why not cut out that step of coding to SNDO entirely, and code only to the *ICD* category." So they did, and "category coding" was born.[10]

In those days of manual coding, without the computer in the picture, the change to *ICD* was indeed a major simplification, and a way to meet the primary demand placed on the record indexing system.

✓ No one foresaw in the mid-1950s that the same codes would be used for all sorts of statistics, for determining payment for care, and for many other purposes.

---

9. In *SNDO, 4th Edition,* the *ICD-6* group for each diagnosis was given at the right margin of the page in the "Nomenclature of Diseases" chapter, and a table showing which *SNDO* codes fell into each *ICD-6* category was provided in an appendix. The 5th, and final, edition of *SNDO* (1961) dropped the *ICD* table and introduced its own "Abridged Statistical Classification for Clinical Indexing" to handle this problem, but it was too late; the switch to *ICD* had already taken place.

10. See "How We Code Today: Category Coding," page 205.

The *International Classification of Diseases* was designed as a way to compare health statistics (primarily mortality statistics) internationally.[11] Clearly its title is a misnomer, because *ICD* is not a classification of diseases, but rather a classification of *persons* — most, but not all, of whom have some disorder, disease, injury, malformation, or other problem.

In addition, the 9th Revision, still in use in the United States, has classifications for external causes of injury (E Codes) and also of "Factors Influencing Health Services and Contact with Health Services" (V Codes). The 10th Revision's universes are broader and even more diverse. For example, the chapter previously entitled "Factors Influencing Health Status and Contact with Health Services" has been expanded to include "Symptoms, Signs, and Abnormal Clinical and Laboratory Findings not Elsewhere Classified."

ICD-9 has a number of different universes in its schema, as has *ICD-10*. This is inevitable, but would present fewer problems if they were used in such a manner that they resulted in a single, compound axis. This is not the case, however. Different axes are used in different sections of the classification. One of its architects, a nosologist at the World Health Organization (which is primarily responsible for *ICD*'s construction), has described *ICD-10* as a "variable multiaxial classification," just as its predecessor (see "Variable Multiaxial Classifications," page 138). This makes it a most complicated instrument into which to classify "cases" — the rules or "conventions" governing the way to take the various attributes of a case into account in deciding its category are awesome. In fact, *ICD-10* devotes its entire Volume 2, the *Instruction Manual*, to the rules for use of the system. So as it turned out, the matter of "coding" with *ICD* — just as with *SNDO* — is not trivial.[12]

---

11. See the appendices, page 347, for more about *ICD*.

12. For more about coding with *ICD*, see "How We Code Today: Category Coding," page 205.

ICD's Primary Purpose: International Health Statistics

For many years, there has been international exchange of statistical information on health. Under the World Health Organization, many nations have agreed by treaty to use the *International Classification* as the format for these statistical exchanges. As *ICD* has been used for more and more detailed categorization of mortality and morbidity information, it has become less and less useful for the broad international statistics. Consequently, for more than fifty years, each revision has carried with it "short lists" of mortality and morbidity groupings into which all the information is collected as the vehicles for the international statistics. The two "Special Tabulation Lists" from *ICD-9* are shown below (the tenth revision has added a list for infant and child mortality). The first column contains the category numbers of the list itself; the second column contains the three-digit *ICD-9* codes (any decimal subdivisions have been ignored). Note that these short lists do not require that all of the categories in *ICD-9* be included in the tabulations. Some are simply omitted as of no interest for the international mortality and morbidity statistics.

Figure 7.1 ICD-9 Special Tabulation List: Mortality (page 1 of 2)

MORTALITY LIST

01-56	All causes of death	001-999
01-07	Infectious and parasitic diseases	001-139
01	Intestinal infectious diseases	001-009
02	Tuberculosis	010-018
034	Whooping cough	033
036	Meningococcal infection	036
037	Tetanus	037
038	Septicaemia	038
041	Smallpox	050
042	Measles	055
052	Malaria	084
08-14	Malignant neoplasms	140-208
091	Malignant neoplasm of stomach	151
093	Malignant neoplasm of colon	153
094	Malignant neoplasm of rectum, rectosigmoid junction and anus	154
101	Malignant neoplasm of trachea, bronchus and lung	162
113	Malignant neoplasm of female breast	174
120	Malignant neoplasm of cervix uteri	180
141	Leukaemia	204-208
181	Diabetes mellitus	250
191	Nutritional marasmus	261
192	Other protein-calorie malnutrition	262, 263
200	Anaemias	280-285
220	Meningitis	320-322
25-30	Diseases of the circulatory system	390-459
250	Acute rheumatic fever	390-392
251	Chronic rheumatic heart disease	393-398
26	Hypertensive disease	401-405
27	Ischaemic heart disease	410-414
270	Acute myocardial infarction	410

— 757 —

Special Tabulation List for Mortality. *International Classification of Diseases, Ninth Edition*, pages 757-58.

Figure 7.2 ICD-9 Special Tabulation List: Mortality (page 2 of 2)

758	**SPECIAL TABULATION LISTS**	
29	Cerebrovascular disease	430-438
300	Atherosclerosis	440
321	Pneumonia	480-486
322	Influenza	487
323	Bronchitis, emphysema and asthma	490-493
341	Ulcer of stomach and duodenum	531-533
342	Appendicitis	540-543
347	Chronic liver disease and cirrhosis	571
350	Nephritis, nephrotic syndrome and nephrosis	500-589
360	Hyperplasia of prostate	600
38	Abortion	630-639
39	Direct obstetric deaths	{ 640-646 651-676
44	Congenital anomalies	740-759
45	Certain conditions originating in the perinatal period	760-779
453	Birth trauma	767
46	Signs, symptoms and ill-defined conditions	780-799
47-56	Injury and poisoning	800-999
47	Fractures	800-829
49	Intracranial and internal injuries, including nerves	{ 850-869 950-957
52	Burns	940-949
53	Poisonings and toxic effects	960-989
E47-E53	Accidents and adverse effects	E800-E949
E471	Motor vehicle traffic accidents	E810-E819
E50	Accidental falls	E880-E888
E54	Suicide	E950-E959
E55	Homicide	E960-E969

Figure 7.3 ICD-9 Special Tabulation List: Morbidity (page 1 of 2)

MORBIDITY LIST

01-56	All causes of morbidity	001-999
01	Intestinal infectious diseases	001-009
02	Tuberculosis	010-018
036	Meningococcal infection	036
042	Measles	055
052	Malaria	084
06	Venereal diseases	090-099
08-14	Malignant neoplasms	140-208
091	Malignant neoplasm of stomach	151
093	Malignant neoplasm of colon	153
094	Malignant neoplasm of rectum, rectosigmoid junction and anus	154
101	Malignant neoplasm of trachea, bronchus and lung	162
113	Malignant neoplasm of female breast	174
120	Malignant neoplasm of cervix uteri	180
141	Leukaemia	204-208
152	Benign neoplasm of uterus	218, 219
180	Diseases of thyroid gland	240-246
181	Diabetes mellitus	250
19	Nutritional deficiencies	260-269
21	Mental disorders	290-319
223	Multiple sclerosis	340
23	Diseases of eye and adnexa	360-379
24	Diseases of ear and mastoid process	380-389
25-30	Diseases of the circulatory system	390-459
251	Chronic rheumatic heart disease	393-398
26	Hypertensive disease	401-405
270	Acute myocardial infarction	410

— 759 —

Special Tabulation List for Morbidity. *International Classification of Diseases, Ninth Edition*, pages 759-60.

Figure 7.4 ICD-9 Special Tabulation List: Morbidity (page 2 of 2)

760	SPECIAL TABULATION LISTS	
29	Cerebrovascular disease	430-438
304	Varicose veins of lower extremities	454
315	Chronic diseases of tonsils and adenoids	474
321	Pneumonia	480-486
322	Influenza	487
323	Bronchitis, emphysema and asthma	490-493
330	Diseases of teeth and supporting structures	520-525
341	Ulcer of stomach and duodenum	531-533
342	Appendicitis	540-543
343	Hernia of abdominal cavity	550-553
35	Diseases of urinary system	580-599
360	Hyperplasia of prostate	600
371	Salpingitis and oophoritis	614.0-614.2
374	Uterovaginal prolapse	618
38	Abortion	630-639
39	Direct obstetric conditions	{ 640-646 651-676
41	Normal delivery	650
43	Diseases of the musculoskeletal system and connective tissue	710-739
44	Congenital anomalies	740-759
47-56	Injury and poisoning	800-999
47	Fractures	800-829
49	Intracranial and internal injuries, including nerves	{ 850-869 950-957
52	Burns	940-949
53	Poisonings and toxic effects	960-989
E47-E53	Accidents and adverse effects	E800-E949
E471	Motor vehicle traffic accidents	E810-E819
E50	Accidental falls	E880-E888
E54	Suicide and self-inflicted injury	E950-E959
E55	Homicide and injury purposely inflicted by other persons	E960-E969

Not only does a clearer picture of international health issues emerge with the broader groupings, but only by such groupings can useful world-wide comparisons be made at all, for the data must be grouped at the level of the lowest common denominator of available data detail. That means that the countries with the more sophisticated data systems must conform their data to the detail which can be achieved by simpler data systems in less developed countries, some of which must rely on "barefoot doctors" for their data collection.

In addition, broader groupings give better pictures for the global purpose. At the World Health Organization Conference which developed *ICD-9*, a specific recommendation read:

> Proposed new [short] lists were presented to the Conference in which totals were shown for groups of diseases and for certain selected individual conditions. Minimum lists of 55 items were recommended for the tabulation of mortality and morbidity [for all countries] and countries could add to these further items from a basic list of 275 categories.

The United States has no problem with placing its statistics into these groupings with *ICD-9-CM*, because *ICD-9-CM* was created under a mandate from the Federal Government that it be completely "collapsible" into the categories of *ICD-9* itself.

Modifications for Clinical Use

The change to using the *International Classification of Diseases* in place of *SNDO* pretty much solved the problem of collecting groups of cases, and meeting the demands for that type of retrieval of hospital medical records. However, from the first such use of *ICD*, which began with its 6th Revision, it was clear that its categories were often too broad to meet the demands of clinicians, and so they were subdivided and modified in order to give more specificity.

The first series of modifications came from the pioneers, Kurtz and Voelker (see page 115), on the basis of their experience in their two hospitals. These subdivisions and modifications were picked up by the fledgling Professional Activity Study (PAS) and issued to the pilot study hospitals — in the form of labels to be pasted into the *ICD* volume.[13]

---

13. PAS was the prototype hospital discharge abstract system; see page 103.

However, even in this highly motivated group of only fifteen hospitals, putting the labels (along with "errata") simultaneously and uniformly into each *ICD* book proved such a challenge that the PAS staff convened a meeting and supervised the task. A valuable lesson was learned about the futility of such a process (and of the similar process of issuing new and replacement pages for looseleaf binders): *don't try it!* It's far better and safer — and cheaper — to just reprint the entire volume.[14] Of course, even at that you haven't solved the problem, since you can't make people buy and look at the new volume.

✓ When changes are adopted at different times by various users, confidence in data quality drops.

After the PAS experience, the United States Public Health Service in 1959 issued *Publication 719*, entitled *International Classification of Diseases — Adapted for Indexing of Hospital Records and Operation Classification*, (commonly referred to as "PHS 719") which collected the subdivisions and modifications which had been developed up to that time into a single hard-backed volume. A revision of this volume appeared in 1962, which expanded the classification and separated it into two volumes: a tabular list and an alphabetic index.

As the adoption of *ICD* for hospital indexing became more widespread, and as the World Health Organization issued succeeding generations of *ICD* (*ICD-7*, *ICD-8*, and *ICD-9*), a series of companion volumes to each of the generations has been issued in the United States. The edition in current use (since about 1978) is *ICD-9-CM*. The tenth revision, *ICD-10-CM*, is being readied for use (see page 166).

Reimbursement: DRGs & ACGs

While *ICD-9-CM* may be seen as our "basic" disease classification, it is not the only one we use. In order to use *ICD-9-CM* for reimbursement, two more classifications were created: DRGs and ACGs.

---

14. Despite this and similar experiences, to this day changes in *ICD-9-CM* are handled by the publication of lists of new codes, new instructions, old codes to be abandoned, and the like. With some delay, a new revision of the entire volume is published, but no information is available on its sales and use. This problem could be solved by having an online reference be the *only* source of information.

✓ The Prospective Payment System (PPS) was introduced in the mid-80s by the Health Care Financing Administration (HCFA) as a method of paying for services provided to Medicare patients.

Under PPS, payment is made for patients according to the patients' "Diagnosis Related Groups" (DRGs). Patients are classified into categories (the DRGs) for which prices are negotiated or imposed on the hospital in advance.[15] Each DRG represents a case ("product") for which a certain, set amount will be paid.[16]

For the Prospective Payment System, the *ICD-9-CM* codes are grouped into Diagnosis Related Groups (DRGs).[17] To receive payment, the hospital must assign each patient to one of about 474 DRGs. This assignment is done in a standard (and auditable) manner by the use of "official" software called GROUPER, which uses the necessary patient attributes and does the actual classification. Each DRG takes into account the patient's principal and secondary diagnoses, whether or not the patient underwent certain surgery, and the patient's age. In the entire DRG assignment process, the *ICD-9-CM* codes serve as the surrogates for the original diagnosis terms.

Payment for care under DRGs has caused great dissatisfaction, because often the payment allowed does not reflect the resources required for the care of the specific patient. Sometimes a category contains one or more diagnoses which are typically much higher in their demands than the

---

15. At present PPS is only applied to hospital care, not physician care, although the idea is the same as a single fixed package fee which includes prenatal care, delivery, and postpartum care for a maternity patient, or the inclusion of preoperative care, operation, and postoperative care for an appendectomy patient within one fixed physician's fee. PPS, while not mandated by federal law for payers other than Medicare, is being applied to patients under other health care plans. PPS is sometimes referred to as the "DRG system."

16. The purpose of DRGs is to have a manageable number of products for which to pay, not to have greater detail or precision in healthcare information. More about DRGs can be found in the appendices; see page 421.

17. DRGs are used for hospital services. DRGs have been found unsuitable in the ambulatory setting, so a classification called Ambulatory Care Groups (ACG) has been defined (even though the diagnoses going into both DRGs and ACGs may be the same).

average for that category. (There will, of course, also be cases which require much less care, but no one believes that there will be enough low-cost cases in a given institution to average the two out.) Furthermore, in many situations, there is complaint that certain patients were demonstrably more ill than the average for the category, and thus should demand more liberal reimbursement.

Attempts to compensate for these situations have resulted in two main approaches:

1. Coding "enhancement" schemes, usually in the form of proprietary computer programs, and

2. Overlaying or supplementing the DRGs with "severity" codes, adding a to each DRG a descriptor code indicating its severity level.

Coding enhancement schemes These have proliferated to "improve" the billing for care. They work by changing the sequences of the codes on the bills, adding (or deleting) codes representing additional conditions, and even preventing the use of certain codes and code combinations which are known to be red flags to the payers. Coding enhancement products tend to be "one-way," in that they work in the direction of providing greater reimbursement, rather than greater accuracy in describing the cases.

Severity levels Because of the objection that within a given DRG there are enormous differences in severity of cases — and as a result, widely varying demands for hospital and physician services and other resources — severity modifiers have been developed. Severity modifiers run counter to the purpose of DRGs, because they give greater detail rather than less.

Both solutions have serious drawbacks.

✓ The root issue — namely that *ICD-9-CM* was never designed for a payment system — is not addressed.

Research & Other Applications

A researcher would logically require quite a different classification to study office practices than for inpatient care. For example, a physician may have a substantial number of patients visit the office with simply the common cold, and wish to identify them as a single unique category. This is possible using *ICD-9-CM*, but patients rarely are hospitalized just for a cold. Although one may wish to find individual cases of the common cold among a hospital population, they would hardly deserve their own independent grouping in the usual hospital statistics, where they are typically grouped together with "upper respiratory diseases."

However, for research and other uses for data classified to *ICD-9-CM*, listed above, no solutions such as those for billing and international statistics have been proposed or provided.

The Tenth Revision of ICD

In 1992, the World Health Organization (WHO) published the tenth revision of *ICD*, entitled, *International Statistical Classification of Diseases and Related Health Problems*, and commonly known as *ICD-10*.

From ICD-9 to ICD-10

Appendix A contains some detail on *ICD-10* and how it compares to *ICD-9* (see page 355). Some of the notable changes from *ICD-9*:

- The format of having the Tabular List in one volume and the Alphabetic Index in another is the same in both *ICD-9* and *ICD-10*, but in *ICD-10*, the Instruction Manual has been placed in a separate volume, Volume 2. In *ICD-9* it preceded the Tabular List in Volume 1. So *ICD-10* is a 3-volume set rather than two.

- One measure of the differences between the two is shown in the table below:

Figure 7.5 Page Counts of ICD-9 and ICD-10

Volume	ICD-9	ICD-10
1: Tabular List	773	1,231
2: Instruction Manual	included in Volume 1	160
3: Alphabetic Index (Volume 2 in ICD-9)	659	750
Totals	1,432	2,141

Numbers of pages devoted to various sections of *ICD-10* compared with *ICD-9*.

- Much of the classification has been reorganized.

- Most of the detail which was added to *ICD-9* to form *ICD-9-CM* was incorporated in *ICD-10*.

- Many categories have been added for "problems" which are not diagnoses or symptoms. Examples are:

  - Occupational exposure to risk-factors

  - General examination and investigation of persons without complaint or reported diagnosis

  - Examination and encounter for administrative purposes

  - Immunization not carried out

- ICD-10 uses alphanumeric codes, with an alphabetic character (any letter but "U") in the first position. It includes the letters "I" and "O" even though these are usually avoided in alphanumeric coding because of the likelihood of confusion with the numerals "1" and "0":

I37	Pulmonary valve disorder
137	Late effects of tuberculosis
O15	Eclampsia
015	Tuberculosis of bones and joints

- Somewhat surprising is the fact that chapters in *ICD-10* do not necessarily start with new alphabetic characters; see the table below.

Figure 7.6 Chapters & Code Formats in ICD-10

Chapter	Title	Code Format
Chapter I	Certain infectious and parasitic diseases	A00 - B99
Chapter II	Neoplasms	C00 - D48
Chapter III	Diseases of the blood and blood-forming organs and certain disorders involving the immune mechanism	D50 - D89
Chapter IV	Endocrine, nutritional and metabolic diseases	E00 - E90
...		
Chapter IX	Diseases of the circulatory system	I00 - I99
...		
Chapter XV	Pregnancy, childbirth and the puerperium	O00 - O99
...		

Chapters and corresponding code formats used in ICD-10, showing use of both alphabetic and numeric characters in the codes. The full table from which this is taken is in the appendices; see page 357.

ICD-10 retains the "dagger and asterisk" dual coding system which was found in earlier generations of the classification, and which was unacceptable for U.S. clinical use (see page 139). *ICD-10-CM*, like *ICD-9-CM*, appears to have eliminated dual coding.

These changes resulted in an increase in categories in the basic volume, *ICD-10*, from roughly 7,000 in *ICD-9* to 13,000.

The Clinical Modification of ICD-10

The United States National Center for Health Statistics (NCHS), the federal agency responsible for the use in the United States of *ICD*, determined that *ICD-10* is not sufficiently detailed for use in the national health information system. So NCHS commissioned the development of a clinical modification "for morbidity purposes," to replace Volumes 1 and 2 of the *International Classification of Diseases, 9th Revision, Clinical Modification (ICD-9-CM)*.[18]

A draft of the Tabular List of the Clinical Modification of *ICD-10 (ICD-10-CM)* was placed on the Internet on 19 November 1997, with an invitation for comments which would contribute to "a more clinically robust classification." The Alphabetic Index was to be completed after response to the request for reactions to the Tabular List. A "crosswalk" between *ICD-9-CM* and *ICD-10-CM* has been written.[19] The Alphabetic Index will be available with the final version. The number of volumes to be required for the final product has not been announced.

Some comparisons of the old and new clinical modifications, *ICD-9-CM* and *ICD-10-CM*, may be of interest.

- In October 1998, the official *ICD-9-CM* contained 12,628 diagnosis codes (categories).

- The draft version of *ICD-10-CM* as posted on the Internet, however, contained approximately 60,000 codes. Although most of the additions are at the 5th and 6th digit levels, there are also changes among the 3rd and 4th digits categories.

✓ The enormous increase in numbers of categories (codes) appears to be primarily the result of an increase in the use of "combination coding."

One type of combination coding is to subdivide a disease or injury category by adding digits, in this case usually 4th and 5th digits, which describe the site of its manifestation.

Combination coding for site was used moderately in *ICD-9-CM*. For example, for several categories of "malignant neoplasms of lymphatic and hemopoietic tissue" *ICD-9-CM* offered 9 last-digit subdivisions in order to show the sites of the disease. These subdivisions were picked up

---

18. Volume 1 of *ICD-9-CM* is the Tabular List and Volume 2 is the Alphabetic Index. Volume 3 , Procedures, will be replaced by the *ICD-10 Procedure Classification System (ICD-10-PCS)*, being developed by the Health Care Financing Administration (HCFA). For more about *ICD-10-PCS*, see page 191.

19. See "Crosswalk to ICD-10-CM," page 299.

by *ICD-10-CM*, and their use can be illustrated with category C81.1, "nodular sclerosis," a subdivision of the Hodgkin's disease category:

> ...
>
> C81.11   nodular sclerosis of head, face, and neck
>
> ...
>
> C81.18   nodular sclerosis of multiple sites
>
> ...

These same site codes are used with the other forms of Hodgkin's disease: "C81.0, Lymphocytic predominance ... ," "C81.3, Lymphocytic depletion ... ," and so on in *ICD-10-CM*.

In the Hodgkin's disease example, there was consistency in the use of the subdivisions, e.g., x.x8 was "unspecified." Later in the classification, such consistency was abandoned, e.g., "unspecified" has different decimal locations here:

> S55.11   Laceration of radial artery at forearm level
>
> > S55.111   Laceration ... right arm
> >
> > S55.112   ... left arm
> >
> > S55.119   ... unspecified arm
>
> S93.2   Rupture of ligaments at ankle and foot level
>
> > S93.20   Rupture ... unspecified side
> >
> > S93.21   ... right ...
> >
> > S93.22   ... left ...

The second kind of combination coding puts several conditions, and perhaps sites, into the same category. This usage and the great number of possible anatomical sites for injury are responsible for the fact that by far the greatest expansion of *ICD-10-CM* over *ICD-9-CM* occurs in the trauma categories. The complexity of the information in individual categories which results is illustrated from the version of *ICD-10-CM* which was on the Internet for comment in November 1997:

S02.974　　　　　　　Open fracture of skull and facial bones, part unspecified with subarachnoid, subdural, and extradural hemorrhage with prolonged [greater than 24 hours] loss of consciousness, without return to pre-existing conscious level, or when an unconscious patient dies before regaining consciousness, regardless of the duration.

(If the patient died in 22 hours, what does the coder do? And when does the clock start — at injury or at hospital admission?)

This code contains 2 fracture sites, 3 kinds of hemorrhage, a time duration (not a diagnosis), a statement about consciousness, and an ambiguous outcome. Each of these items of "diagnostic" information (entities) must be retrieved from the medical record and assembled in order to code (classify) the case.

If this approach, i.e., concatenation of entities into single categories to describe the entire case, were to be rigorously applied throughout the classification, the classification would be expanded by several orders of magnitude. Furthermore, consider the problem of retrieval of information.

Anyone wishing to find all cases with, for example, open fracture of the facial bones, would have to add this code (S02.974), and all other category codes in which the diagnosis of open fracture of the facial bones had been included, into the search criteria along with the code for the facial bone fracture alone, a category which surely exists. The same would be true, of course, for open fracture of the skull, the 3 kinds of hemorrhages, or coma.

✓ Designing searches in systems with combination categories is a nightmare.

It is this problem which has been solved in modern informatics by implementing the relational approach. This avoids having to repeat the same information, for example, site, for each diagnosis in which site is a necessary component. For additional information, see "Database 101," below.

Background   ## Database 101

A *database* is any collection of data or information organized with some type of structure, such as records (rows) and fields (columns). A collection of records, all sharing the same structure, may be referred to as a table. A database record, or a single row in a table, is group of information items logically related in some fashion (e.g., name, address, phone number of one individual). Rows are typically subdivided into columns — smaller units of data known as data elements or fields. For example, a telephone book is a database (table), each person or company listing being one row. Each row in the telephone book is further subdivided into three data elements or columns: name, address, and telephone number. While today it seems that databases only exist in computers, it should be remembered that people have created and managed databases since long before the advent of computers.

The word "database" also describes a type of *software* application or language used to store and manipulate such data on computer systems. In this context, it is more appropriately referred to as a database management system (DBMS). In its simplest form, a DBMS is a computerized filing system. In more elaborate forms, it relates information from different files together to produce new files, reports, and detailed analyses. Different DBMSs also tend to have their own languages with which they can be programmed for specific purposes, such as automatically performing certain functions when certain types of data are entered. The actual DBMS is frequently hidden from the user by a user-friendly interface (menus and/or dialog boxes) which prompts and guides the user every step of the way.

At the beginning of the twenty-first century, the *relational database* is the most common type in use. It is characterized by having two or more tables, each of which is "related" to one or more of the other tables by means of primary and (optionally) secondary "keys." The keys are simply columns of the same information which appear in all the tables that are related to each other, and thus allow one row in one table to be linked to a companion row in another table. As you might guess, when selecting a key you need to chose a column whose values are unique (no duplicates allowed). In a hospital's database, for instance, a unique patient identifier number (PatientID) is likely to be used as a primary key, as would a unique physician identifier number (PhysicianID).

Like a phone book, one table might be all of that hospital's patients — one row per patient. Another table may be all of the physicians who are on the hospital's staff. The patient table would include one column for PatientID and probably at least one column for PhysicianID, allowing a "relation" between each patient and at least one physician. This DBMS would be able to answer the question, "Who is Mr. Jones' doctor?" as well as "Who are Dr. Smith's patients?"

A major advantage to a DBMS that uses relational database technology is the elimination of duplicate data. If correctly designed *("normalized")*, a relational database will contain only one copy of any data element, such as a patient's address. Any other table that needs the patient's address will simply be linked to it via a key common to both tables. Changing a patient's address requires a change in only one place. In real life, of course, design and normalization of a relational database can become quite complex, but the idea behind it has been fairly constant since this technology's invention in the 1970s.

The other key ingredient in a DBMS, other than the database itself, is the language used to manage it. By far the most accepted language used with relational databases is known as SQL, which stands for "Structured Query Language." SQL is usually pronounced as 'sequel' or S.Q.L. Its widespread acceptance is largely due to its maturity and standardization across varying computer platforms, from microcomputers to mainframes. The language itself, such as "SELECT lastname FROM providers WHERE specialty = 'Surgery'," is often hidden from users by using front end programs which give the user a fill-in-the-form type of interface.

SQL was invented by IBM in the 1970's, and was actually called SEQUEL in its early years. The American National Standards Institute (ANSI) and International Organization of Standardization (ISO) published an official standard for SQL in 1986, and significantly expanded it in 1992 (SQL-92). The U. S. version (ANSI SQL) and the international version (ISO SQL) are identical, a factor which contributes to SQL's widespread acceptance.

It is clear that the modus operandi for coding employed in past versions of the classification, i.e., consulting the alphabetic index and then the tabular list, is expected to continue with *ICD-10-CM*. It is intriguing to speculate on the format and conventions which will have to be employed in creating the alphabetic index. Clearly, there is little likelihood of users memorizing many codes. Data management, i.e., coding and classifying, of this complexity demands computerization rather than education and monitoring of several hundred thousand "coders."

8

Procedure Classifications

IN MEDICINE, a "procedure" is something which is done or carried out for a patient by a physician or other caregiver. A procedure is usually discrete, and a relatively short time is required for its execution. Procedures are generally either diagnostic or therapeutic. For example, a diagnostic procedure might be the taking of an x-ray or blood pressure, or a cardiac catheterization or biopsy, while a therapeutic procedure (treatment) might be anything from removing a splinter from a finger to an extensive operation such as a heart transplant.

A given surgical operation, which sometimes is called "a procedure," is often actually several procedures, and the array of procedures which make up a given operation will vary from patient to patient. For example, cholecystectomy (gall bladder removal) for one patient may include exploration of the common bile duct, while for another patient, this procedure may be omitted. For this reason, a proper description of an operation requires that its specific procedures be listed. Those interested in the description of procedures in detail should see the material on *ICD-10-PCS* below (page 191).

History

Procedure classifying has been approached in the United States in quite a different manner than disease classifying. As a matter of fact, "procedure" classifying is an expansion of "operation" classifying. There were several purposes behind its development, including:

Publications Surgeons, like other physicians, wanted to collect series of cases in order to evaluate and publish on the pros and cons of various techniques. The information on these techniques was derived from the medical records of the cases.

Credentials In applying for certification as experts in their fields, surgeons had to provide evidence of their experience and success. For this, they reported from the medical records of cases on which they had operated.

This, like publication, required an indexing system for retrieval of medical records according to the operations performed by the applicant surgeon.

Quality Management Systematic evaluation of the quality of patient care originally began with evaluation of operations by the hospital Tissue Committee, established by the American College of Surgeons. Evaluation of patients on the basis of the management of various diagnoses and other factors followed later. Quality evaluation required indexing and grouping so that patterns of care could be seen.

Payment With the advent of healthcare insurance, operations were reported by categories; the insurer wasn't interested in fine detail such as, for example, surgical approach. The payment was for the operation and the normal preoperative and postoperative care. This led to the development of a classification specifically for this purpose, in addition to the classification used for indexing hospital records according to operation and procedure.

Procedure Classifications for Hospital Use

The first three motivations listed above were more or less simultaneous, and hospitals desiring accreditation were required, beginning in the 1930s, to index their medical records. The nomenclature in use — the *Standard Nomenclature of Diseases and Operations (SNDO)* — was a system in which topography was the base of both disease and operation nomenclature. For disease, topography was supplemented by information as to cause (etiology) and manifestations. For operations, topography was supplemented by one of several types of procedures. For example, in the Fourth Edition of *SNDO* (1952), nine classes of procedures were used:

        -0   Incision
        -1   Excision
        -2   Amputation
        -3   Introduction
        -4   Endoscopy
        -5   Repair
        -6   Destruction
        -7   Suture
        -8   Manipulation

Each of these major classes of procedure was, of course, further subdivided and expanded by adding digits. For example

   1   Excision,
         11   local incision of lesion of organ
            111 partial incision of lesion

   3   Introduction
         30 injection
            300 injection of serum, immunizing

   5   Repair
         50 plastic repair, generally or unspecified (suffix -plasty)
            500 plastic repair, lengthening
               5001 plastic repair, lengthening,
               by oblique transection and resuture

The resulting classification in *SNDO* was more detailed than hospitals required for indexing, since their goal was to retrieve series of cases for review. So when the switch was made to *ICD* for indexing of diseases in hospitals, a companion "Classification of Operations and Treatments" was included in the 1959 United States Public Health Service Publication, *International Classification of Diseases Adapted for Indexing of Hospital Records and Operation Classification*, a volume usually referred to simply as "*PHS 719*"(although on its spine it was called, simply, "Diagnostic Index"!). The procedure classification in PHS 719 (developed by the Commission on Professional and Hospital Activities at the request of the federal government) was quite different from that of *SNDO*. It required only three digits. The concept is illustrated in the figure below.

Figure 8.1 PHS 719, Classification of Operations and Treatments

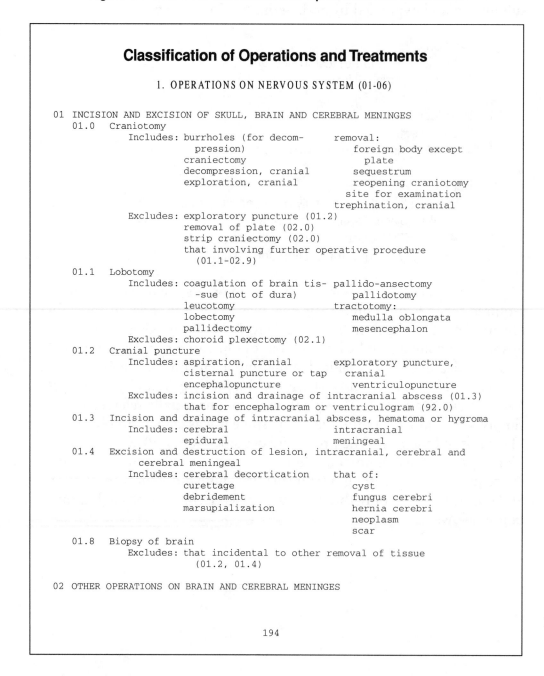

Classification of Operations and Treatments

1. OPERATIONS ON NERVOUS SYSTEM (01-06)

```
01 INCISION AND EXCISION OF SKULL, BRAIN AND CEREBRAL MENINGES
   01.0   Craniotomy
          Includes: burrholes (for decom-    removal:
                      pression)                foreign body except
                    craniectomy                  plate
                    decompression, cranial     sequestrum
                    exploration, cranial       reopening craniotomy
                                               site for examination
                                               trephination, cranial
          Excludes: exploratory puncture (01.2)
                    removal of plate (02.0)
                    strip craniectomy (02.0)
                    that involving further operative procedure
                      (01.1-02.9)
   01.1   Lobotomy
          Includes: coagulation of brain tis- pallido-ansectomy
                      -sue (not of dura)        pallidotomy
                    leucotomy               tractotomy:
                    lobectomy                  medulla oblongata
                    pallidectomy               mesencephalon
          Excludes: choroid plexectomy (02.1)
   01.2   Cranial puncture
          Includes: aspiration, cranial     exploratory puncture,
                    cisternal puncture or tap  cranial
                    encephalopuncture          ventriculopuncture
          Excludes: incision and drainage of intracranial abscess (01.3)
                    that for encephalogram or ventriculogram (92.0)
   01.3   Incision and drainage of intracranial abscess, hematoma or hygroma
          Includes: cerebral                intracranial
                    epidural                 meningeal
   01.4   Excision and destruction of lesion, intracranial, cerebral and
            cerebral meningeal
          Includes: cerebral decortication  that of:
                    curettage                 cyst
                    debridement               fungus cerebri
                    marsupialization          hernia cerebri
                                              neoplasm
                                              scar
   01.8   Biopsy of brain
          Excludes: that incidental to other removal of tissue
                      (01.2, 01.4)

02 OTHER OPERATIONS ON BRAIN AND CEREBRAL MENINGES
```

194

Page 194, Classification of Operations and Treatments, from *International Classification of Diseases Adapted for Indexing of Hospital Records and Operation Classification (PHS 719)*. United States Public Health Service Publication, 1959.

Subsequent volumes in the *ICD* series as used in the United States — i.e., the various adaptations of *ICD-7* and *ICD-8*, and *ICD-9-CM* — carried expansions of this same classification schema, although greater detail was added by using a second digit to the right of the decimal point. The procedure classifications were placed at the end of the Disease List in the first volume of each series, and indexed alphabetically in the second volume until the publication of *ICD-9-CM* in 1978, when both the procedures list and its alphabetical index occupied Volume 3 of the set.

Following publication of *ICD-9*, the World Health Organization published its *International Classification of Procedures in Medicine* (also in 1978) as a softbound, trial volume. It never achieved permanent status, however, and no similar volume accompanies *ICD-10*. To bridge this gap, the Health Care Financing Administration (HCFA) contracted for a procedure *coding* system — *ICD-10-Procedure Coding System* (see page 191).

To the present, hospitals typically use the procedures list in Volume 3 of *ICD-9-CM* for their indexes of procedures, for their statistical tabulations, and for reporting procedures in the Uniform Hospital Discharge Data Set (UHDDS) for reimbursement under Medicare and Medicaid. Although it is far from as detailed as many would like, it has been expanded periodically in the same fashion as the rest of *ICD-9-CM* in order to accommodate new procedures and new thinking. *ICD-10-PCS*, because of its exquisite detail, does not appear to be suited to these uses.

Procedure Classifications for Physician Use

Meanwhile, the classifying and coding of procedures for billing by physicians and other caregivers (excepting hospitals, for hospital care) proceeded along a different path, because the hospital classification was deemed inadequate for the task. Surgeons, pathologists, and radiologists in particular contended that they should be paid in proportion to the resources expended, including the time, and also the skill required.

Relative Value

The result was to develop schemes for comparing the relative resources required for different services, procedures and others, and this was called the "relative value" approach. Soon anesthesiologists and primary care physicians were also given terminology and codes for their services. Then it was realized that a good portion of physicians' "procedures," regardless of specialty, were "general evaluation and management" (E&M), so relative values for these services were developed as well.

In response to the demand for a system which accounted for resource consumption, the idea of a *relative value scale* emerged.

Background

Relative Value Scale (RVS)

A relative value scale (RVS) is a numerical system designed to permit comparisons of the resources needed (or appropriate prices) for various units of service. The RVS is the compiled table of the relative value units (RVUs) for all the objects in the class for which it is developed. An RVS takes into account labor, skill, supplies, equipment, space, and other costs into an aggregate cost for each procedure or other unit of service. The aggregate cost is converted into the relative value unit (RVU) of the procedure or service by relating it to the cost of a procedure or service selected as the base unit.

For example, the developer of the RVS for laboratory work might decide to use the cost of a red blood count as the base unit. Its actual cost might be $5.00, but, as the base, its RVU would arbitrarily be set at 1.0. If a blood sugar estimation, then, actually cost $25.00, it would have an RVU value of 5.0 ($25.00 divided by $5.00). If a urinalysis cost $3.00, it would have an RVU of 0.6 ($3 divided by $5). (The illustrations are imaginary as to the prices given.)

The California Medical Association developed (and in 1956 published) the *California Relative Value Schedule (CRVS)*, the first of a series later called *Relative Value Studies*. The tables reproduced below show generally how the CRVS was originally set up.

Figure 8.2 Tables from *California Relative Value Schedule,* 1956

TABLE 1.— *Illustrating relative values in the "MEDICAL SERVICES" section of the Report.*

Procedure No.	Procedure	Relative Value in Units
001	Office visit (first call—routine history and necessary examination)	2.0
002	Hospital visit	1.0
003	First home visit	2.0
004	Home visit (11 p.m. to 8 a.m.)	2.5
005	Home visit—each additional member, same household	.8
006	Follow-up office visit	1.0
007	Follow-up home visit	1.5
008	Mileage—per mile, one way, beyond radius of 10 miles, office or home	.2

TABLE 2.— *Illustrating the conversion of relative values in the "SURGERY" section of the Report into dollars.*

Procedure No.	Procedure	Relative Value		Your Conversion Factor	Fee (Nearest Even $)
3261	Appendectomy	35	X	571%	$200.00
4801	Classic Cesarean section	50	X	571%	285.00
4318	Prostatectomy retropubic	70	X	571%	400.00
4613	Hysterectomy	50	X	571%	285.00
2992	Tonsillectomy	15	X	571%	86.00

TABLE 3.— *Illustrating the conversion of relative values in the "MEDICAL SERVICES" section of the Report into dollars.*

Procedure No.	Procedure	Relative Value		Your Conversion Factor	Fee
001	Office visit (first call—routine history and necessary examination)	2.0	X	400%	$8.00
002	Hospital visit	1.0	X	400%	4.00
003	Home visit	2.0	X	400%	8.00
004	Home visit (11 p.m. to 8 a.m.)	2.5	X	400%	10.00
005	Home visit—each additional member, same household	.8	X	400%	3.20
006	Follow-up office visit	1.0	X	400%	4.00
027	Consultation requiring complete examination, office, hospital or home	7.0	X	400%	28.00
	(etcetera)				

Illustrative tables from the *California Relative Value Schedule,* California Medical Association, 1956.

TABLE 4.— *Illustrating the conversion of relative values in the "PATHOLOGY" section of the Report into dollars.*

Procedure No.	Procedure	Relative Value		Your Factor	Fee
8628	Complete blood count	1.0	X	500%	$5.00
8636	Bone marrow, examination of material	3.0	X	500%	15.00
8658	Coagulation time (Lea & White)	.6	X	500%	3.00
8710	Prothrombin utilization	1.5	X	500%	7.50
8930	Urine — routine chemical qualitative	.2	X	500%	1.00

(etcetera)

TABLE 5.— *Illustrating the use of the Report to test an existing fee schedule.*

Procedure	Insurance Company Indemnity	Relative Value		Factor	On Basis of Relative Values if Appendectomy Is $150, Indemnity Should Be
Appendectomy	$150.00	35	X	428%	$150.00
Amputation of finger	37.50	12.5	X	428%	53.50
Simple mastectomy	150.00	30	X	428%	128.40
Laryngectomy	300.00	80	X	428%	428.00
Hemorrhoidectomy:					
External	37.50	5	X	428%	21.40
Internal	75.00	25	X	428%	107.00
Complete blood count	225.00	60	X	428%	256.80
Complete blood count	45.00	15	X	428%	64.20

TABLE 6.— *Illustrating why relative values in one section of the Report should not be related to values in any other section.*

Procedure No.	Procedure	Relative Value	Fee	Fee	Fee	Fee
006	Follow-up office visit	1.0	$ 3.00	$ 4.00	$ 5.00	$ 6.00
2114	Total gastrectomy	100.0	300.00	400.00	500.00	600.00

TABLE 7.— *Illustrating the injustice of across-the-board changes in fee schedules.*

	Fee Schedule	Required Overhead	Net to Physician	Decrease Fee 20 Per Cent	Net to Physician	Decrease in Net to Physician
Procedure X	$25.00	50%	$12.50	$20.00	$ 7.50	40%
Procedure Y	25.00	25%	18.75	20.00	13.75	26%

Current Procedural Terminology

Soon the American Medical Association obtained permission to use the CRVS as the basis for a national classifying and coding scheme for billing for procedures, and in 1966 published its first *Current Procedural Terminology (CPT).* With the second edition in 1970, the cover bore the title *Current Procedural Terminology for Naming-Coding-Reporting Diagnoses and Treatment.* The third edition (1973) was called *Physicians' Current Procedural Terminology for Naming, Coding, and Reporting Medical Services.* The fourth edition appeared in 1977, with revisions each year for the next four years.

In 1984, although the volume was still designated as the fourth edition, the name changed to *CPT-1984,* and *CPT* continued to be revised annually, with each year's version bearing the label *CPT* plus the year. To date there have been something like 20 publications in the series. In addition to the "master" *CPT,* the American Medical Association also issues a number of specialized "mini" versions, such as editions for various medical specialties.

CPT is in the hands of an editorial panel of about 15 physicians, with an advisory committee of another 75 physicians, and with its own "AMA *CPT* Health Care Professionals Advisory Committee" (HCPAC) of about 10 individuals representing such professions as nursing, social work, optometry, physical therapy, and podiatry.[1]

---

1. In 1998, AMA announced the mobilization of a substantial effort to "reinvent its CPT system for the 21st century," in an effort to upgrade its physician procedure coding "to a CPT-5 coding system that would:

    Maintain its position as the authority on procedure coding
    Enhance CPT's use by physicians
    Address the needs of nonphysician providers
    More appropriately address different sites of service
    Better serve the needs of researchers, managed care and the international community
    Improve the timeliness and open information exchange of the maintenance and editorial process
    Bolster the structure to allow greater code specificity and computerized patient records"
    Six working groups were to report to an advisory panel in early 1999, which in turn will report to the *CPT* editorial panel in early 2000.

The 1998 *CPT* volume is divided into six sections, as shown in the table below.

Figure 8.3 CPT-98: Schema

Section	Codes
Evaluation and Management	99201 to 99499
Anesthesiology	00100 to 01999 99100 to 99140
Surgery	10040 to 69979
Radiology, including Nuclear Medicine and Diagnostic Ultrasound	70010 to 79999
Pathology and Laboratory	80002 to 89399
Medicine (except Anesthesiology)	90701 to 99199

Organization of *CPT-98*, published by the American Medical Association.

Other features of *CPT-98:*

- Each section is introduced by specific "Guidelines" for its use; these are often quite complex.

- Explanatory material is found throughout the volume as well.

- The base codes are 5 digits in length.

- Code meanings may be modified by

   - Adding a suffix to the base five digit code, e.g., -62 = "plus a second surgeon"; or

   - Adding a second 5-digit code, e.g., "AND 09962." This is an alternative way to give the same information as with the suffix; it also means "plus a second surgeon."

   - Supplementing with a special report.

- A group of codes is provided within each section that the physician may use for reporting unlisted procedures relevant to that section. These codes are to be accompanied by narrative explanations when they are submitted.

- Throughout the volume, special symbols are attached to codes which have been revised and to new codes.

- An alphabetic index is included.

- As a general principle, codes represent "package prices" for the services described. An exception is found in the Surgical Section, where one finds certain "Starred (*) Procedures or Items." These are described as procedures which are small and readily identifiable, but for which the preoperative and postoperative services vary with the patient. For starred procedures, the procedure itself is coded and billed for, billing separately for the preoperative and postoperative services is permitted, and special rules are provided for other situations, such as when a starred procedure is done incidentally along with, say, a comprehensive history and physical examination. Clinical examples are provided.

The illustration below shows the coding section in *CPT-95* for 99213, "Office or other outpatient visit."[2] After the code description, *CPT* provides several examples of cases which would use this code; these are shown on page 187.

---

2.   American Medical Association, *Physicians' Current Procedural Terminology, CPT 1995*, p. 12

Figure 8.4 CPT Coding for Office Visit

Established Patient

99213   Office or other outpatient visit for the
evaluation and management of an established
patient,which requires at least two of these
three key components:

- **an expanded problem focused history;**

- **an expanded problem focused
  examination;**

- **medical decision making of low
  complexity.**

Counseling and coordination of care with other
providers or agencies are provided consistent
with the nature of the problem(s) and the
patient's and/or family's needs.

Usually, the presenting problem(s) are of low
to moderate severity. Physicians typically
spend 15 minutes face-to-face with the patient
and/or family.

An example from *CPT-95* showing the code for a 15-minute office visit with an
established patient. American Medical Association, 1995.

Figure 8.5 Examples of Office Visits for CPT 99213

Examples

Office visit with 55-year-old male, established patient, for management of hypertension, mild fatigue, on beta blocker/thiazide regimen. (Family Medicine/Internal Medicine)

Outpatient visit with 37-year-old male, established patient, who is 3 years post total colectomy for chronic ulcerative colitis, presents for increased irritation at his stoma. (General Surgery)

Office visit for a 70-year-old diabetic hypertensive established patient with recent change in insulin requirement. (Internal Medicine/Nephrology)

Office visit with 80-year-old female established patient, for follow-up osteoporosis, status-post compression fractures. (Rheumatology)

Office visit for an established patient with stable cirrhosis of the liver. (Gastroenterology)

Routine, follow-up office evaluation at a three-month interval for a 77-year-old female, established patient, with nodular small cleaved-cell lymphoma. (Hematology/Oncology)

Quarterly follow-up office visit for a 45-year-old male established patient, with stable chronic asthma, on steroid and bronchodilator therapy. (Pulmonary Medicine)

Office visit for 50-year-old female, established patient, with insulin-dependent diabetes mellitus and stable coronary artery disease, for monitoring. (Family Medicine/Internal Medicine)

An example from *CPT-95* showing examples for code 99213. American Medical Association, 1995.

HCFA Common Procedure Coding System

The Health Care Financing Administration (HCFA) found that, while *CPT* was adequate for the area of procedures and services it covered, a great many items for which bills could be submitted (or for which coverage under Medicare was not provided, but billing might be attempted) were not included. Consequently, it produced the *Health Care Financing Administration Common Procedure Coding System* (HCPCS) ("HickPicks"), a list with codes of some 3,000 items.

As a result, the following three-level nomenclature was introduced:

Level 1: *CPT* Level 1 of HCPCS is *CPT* itself.

Level 2: National Codes Level 2 of HCPCS is the supplement to *CPT* which is called "National Codes." Most of the codes in the National system are for durable items, but a substantial number are for injections, chemotherapy drugs, medical and surgical supplies, etc. Level 2 codes are distinguishable from *CPT* codes because, although they are also 5 characters in length, they are alphanumeric, with the first character alphabetic (restricted to the letters A, B, D, E, H, J, K, L, M, P, Q, R, V) and the last four characters numeric. K and Q codes are under the sole control of HCFA, while the other alphabetic codes are controlled by a panel. Modifiers are also used in the National Codes, and they also are alphanumeric.

Level 3: Local Codes Level 3 of HCPCS contains "Local Codes" which may be created and used by each Medicare carrier individually. Level 3 codes are allocated the letters W, X, Y, and Z, and their modifiers are also restricted to these four alphabetic characters.

Toward a Single Procedure Classification

It should be clear that the process for coding and reporting procedures is extremely complex.

- Volume 3 of *ICD-9-CM* is *used by hospitals* for indexing and in the Uniform Hospital Discharge Data Set (UHDDS), the core of billing for Medicare and Medicaid hospital services.

- HCPCS (Levels 1, 2, and 3) is *used by physicians* and other providers for billing for their services.

Thus many coders are forced to learn and use up to four different procedure classifying, terminology, and coding systems. It is not surprising that there is a substantial movement to simplify the system, and it is quite predictable that the proposed solution is to create yet another, but single (all-purpose), procedure classification.

The United States National Committee on Vital and Health Statistics (NCVHS)[3] went on record in 1986 recommending "moving to a single classification system." In 1992 it charged its Subcommittee on Medical Classification Systems to again look at the problems of procedure "coding" and of achieving a single classification, and in 1993 NCVHS made the following formal recommendations to the Secretary of Health and Human Services:

Recommendations

- The National Committee on Vital and Health Statistics recommends development and adoption of a single system for classification of health services and procedures to be used in all settings in which healthcare is delivered in the United States.

- The Secretary of the Department of Health and Human Services should assume the responsibility for the development and maintenance of a single classification system as a collaborative effort involving those who have an interest or stake in a new system.

- Development of a single procedure classification system should be given immediate priority, and implementation should be coordinated with national health reform.

- The Secretary should ensure that the system is easy to use, comprehensive, hierarchical, flexible, and serves present and future needs in the public and private sectors of healthcare.

- Adequate resources must be provided to support all aspects of development, implementation, evaluation, education, and maintenance.

---

3. The National Committee on Vital and Health Statistics (NCVHS) is an independent, nonprofit organization which serves as the statutory public advisory body to the Department of Health and Human Services (DHHS) on health data, statistics and national health information policy. Its mandate includes being a national forum on health data and information systems. Their website is http://www.ncvhs.hhs.gov. See also "Standards for Health Information," page 247.

The NCVHS made specific recommendations of the desirable attributes of a procedure classification system; these may be found on page 545. The entire recommendation, Appendix V to the *1993 Annual Report of the National Committee on Vital and Health Statistics,* is also included (see page 533). It is worth reading, with its discussion of the problems presented by having "two" classifications (*ICD-9-CM* and HCPCS), neither entirely satisfactory (even for its own purpose), its presentation of the pros and cons of creating a new classification as perceived by various segments of the healthcare system, recital of the tasks involved in developing a new classification, and statement of some of the problems which would have to be solved to implement a new classification.

It seems clear that some of the "characteristics" recommended by the NCVHS are mutually exclusive if they are considered as attributes of a classification, such as *CPT* or *ICD-9-CM,* or the desired successor which would replace them both. For example,

- "ability to aggregate data from individual codes into larger categories"

This is possible, but limited, in the required hierarchical structure.[4] Even so, it would not be possible to do some of the aggregation implied by the requirement that the classification be multiaxial. That requirement imposes the need for different kinds of, or "secondary," hierarchical trees. For example, a user might want to see all procedures for each body system separately, a view which would be impossible if there were only one hierarchical route for the aggregation; someone else might want to see only the uses of specific implants.

- "each code has unique definition forever — not reused"

This statement acknowledges the importance of this fundamental of proper data management but, of course, it is not possible if there is to be

---

4. "Hierarchical" in a classification is most easily described by the terminology employed by the National Library of Medicine (NLM) in connection with the "Unified Medical Language System" (UMLS). UMLS uses the term "isa," formed by combining the two words "is" and "a," to refer to the link in a hierarchical, "one way," network. To illustrate: a dog *isa* animal *isa* living organism. But not all living organisms are animals, and not all animals are dogs. All objects linked to "animal" by "isa" are animals, all "animals" linked to "living organism" by "isa" are living organisms.

flexibility to incorporate new procedures and technologies (empty code numbers or unlimited code length; "forever" is implied). When, over time, an empty code area overflows, subsequent codes would have to be renumbered, and thus the code would in fact be reused.[5]

The current situation in procedure classifying — having to use several different classifications, described above — makes it easy to see the forces urging simplification in handling data about procedures.

ICD-10-PCS — A New Coding System

The Health Care Financing Administration (HCFA) is responsible for the procedure coding system used for Medicare and Medicaid inpatient procedures. HCFA contracted with 3M Health Information Systems to develop a new procedure coding system, to be used along with the new disease classification, *ICD-10-CM*. The new system, called *ICD-10 Procedure Coding System (ICD-10-PCS)*, may be put into use in the near future.

ICD-10-PCS does not have "International Classification of Diseases" in its name, but simply *"ICD-10"*. This title was adopted presumably to link the procedure coding system to the disease classification, *ICD-10-CM*. Unlike the *ICD-10-CM*, which is a modification of the "parent" *ICD-10*, *ICD-10-PCS* is an entirely free-standing coding system. There is no "international" procedure classification to modify or with which to maintain a relationship.

✓ Note that *ICD-10-PCS* is clearly labeled to be used for *coding*, i.e., compressing a description of a procedure into a seven-character representation. *ICD-10-CM*, in contrast, is a classification, or grouping system (see "The Tenth Revision of ICD," page 166).

The comments which follow are based on the draft of *ICD-10-PCS* placed on the Internet in June 1998. The documents (which will be referred to here as the [3M HIS] "Working Paper") consist of:

- "Development of the ICD-10 Procedure Coding System (ICD-10-PCS)"

---

5. Only by abandoning the dual use of a code — for sorting and for carrying clinical meaning — could this requirement be met. See "Codes & Coding," page 117.

- Training Manual
- Tabular List
- Alphabetic Index

The four objectives stated as followed in developing *ICD-10-PCS* were:

- Completeness
- Expandability
- Multiaxial structure, here defined as "each code character having the same meaning within a specific procedure section and across procedure sections to the extent possible"
- Standardized terminology

Additional constraints noted by the authors are that:

- Diagnostic information is not included in the procedure description
- Not Otherwise Specified (NOS) option is not provided
- There is limited use of the Not Elsewhere Classified (NEC) option
- All possible procedures can be described

ICD-10-PCS is a modular code. The codes are alphanumeric, with 7 characters, each with 34 possible values: digits 0-9 and 24 alphabetic characters. Unlike *ICD-10* and *ICD-10-CM*, the characters "I" and "O" are not used because to use them would present confusion with the numerals "1" and "0". Each procedure is expressed by the full 7 characters. The Working Paper states that the term "procedure is used to refer to the complete specification of the seven characters," and goes on to state that the Tabular List

> … contains only combinations of characters that represent a valid procedure. Combinations of characters that do not constitute a valid procedure are not contained in the Tabular List.

ICD-10-PCS then has the building blocks for 52,000,000,000 (billion) procedure codes (and terms). As will be seen, not all have been used; not all 34 possible values are always available, but it may well be more than are really needed.

Procedures are found in sixteen Sections, shown below. The character designating the Section is the first character in a procedure code:[6]

Code	Title
0	Medical and Surgical (31 sections)
1	Obstetrics
2	Placement (2 sections)
3	Administration (2 sections)
4	Measurement and Monitoring
5	Imaging
6	Nuclear Medicine
7	Radiation Oncology
8	Osteopathic
9	Diagnostic Audiology and Rehabilitation
B	Extracorporeal Assistance and Performance
C	Extracorporeal Therapies
D	Laboratory (8 sections)
F	Mental Health
G	Chiropractic
H	Miscellaneous

Each of the seven characters which form a procedure code has the same meaning within a Section, but may have different meanings in different Sections, as shown in table below.[7]

---

6. From *ICD-10 Procedure Coding System (ICD-10-PCS)*, published by the Health Care Financing Association, 1999.

7. The table was developed by the authors from the Final Drafts of the *ICD-10-PCS* Introduction, Training Manual, and Tabular List, HCFA, Internet, Summer 1998.

Figure 8.6 ICD-10-PCS Code Character Meaning, by Section

Code & Name of Section	Characters					
	2	3	4	5	6	7
0 = Medical & Surgical	Body System	Root Operation	Body Part	Approach	Device	Qualifier
1 = Obstetrics	Body System	Root Operation	Body Part	Approach	Device	Qualifier
2 = Placement	Anatomical Regions/ Orifices	Root Operation	Body System/ Region	Approach	Device	Qualifier
3 = Administration	Physiological Systems Anatomical Regions	Root Operation	Body System/ Region	Approach	Substance	Qualifier
4 = Measurement & Monitoring	Physiological Systems	Root Operation	Body System	Approach	Function	Qualifier
5 = Imaging	Body System	Root Type	Body Part	Contrast	Contrast/ Qualifier	Qualifier
6 = Nuclear Medicine	Body System	Type	Body Part	Radionuclide	Radiopharmaceutical	Qualifier
7 = Radiation Oncology	Body System	Modality	Treatment Site	Ports/ Isotopes	Equipment	Qualifier/ Risk Structure

Meaning of each code character, within each section, of *ICD-10 Procedure Coding System (ICD-10-PCS)*.

Figure 8.7 ICD-10-PCS Code Character Meaning, by Section *(continued)*

Code & Name of Section	Characters					
	2	3	4	5	6	7
8 = Osteo-pathic	Anatomical Regions	Root Operation	Body Region	Approach	Method	Qualifier
9 = Diagnostic Audiology & Rehab-ilitation	Type	Test / Method		Body Part	Equipment	Qualifier
B = Extracor-poreal Assistance & Performance	Physiolo-gical Systems	Root Operation	Body System	Duration	Function	Qualifier
C = Extracor-poreal Therapies	Physiolo-gical Systems	Root Operation	Body System	Duration	Qualifier	Qualifier
D = Laboratory	Type of Laboratory	Analyte		Specimen Source		Method
F = Mental Health	Type	Type Expansion	Qualifier	Qualifier	Qualifier	Qualifier
G = Chiropractic	Anatomical Regions	Root Operation	Body Region	Approach	Method	Qualifier
H = Miscellan-eous	Body System	Root Operation	Body Region	Approach	Method	Qualifier

For the Medical and Surgical Section, as an example:

- The Table of Body Systems (Character 2) shows 29 systems.
- The Table of Root Operations (Character 3) shows 28 possibilities.
- Approaches (Character 5) listed are 13.

The Tabular Listing is in the form of a grid, the top portion of which contains the first two or three characters of the procedure code (and their translations) along with a description of the procedure. For example, the box at the top of the grid is illustrated in the Working Paper:[8]

Tabular Listing	
Character 1 Character 2 Character 3	0: Surgical 9: Ear, Nose, Sinus 5: Dilation: Expanding the orifice or the lumen of a tubular body part

Below this header box, the remainder of the grid gives the remaining characters available ("legal") for the characters in the header. The illustration for code "095," above, is:

Character 4 Body Part	Character 5 Approach	Character 6 Device	Character 7 Qualifier
H: Eustachian Tube, Right J: Eustachian Tube, Left	1: Open Intraluminal 2: Open Intraluminal, endoscopic B: Transorifice Intraluminal C: Transorifice Intraluminal Endoscopic	D: Intraluminal Device Y: Device NEC Z: None	Z: None

Accompanying this grid is the Table of Codes which shows some of the codes which can legally be constructed from the offerings in the grid for "095" (examples are from the surgical procedures in the illustrations above):

---

8.   This and the following grids were developed from the *ICD-10 Procedure Coding System (ICD-10-PCS) Working Paper.*

Table of Codes	
095H1DZ	Dilation, Eustachian Tube, Right, Open Intraluminal, Intraluminal Device, No Qualifier
095H1DZ	Dilation, Eustachian Tube, Right, Open Intraluminal, Endoscopic, Intraluminal Device, No Qualifier
... and so on	

In this illustration (i.e., for code "095"), 24 legal codes would be possible (2 x 4 x 3 x 1).

The Tabular List for the Medical and Surgical Procedures (Character 1, code 0) for the Male Reproductive System, code "0W... ," looks like:

Male Reproductive System "0W"				
Character 1 Character 2	0: Medical and Surgical W: Male Reproductive System			
Character 3 Root Operation	Character 4 Body Part	Character 5 Approach	Character 6 Device	Character 7 Qualifier
Codes: 19 possible; Bypass Change etc.	Codes: 22 possible; Prostate Seminal vesicle, right etc.	Codes: 10 possible; Open Open, intraluminal etc.	Codes: 12 possible; Drainage device Radioactive element etc.	Codes: 4 possible; Vas deferens, right Vas deferens, left etc.

The product of these possibilities (19 x 22 x 10 x 12 x 4) is 200,640 — the number of codable procedures for the male reproductive system.

The corresponding table for the Female Reproductive System, code "0V... ," is:

Female Reproductive System "0V"				
Character 1 Character 2	0: Medical and Surgical V: Female Reproductive System			
Character 3 Root Operation	Character 4 Body Part	Character 5 Approach	Character 6 Device	Character 7 Qualifier
Codes: 23 possible; Bypass Change etc.	Codes: 25 possible; Ovary, right Ovary, left etc.	Codes: 10 possible; Open Open, intraluminal etc.	Codes: 14 possible; Drainage device Radioactive element etc.	Codes: 6 possible; Vaginally Fallopian tube, right etc.

Here, the arithmetic is 23 x 25 x 10 x 14 x 6, yielding 482,000 procedures.

It is probable that not all of these combinations are clinically feasible or likely, but it may not be practical to eliminate all "impossible combinations" in order to produce a computer-processible list of legal (valid) codes to be used in editing the data.

In addition to the Tabular Listing of procedures, *ICD-10-PCS* has an alphabetic index and a list of codes. There is no intent that coding can be done from the Alphabetic Index; the user must always refer to the Tabular Listing. An example of the result of this process is as follows.

Coding an Appendectomy

The user looks up "appendectomy" and finds:

> ...
>
> Appendectomy
> - *see* Excision, gastrointestinal system 0D8 ...
> - *see* Resection, gastrointestinal system 0DR ...
> Appendicectomy
> - *see* Excision, gastrointestinal system 0D8 ...
> - *see* Resection, gastrointestinal system 0DR ...

Stedman's Medical Dictionary, as well as *Dorland's* and *Taber's* dictionaries, consider appendectomy and appendicectomy as simply spelling variants. As to the distinction between excision and resection, the issue is not as clear. *Dorland, Stedman,* and *Taber* favor excision as the complete removal of a structure, and resection as the removal of a part of a structure, and in fact include under resection, *wedge resection* (removal of a triangular piece of tissue), *transurethral resection* (a portion of the prostate), and *gastric resection* (part of the stomach). *ICD-10-PCS*, however, reversed the meanings, at least in the version on the Internet in 1998 as shown in the tables below.

And *ICD-10-PCS* offers many more choices than we usually consider for appendectomies. Most of us think of them as "primary," meaning the reason for the operation was to remove the appendix, and "incidental," meaning done prophylactically while the surgeon is in the abdomen anyway (sometimes these are called *en passant* — "in passing").

Reference to the Tabular List finds 35 pages (grids) for "0D." The portion of the grid for code "0D8..." which concerns "excision" of the appendix is reproduced here. The first 3 characters of the code are in the top box:

Coding Appendectomy with ICD-10-PCS				
Character 1 0: MEDICAL AND SURGICAL Character 2 D: GASTROINTESTINAL SYSTEM Character 3 **8: EXCISION**: Cutting out or off, without replacement, ***a portion of*** a body part.				
Character 4 Body Part	Character 5 Approach		Character 6 Device	Character 7 Qualifier

0 Esophagus
1 Esophagus, Upper
2 Esophagus, Middle
3 Esophagus, Lower
4 Esophagogastric Junction
6 Stomach
7 Stomach, Pylorus
9 Duodenum
A Jejunum
B Ileum
C Ileocecal Valve
D Large Intestine
F Large Intestine, Right
G Large Intestine, Left
H Cecum
J Appendix
K Ascending Colon
L Transverse Colon
M Descending Colon
N Sigmoid Colon
P Rectum
	0 Open
	1 Open Intraluminal
	2 Open Intraluminal Endoscopic
	3 Percutaneous
	4 Percutaneous Endoscopic
	5 Percutaneous Intraluminal
	6 Percutaneous Intraluminal
	   Endoscopic
	B Transorifice Intraluminal
	C Transorifice Intraluminal
	   Endoscopic
			Z None	Z None

Q Anus R Anal Sphincter	0 Open 3 Percutaneous 4 Percutaneous Endoscopic D Intraorifice		Z None	Z None
S Greater Omentum T Lesser Omentum V Mesentery W Peritoneum	0 Open 3 Percutaneous 4 Percutaneous Endoscopic B Intraorifice Intraluminal C Intraorifice Intraluminal Endoscopic		Z None	Z None

So a partial appendectomy, cutting off a portion of a body part, could be coded 18 different ways, depending on which of the 9 approaches offered in Character 5 were used and whether the surgery was specified as diagnostic or not in Character 7. Thus:

- Code "0D8J[Character 5]ZX" would have 9 possibilities for a diagnostic partial appendectomy

- Code "0D8J[Character 5]ZZ" would have 9 possibilities for a therapeutic partial appendectomy

To illustrate:

- Code "0D8JCZX" would decode to a diagnostic subtotal appendectomy done by a transorifice intraluminal endoscopic approach.

Character		Meaning
Number	Value	
1	0	Medical and surgical
2	D	Gastrointestinal system
3	8	Excision (partial removal)
4	J	Appendix
5	C	Transorifice Intraluminal Endoscopic
6	Z	No device
7	X	Diagnostic

Reference to the Tabular List for "resection" of the appendix, "0DR … ," yields this grid:

Character 1 0: MEDICAL AND SURGICAL			
Character 2 D: GASTROINTESTINAL SYSTEM			
Character 3 **R: RESECTION**: Cutting out or off, without replacement, ***all of*** a body part.			
Character 4 Body Part	Character 5 Approach	Character 6 Device	Character 7 Qualifier

. . .
 	
 J Appendix
 . . .
	0 Open
	 1 Open Intraluminal
	 2 Open Intraluminal Endoscopic
	 3 Percutaneous
	 4 Percutaneous Endoscopic
	 5 Percutaneous Intraluminal
	 6 Percutaneous Intraluminal
	    Endoscopic
	 B Transorifice Intraluminal
	 C Transorifice Intraluminal
	    Endoscopic
		Z None	Z None

There is no option for diagnostic total appendectomy. With 9 approaches offered for Character 5,

- Code "0DRJ[Character 5]ZZ" would have 9 possibilities for a total appendectomy.

✓ It appears possible to code a total of 27 different kinds of appendectomies, and a given individual would be a candidate for 3 operations, one of each kind.

It seems unlikely that coders will memorize codes.

ICD-10-PCS *does* code procedure *entities* for its universe, rather than forcing procedures to be grouped. However, it differs from the entity coding envisioned in this book in that the string of modular terms which is the product of the coding — just as with any modular coding system — sounds nothing like the language used in everyday practice. The alphabetic index to *ICD-10-PCS* is a kind of translation of the codes into clinical English. But true entity codes must decode back to the original clinical input language.

In the past, in the face of coding systems of such intricacy, abbreviated versions have been forthcoming, usually for a specialty, such as general surgery or ophthalmology, containing only the categories (codes) the author believes will be used by that particular group of users. These specialized versions have been greeted eagerly because of the expectation that (1) only the procedures really done are there and (2) the codes which will give trouble in the reimbursement system have been left out. The down side is that most specialists will occasionally need to code some procedures outside of their specialties, and those codes would not be available to them. The result is that information is left out, and that often procedures must be coded to "the nearest thing."

Finally, at this writing, no information is available as to just how the exquisitely-detailed coded information will be used, either in the payment system or for other purposes. It can be predicted that grouping of procedures will be required for reimbursement and for analysis of patterns of health care. HCFA itself is unlikely to want to cope with the 482,000 different procedures on the female reproductive system. Hospitals certainly don't want that dispersion of informaton as they try to plan and manage facilities. And medical educators will find it more useful to put the procedures into classes as they plan their curricula.

9

How We Code Today: Category Coding

MOST OF US think of coding as simply looking something up in a list of codes and getting the code, much as we look up telephone numbers in a phone book. Of course, we also expect the phone number to take us unambiguously to the customer or the name. Coding healthcare information today is nothing like that process.

The coding system used today in the health information system is "category" coding — diagnoses and procedures (and the cases in which they occur) are dropped directly into the categories of the classifications employed. In the case of diagnoses, the classification is the *International Classification of Diseases, 9th Revision, Clinical Modification (ICD-9-CM)*. For procedures, several classifications are used: *ICD-9-CM*, *Physicians' Current Procedural Terminology (CPT)*, and the *Health Care Financing Administration's Common Procedure Coding System* (HCPCS) (two and sometimes three levels).

It is essential that this approach to coding — category coding — be thoroughly examined.

How "Category Coding" Works

Remember that category coding is actually a *classifying* process (one of classifying *cases*) — not a coding process at all. A good deal of misunderstanding has resulted from our calling it "coding."[1] In contrast, "pure" coding is simple — a code (usually alphanumeric) is exchanged for a term in a one-to-one relationship. Entity coding is such a process; it will be discussed in the next chapter. Category coding, a process of classifying, is quite different.

The best way to understand how we "code" today is to walk through the process of category coding diagnoses to *ICD-9-CM*. Using as an

---

1. See "Category Coding," page 124.

example a diagnosis of polyneuropathy,[2] the following discussion describes a process all too familiar to medical record professionals and physicians' office personnel.[3]

Walking Through: Coding "Polyneuropathy" with ICD-9-CM

In the medical record, the physician records each diagnosis or problem as a statement — a string of words. We will call the physician's statement of a diagnosis or problem the original *term* used in the medical record. Here's what it's like to code a diagnosis using *ICD-9-CM*.

If you were the coder, you would first have to look up the term in the *second* volume of *ICD-9-CM*, the Alphabetic Index (about 900 pages). There are two possibilities: either (1) you will, or (2) you won't, find the exact term used by the physician. Here's what the physician wrote in the medical record as the patient's primary diagnosis: "polyneuropathy." Here's what you find in the Alphabetic Index:

> **Polyneuropathy** (peripheral[4]) 356.9[5]
>   alcoholic 357.5
>   amyloid 277.3 *[357.4]*
>   arsenical 357.7
>   diabetic 250.6 *[357.2]*
>   due to
>   antitetanus serum 357.6

---

2.   Polyneuropathy is defined in *Taber's* as a "term applied to any disorder or affection of peripheral nerves, but preferably restricted to those of a noninflammatory nature. SYN: neuritis, multiple; polyneuritis." *Taber's Cyclopedic Medical Dictionary*®.

3.   A great many computer programs are offered to aid in the coding process, but they may obscure the actual steps which are taken. Therefore, in this discussion, the process is described as entirely a manual one.

4.   Do you know whether the polyneuropathy is "peripheral"? A trip to the dictionary defines polyneuropathy as peripheral. So the first entry seems to give the necessary code. Why are there 60 other lines of entries under the term?

5.   The code numbers after each term refer to the Tabular List. To understand the second number (in italics after the first number with some terms), the coder must know the "conventions" of *ICD-9-CM*. Those for the Alphabetic Index are found in the introduction to the volume. The first code recorded should represent the etiology and the second the manifestation (the polyneuropathy); they must be recorded in this sequence. But some entries under "due to" have only one code; this also is covered in the introduction.

    arsenic 357.7
    drug or medicinal substance 357.6
        correct substance properly administered
            357.6
        overdose or wrong substance given or
            taken 977.9
            specified drug — *see* Table of drugs and chemicals
    lack of vitamin NEC 269.2 *[357.4]*
    lead 357.7
    organophosphate compounds 357.7
    pellagra 265.2 *[357.4]*
    porphyria 277.1 *[357.4]*
    serum 357.6
    toxic agent NEC 357.7
hereditary 356.0
idiopathic 356.9
    progressive 356.4
in
    amyloidosis 277.3 [357.4]
    avitaminosis 269.2 [357.4]
        specified NEC 269.1 *[357.4]*
    beriberi 265.0 *[357.4]*
    collagen vascular disease NEC 710.9
        [357.1]
    deficiency
        B-complex NEC 266.2 [357.4]
        vitamin B 266.9 *[357.4]*
        vitamin B 266.1 *[357.4]*
    diabetes 250.6 *[357.2]*
    diphtheria (*see also* Diphtheria) 032.89
        [357.4]
    disseminated lupus erythematosus 710.0
        [357.1]
    herpes zoster 053.13
    hypoglycemia 251.2 *[357.4]*
    malignant neoplasm (M8000/3) NEC 199.1
        [357.3]
    mumps 072.72
    pellagra 265.2 *[357.4]*
    polyarteritis nodosa 446.0 *[357.1]*
    porphyria 277.1 *[357.4]*
    rheumatoid arthritis 714.0 *[357.1]*
    sarcoidosis 135 *[357.4]*
    uremia 585 *[357.4]*
lead 357.7
nutritional 269.9 *[357.4]*
    specified NEC 269.8 *[357.4]*
postherpetic 053.13
progressive 356.4
sensory (hereditary) 356.2

If you do find the exact term — "polyneuropathy" — you will be tempted to simply use the code which is shown beside the term. But that's wrong.

If you have been trained in coding, you know that there are number of coding rules and conventions which go along with ICD-9-CM. See the boxes on the following pages — "Guidance in the Use of ICD-9-CM" and "Conventions Used in the Tabular List" — for an introduction to these.

The next proper step is to look up the codes in Volume 1 of *ICD-9-CM*, the Tabular List (about 1200 pages). There, each code is accompanied by the label of the category, along with a list of the diagnoses included in that category. Two of the codes given for polyneuropathy in the Alphabetic Index — 356 and 357 — are shown here as they look in the Tabular List:

356 Hereditary and idiopathic peripheral neuropathy
   356.0   Hereditary peripheral neuropathy
             Déjérine-Sottas disease
   356.1   Peroneal muscular atrophy
             Charcôt-Marie-Tooth disease
             Neuropathic muscular atrophy
   356.2   Hereditary sensory neuropathy
   356.3   Refsum's disease
             Heredopathia atactica polyneuritiformis
   356.4   Idiopathic progressive polyneuropathy
   356.8   Other specified idiopathic peripheral neuropathy
             Supranuclear paralysis
   356.9[6] Unspecified
357 Inflammatory and toxic neuropathy
   357.0   Acute infective polyneuritis
             Guillain-Barré syndrome
             Postinfectious polyneuritis
   357.1   Polyneuropathy in collagen vascular disease
             Code also underlying disease, as:
                  disseminated lupus erythematosus (710.0)
                  polyarteritis nodosa (446.0)
                  rheumatoid arthritis (714.0)

---

6.   The first code to which you are referred, 356.9, doesn't contain the word *polyneuropathy.*

GUIDANCE IN THE USE OF ICD-9-CM

To code accurately, it is necessary to have a working knowledge of medical terminology and to understand the characteristics, terminology, and conventions of the ICD-9-CM. Transforming verbal descriptions of diseases, injuries, conditions, and procedures into numerical designations (coding) is a complex activity and should not be undertaken without proper training.

Originally coding was accomplished to provide access to medical records by diagnoses and operations through retrieval for medical research, education, and administration. Medical codes today are utilized to facilitate payment of health services, to evaluate utilization patterns, and to study the appropriateness of health care costs. Coding provides the bases for epidemiological studies and research into the quality of health care.

Coding must be performed correctly and consistently to produce meaningful statistics to aid in the planning for the health needs of the Nation.

Basic steps in coding diagnoses/diseases:

1.   Always consult Volume 2, Alphabetic Index to ICD-9-CM first.

   Locate the main entry term. The Alphabetic Index is arranged by condition. Conditions may be expressed as nouns, adjectives, and eponyms. Some conditions have multiple entries under their synonyms. Select the appropriate code.

2.   Refer to Volume 1 of the ICD-9-CM locating the selected code.

   Be guided by any exclusion notes or other instructions that would direct the use of a different code from that selected in the Index for a particular diagnosis, condition, or disease.

3.   Read and be guided by the conventions used in the Tabular List (Volume 1, ICD-9-CM).

As reference for use by researchers and to maintain comparability with its parent, the ICD-9, a list of three-digit ICD-9-CM categories is given in Appendix E. While these categories form natural statistical groupings, they cannot substitute for the required five-digit ICD-9-CM code.

From the Introduction to the CD-ROM verson of the sixth edition of the *International Classification of Diseases, 9th Revision, Clinical Modification (ICD-9-CM)* (U. S. Government publication, 1997).

CONVENTIONS USED IN THE TABULAR LIST

The ICD-9-CM Tabular List for both the Disease and Procedure Classification makes use of certain abbreviations, punctuation, and other conventions which need to be clearly understood.

Abbreviations

NEC   Not elsewhere classifiable. The category number for the term including NEC is to be used only when the coder lacks the information necessary to code the term to a more specific category.

NOS   Not otherwise specified. This abbreviation is the equivalent of "unspecified."

Punctuation

[ ]   Brackets are used to enclose synonyms, alternative wordings, or explanatory phrases.

( )   Parentheses are used to enclose supplementary words which may be present or absent in the statement of a disease or procedure without affecting the code number to which it is assigned.

:   Colons are used in the Tabular List after an incomplete term which needs one or more of the modifiers which follow in order to make it assignable to a given category.

Other Conventions

Format: ICD-9-CM uses an indented format for ease in reference.

Instructional Notations

Includes   This note appears immediately under a three-digit code title to further define, or give example of, the contents of the category.

Excludes   Terms following the word "excludes" are to be coded elsewhere. The term excludes means "DO NOT CODE HERE".

Use additional   This instruction is placed in the Tabular List in those categories where the user will need to add further information (by using an additional code) to give a more complete picture of the diagnosis or procedure.

Code first underlying disease   This instructional note is used for those codes not intended to be used as a principal diagnosis, or not to be sequenced before the underlying disease. The note requires that the underlying disease (etiology) be recorded first and the particular manifestation recorded secondarily. This note appears only in the Tabular List.

From the Introduction to the CD-ROM version of the sixth edition of the *International Classification of Diseases, 9th Revision, Clinical Modification (ICD-9-CM)* (U. S. Government publication, 1997).

357.2 Polyneuropathy in diabetes[7]
      Code also underlying disease (250.6)
357.3 Polyneuropathy in malignant disease
      Code also underlying disease (140.0-208.9)
357.4 Polyneuropathy in other diseases classified elsewhere
      Code also underlying disease, as:
            amyloidosis (277.3)
            beriberi (265.0)
            deficiency of B vitamins (266.0-266.9)
            diphtheria (032.0-032.9)
            hypoglycemia (251.2)
            pellagra (265.2)
            porphyria (277.1)
            sarcoidosis (I 35)
            uremia (585)
      Excludes: polyneuropathy in:
            herpes zoster (053.13)
            mumps (072.72)
357.5 Alcoholic polyneuropathy
357.6 Polyneuropathy due to drugs
      Use additional E code to identify drug[8]
357.7 Polyneuropathy due to other toxic agents
      Use additional E code to identify toxic agent
357.8 Other
357.9 Unspecified

Here again there are two possibilities: either you will find the exact diagnosis term the physician used, or you won't. Interestingly enough, the term used in the medical record, *and* which you found in the Alphabetic Index, may not even be in the Tabular List! If it is in the Tabular List, you will then be expected to study and follow the instructions in the book under headings such as "exclusion notes," "inclusion note," "code also," and more. So far, this has not been a simple process, even if you were lucky and found the exact term in both indexes, and had no further coding instructions.

---

7. "In diabetes" is found in both the Alphabetic Index and the Tabular List to require also code 250.6. But "diabetes mellitus" is given elsewhere as simply 250.0. A trip to 250.0 adds the instruction that ".0" actually means "without mention of complication," that the ".6" adds "with neurological complication," and there is also a note that a 5th digit should be used to tell whether the diabetes is "adult-onset, juvenile, or unspecified."

8. "E codes" are in a separate section of the Tabular List and refer to "External Causes."

Note that we never did give you a clear answer as to how to code the term you started with, polyneuropathy. And that end result of a coding effort is all too common.

Now, what if the Tabular List, the "coding book," doesn't even list the term to be coded? If you can't find the desired exact diagnosis at any step along the way, you must become an *expert classifier.* That means knowing a lot more than enough to look up the given term:

- What does the diagnostic term mean?

- What are possible valid alternative terms?

- Are there other diagnoses which should always be sought in conjunction?

- How does the classification "work?" — i.e., how were its designers thinking when they put it together?

- What is its schema of organization? By parts of the body? By body systems?

- Do diseases of infectious origin always go in the infection chapter?

- Does the patient's age put it somewhere else?

- Where can you get answers? Can you go back to the physician for further explanation and possibly another statement of the diagnosis?

- Do you have time to do more than guess at the closest likely category?

This is quite a burden to put on an individual usually thought of as having a simple, "look-up" job.

As though this isn't complicated enough, you probably are using an "annotated" version of the code books, designed to decrease the likelihood of the patient's bill being questioned. These books use color coding to inform which diagnoses may safely be listed first, for example, and which, if shown at all, must be secondary. Coding has become increasingly important in ensuring proper reimbursement.

It should be clear by now that coding the term "polyneuropathy" is not a clerical matter at all; it is a classifying task.[9] The problem would be even

---

9. See "The Process of Classifying," page 144.

more complicated if the polyneuropathy was due to HIV infection. Only in some versions of *ICD-9-CM*, published after 1986, are the codes for HIV even included, and the alphabetic indexes rarely, if ever, carry all the cross-references.[10]

Yet this classifying task has to be performed daily by several hundred thousand persons, only a relatively few of them adequately trained. And there is ample evidence that even fully qualified, credentialed, and conscientious *ICD-9-CM* "coders" (really classifiers, of course) can logically arrive at different coding decisions, as shown later in this chapter (page 216).

The category coding process is illustrated by the flow chart on the following pages.

---

10. Changes in *ICD-9-CM* are officially published annually as errata, with instructions as to what to write in where, a process rarely followed carefully. All the volumes in a given coding section have to be edited by hand, and this is likely to be a low priority. Of course, annual editions of the books are also for sale, but most budgets are unlikely to allow for replacement of all copies every year. In addition, coders usually have their own penned-in notations which they are reluctant to transfer to a new volume. Updating the *ICD* books for coders has always been a problem; see "Modifications for Clinical Use," page 162.

Figure 9.1 Coding Diagnoses with 'Category Coding'

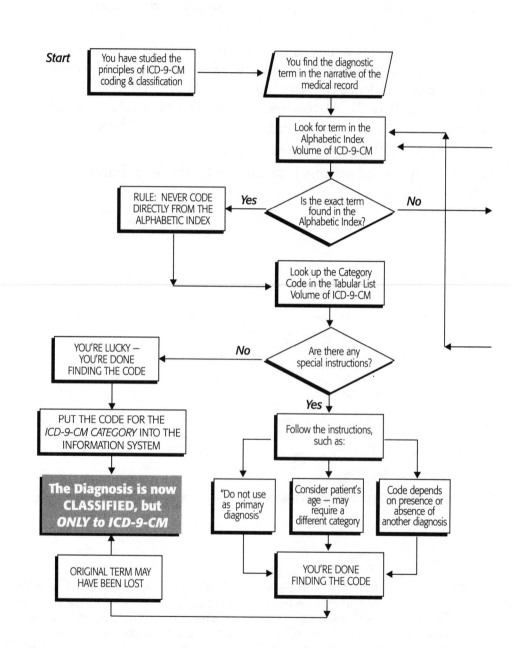

A flow chart showing the "Category Coding" process (by the authors).

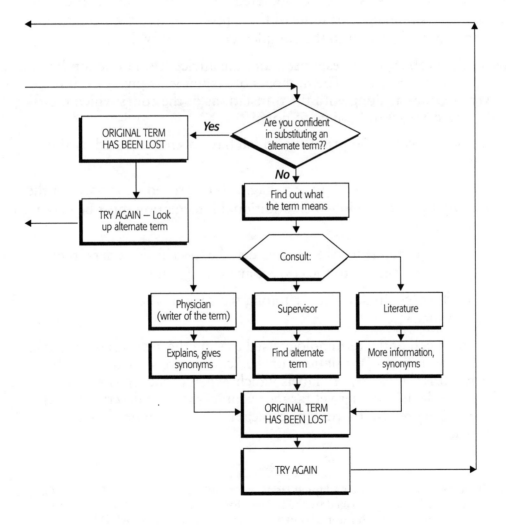

Examples from the Real World

The example above was of the simple task of finding where to put a single diagnosis. Let's consider some examples from the real world.

The Society for Clinical Coding (SCC), an affiliate of the American Health Information Management Association (AHIMA), publishes a bimonthly newsletter, *CodeWrite*. In each issue a set of challenging coding problems is offered, "CodeWrite Back." Interested members submit their answers, which are tabulated and published in a subsequent newsletter. Examination of some of these problems and their treatment by experts gives insight into the complexity of category coding.

Five of the problems, the responses, and the advice from or action by SCC are shown below.[11] The numbers of respondents giving each answer are shown, along with the translations of the codes which they used. There are several points to note:

- These are real world problems which have been submitted by the readers.

- The issue is not the coding of a diagnosis or procedure per se, but the *classifying of a case* in which additional information must be taken into account.

- Since the respondents can be considered experienced coders, their lack of unanimity as to the correct answers is impressive.

- The effort required to decide among the various choices is substantial.[12]

Note how much of the terminology used to state the case has been lost in the category coding. Translations of the "codes" are shown for each problem. It is these category labels which, when decoding is attempted, will replace the far simpler yet far more comprehensive descriptions of the cases as expressed in ordinary clinical narrative language by the physician.

---

11. These examples have been adapted from five problems published in *CodeWrite*, March-April 1997, published by the Society for Clinical Coding (SCC), an affiliate of the American Health Information Management Association (AHIMA).

12. Four large reference volumes were required — the latest version of *ICD-9-CM* for the diagnoses (Volumes 1 and 2), *ICD-9-CM* procedures in Volume 3, and *CPT-4* for the procedures in the problem where that coding was called for.

Figure 9.2 Hemoperitoneum & Traumatic Laceration

Scenario	A patient suffers a hemoperitoneum resulting from a traumatic laceration of the liver. Should 868.03, "Injury to other intra-abdominal organs, with mention of open wound into cavity, peritoneum," be coded as a secondary diagnosis?	
Responses	**Answer given**	**Number of responses**
	Yes	56
	No	85
Advice from the Society for Clinical Coding (SCC)	"Official Coding Guidelines state that 'conditions that are integral to the disease process should not be assigned as additional codes.' Hemoperitoneum is defined as blood in the peritoneal cavity which is an expected result of a liver laceration. 868.03 would not be assigned as a secondary diagnosis in this case."	

Figure 9.3 Breast Biopsy & Needles

Scenario	How would you code (CPT4) an incisional breast biopsy when needles are placed to identify the location prior to surgery?		
Responses	**Answer given**	**Number of responses**	**Meaning of code**
	19125	26 coded	Excision of breast lesion identified by pre-operative placement of radiological marker; single lesion
	19125 & 19290	57 coded	above, plus preoperative placement of needle localization wire, breast
	19101 & 19290	53 coded	Incisional biopsy of breast; needle core (separate procedure), plus preoperative placement of needle localization wire, breast.
Action by SCC	"This question will be sent to the SCC Board for submission to AMA [responsible for CPT4]. CPT Assistant gave specific guidelines on the use of Breast Biopsy Codes. Our question will address the issue of how to code an incisional biopsy (entire lesion not removed) with placement of needle localization wire, 19101 & 10290 or 19125 & 19290."		

Figure 9.4 Hematuria & Coumadin

Scenario	A patient is admitted to the hospital with hematuria. The patient is over-anticoagulated on Coumadin; the doctor states she has coagulopathy secondary to Coumadin. The patient is treated with fresh-frozen plasma and Vitamin K.		
Responses	**Answer given**	**Number of responses**	**Meaning of code**
	Code 599.7	73 coded	Hematuria
	Code 286.7	21 coded	Acquired coagulation factor deficiency
	Code 286.9	15 coded	Other and unspecified coagulation defects
	Code 286.5	13 coded	Hemorrhagic disorder due to circulating anticoagulants
	Code 995.2	4 coded	Unspecified adverse effect of drug, medicinal and biological substance.
Advice from SCC	"As with any case where there is confusion on the correct assignment of codes, the case should be referred to the attending physician. In this case, did the patient actually have coagulopathy, a disease affecting the coagulation of blood, or an adverse reaction to the Coumadin? If the physician indicates this is an adverse effect and not a poisoning, a code for the bleeding, hematuria, should be assigned as the principal diagnosis and the appropriate E code [External cause] for the Coumadin should also be assigned."		
Comment	Only 58% of the respondents coded the hematuria, although apparently all should have. The scenario only asked for the principal diagnosis, so no information is available on whether or not the E code would have been forthcoming.		

Figure 9.5 Falls & Rollerblades

Scenario	What is the appropriate E-code [External cause] for fall off a skateboard or fall while rollerblading? Note that skateboards and rollerskates are considered pedestrian conveyance devices, according to the definitions related to transport accidents (definition q.) at the beginning of the E-code tabular list.		
Responses	**Answer given**	**Number of responses**	**Meaning of code**
	E888	36 coded	Other and unspecified fall.
	E848	24 coded	Accidents involving other vehicles, not elsewhere classifiable.
	E886.9	7 coded	Fall on same level from collision, pushing, or shoving, by or with another person, other and unspecified.
	E885	7 coded	Fall on same level from slipping, tripping, or stumbling.
Action by SCC	*"This question will be sent to the SCC Board for submission to the AHA Editorial Advisory Board."*		
Comment	This scenario demonstrates the difficulty of doing specific research, such as attempting to discover the true number of injuries resulting from the use of skateboards.		

Figure 9.6 Labor & Delivery Complications

Scenario	What diagnosis and procedure code assignments would apply to this situation? She had a second stage of approximately an hour and 10 minutes and required a vacuum assist outlet forceps vaginal delivery because of deep epidural block and inability to push correctly. She required a midline episiotomy that was repaired.		
Responses	**Answer given**	**Number of responses**	**Meaning of code**
	662.21	43 coded	Obstruction caused by malposition of fetus at onset of labor, prolonged second stage.
	668.81	19 coded	Other complication of anesthesia or other sedation in labor and delivery, delivery without mention of antepartum condition.
	662.21 & 668.81	16 coded both	
	Procedure code 72.1	52 coded	Low forceps operation with episiotomy.
	Procedure code 72.71	41 coded	Vacuum extraction with episiotomy.
	Procedure codes 72.1 & 72.71	29 coded both	
Action by SCC	"This question will be sent to the SCC Board for submission to the AHA Editorial Advisory Board."		

Background

The coding "industry"

Coding has become increasingly important in recent years — especially for ensuring proper reimbursement — and healthcare providers are investing great sums in recruiting and training medical information personnel to perform the task. Furthermore, a coder today can get specialized training and can become credentialed, for example, in hospital (inpatient) or ambulatory care (outpatient) coding.

In view of the complexity of category coding, it is not surprising that a huge industry has developed to support it. The classifications *ICD-9-CM*, *CPT*, and HCPCS are published in annual editions. Various publishers offer different formats, employing color-coding and other aids to help ensure that reimbursement rules are followed (that certain codes are never shown as primary, for example). The American Medical Association offers annual updates to its coding manuals.

Computer programs are available for assisting in coding. The major public accounting firms offer software to help providers ensure that their coding obtains the maximum defensible reimbursement. Expert consultants are kept busy.

Teaching materials have been developed. Instruction books on coding in general, and for each of the classifications specifically, have been published, and revised with each revision of the classifications. Coding is taught in the curriculums of information technology schools and short courses are offered throughout the country. In addition, hospitals provide inservice training, and coders may attend continuing education sessions.

The American Health Information Management Association (AHIMA) is a major resource for coding and coders. The AHIMA Resources Catalog is perhaps the best single source of educational materials. A table listing its 1996 coding aids, with their formats and prices, is included in the appendices on page 551. Buying one copy of each of the aids would cost a little over $10,000 (admittedly, more than one volume and type of product may cover the same subject area). In addition, AHIMA offered a home study course in coding for $1,200 and independent study modules at $200 each.

Section 3: Problems & Solutions

Getting the Most from Our Health Information System

10

Preserving Truth in Medical Records

EARLIER CHAPTERS have stressed the importance of having truthful information in our medical records — and the futility of having a system based on them if we can't trust the information in them.

Medical records are created during the course of patient care. We assume that the physicians and other caregivers involved will put into each record all essential information needed to:

- Serve as "memory" of what is going on.

- Communicate to other caregivers what they will need to know.

However, there are influences, old and new, which interfere with getting the "whole truth" into medical records. These factors can bias the information, constrain it, skew the accuracy, and even interfere with the process of care.

Biasing factors include reimbursement, federal rules and regulations, and security fears. The limitations and constraints of the electronic medical record (EMR) also strongly influence our health information. The design of the EMR can drastically affect what gets into the medical record. This is discussed in detail in "Optimizing the Electronic Medical Record," page 237. The other factors are discussed further here.

The "System" Encourages Distortion of Information

The information in the medical record can be distorted (1) as it is being recorded, and (2) as it is being coded (for billing, for example). Both of these points are vulnerable to being biased by outside influences.

Some of the serious threats to medical record accuracy were well stated in a contribution placed on the World Wide Web by a physician in late 1996:

> Sometimes, I think advocates of evidence-based medicine are not being realistic about what can be accomplished in the real world. Medical records and charts, computerized or not, at least in the U.S., are bound to be deliberately inaccurate, for at least two reasons:

1.   Fear of doctors concerning what insurers or others with access to medical records will do with sensitive information about their patients which leads to omissions, if not downright lies, within the records, and

2.   The physician's desire to get services paid for by insurance that would not (or the physician thinks would not) normally be covered. For example, insurers will always cover an ultrasound to determine gestational age of a fetus, so if a pregnant woman wants an ultrasound, physicians justify the procedure to insurers by coding gestational age as the reason, even if gestational age was known.

These are salutary warnings — our [British] NHS [National Health Service] system is not yet so distorted by financial incentives and fear of litigation that medical records are systematically falsified, but the pressures of the "internal market" are fast moving it in that direction.

✓ "If medical records are being increasingly computerised and coding is becoming part of everyday clinical life, though, *wouldn't it be nice to have a system which reflects the uncertainties of clinical practice* rather than the unrealistic tidiness of the manager's business plan or the insurer's/purchaser's contract?" [Emphasis added.]

If clinicians are forced to make arbitrary choices between diagnostic codes, why shouldn't they go one step further and record false ones?

I'm sure it would encourage greater honesty and ultimately be more useful to both clinicians and managers if uncertainty was acknowledged and catered for within the system. With these kinds of things [inaccuracy] going on routinely, it would appear that there is very little hope of using medical records and charts with any validity for research, without adjusting for all this maneuvering. I don't think "proper" research was ever suggested as the main aim, but one of the advantages of formalizing the recording of uncertainty would be to encourage clinicians to develop a more questioning attitude, treating each patient as a diagnostic challenge and auditing their performance against the final answers![1]

---

1.   Professor David Barer (d.h.barer@newcastle.ac.uk), Dept of Medicine of the Elderly, Newcastle General Hospital Newcastle upon Tyne NE4 6BE UK (England), written at 10:03 27/09/96 as a message in mail list http://www.mailbase.ac.uk/lists-a-e/evidence-based-health/.

Security and Confidentiality

Doctor Barer brings up first the question of security. There has always been reluctance to record sensitive information — about mental illnesses and sexually-transmitted diseases, for example — because of fear that it would be read by someone who has no business in the record or someone whose discretion cannot be trusted. This fear has been exacerbated with the coming of the electronic medical record (EMR), even though great efforts are under way to protect its confidentiality, and it is easier to provide security in the electronic medium than in the ordinary hospital's or office's paper-based systems. Still, the fear is there, and it can inhibit truthful recording.

Negative Effects of the Payment System

The current payment system biases medical record content in an unhealthy manner. It requires providers to report, as diagnoses and procedures, all the categories into which a given patient can be classified, on the basis of those diagnoses and procedures which are taken into account in determining payment for care. Certain diagnoses, though present, and procedures, though performed, are to be left out because they (1) do not affect the payment or (2) might conflict with the payment algorithm or otherwise confuse the issue. Such payment rules do not improve the quality of information about the patient.[2]

Example

> **Coding creep**
>
> After the Prospective Payment System (PPS) was instituted by Medicare, the term "DRG creep" was coined for the phenomenon that changes started appearing in hospital statistics as a result of "upcoding." In PPS, the specific diagnosis codes reported and their sequences in the bills began to make significant differences in hospital payments. Were there actual changes in the patterns of patients' problems, or were these artifacts caused in the system by attempts to enhance revenue in response to PPS rules? Often, the changes simply represented a systematic improvement in record-keeping and coding. For more about DRGs, see "Reimbursement: DRGs & ACGs," page 163, and the appendices on page 421.

---

2.   *See* McMahon, Jr., L.F. and Smits, H.L., "Can Medicare Prospective Payment Survive the ICD-9-CM Disease Classification System?" *Ann Intern Med*, 1986; 104:562-566.

The demands of the reimbursement system have introduced at least two types of artifacts into our healthcare information:

- *Coding enhancement schemes* which influence the entry of information in order to obtain the optimum payment. This often results in distortion of the true picture presented by the patient. And it may keep clinically relevant information out — "coding aids," which list diagnoses and procedures (and their combinations) which should *never* be put on bills, are best sellers.[3]

- *Recording rules* which do not make sense. A classic example is the 1985 "rule out" rule, which stated that the diagnoses the physician wished to "rule out" were to be treated as though present.[4]

"Enforced" Truthfulness

The clinical documentation is further influenced by the "Documentation Guidelines for Evaluation and Management Services" (E&M) requirements of the Health Care Financing Administration (HCFA). These tell quite precisely what array of information must be in the medical record for each encounter to support a claim that a given level of service has been rendered.

A portion of the 1997 Guidelines is shown on page 230. This shows some of the detail and complexity of the requirements.

Penalties for failure to adhere to these requirements are severe. Software is appearing which can check the medical record against these requirements, assign the proper level, and thus protect the physician against violations. Such software will certainly influence the medical record content (and clinical care and cost), because it can be put to

---

3. For example, a January 1998 advertisement offered a computer disk which allowed users to search for over 80,000 "improper coding combinations" — improper in that for these combinations, payment would be denied under Medicare Part B.

4. *Coding Clinic for ICD-9-CM*, March-April 1985. Physicians normally make a "rule out" list, a list of the diagnoses the patient may have, with a note that says "[I must] Rule Out: [the following listed possibilities]." In fact, often the sole reason for a procedure may be to "rule out" a disease or injury. Yet, under the rule at that time, even if the test turned out negative, that disease had to be coded as the patient's diagnosis! This can greatly skew clinical data. *See* Iezzoni, *Risk Adjustment for Measuring Health Outcomes*, pp. 198-199.

another use, which might be called a "reverse" use: to tell what must be done (and documented) for the patient in order to achieve each service level. One software vendor agreed with pride that its E&M product was designed to produce "bullet-proof bills."

The regulations were promulgated to make it easier for surveillance to be maintained over the care given and to avoid fraudulent claims and abuse of the payment system by finding medical records which were billed without the proper documentation. It is more likely that the requirements will, with the computer's assistance, simply insure that "cleaner" claims are submitted, and the initial intent will be thwarted. (Fraud and abuse will be detected more readily by examining the data for aberrant patterns of care, unusual numbers of diagnoses and procedures, uncommon treatments for various conditions, and similar events.)

Figure 10.1 E&M Regulations (excerpt)

C.   DOCUMENTATION OF THE COMPLEXITY OF MEDICAL
      DECISION MAKING

The levels of E/M services recognize four types of medical decision making
(straight-forward, low complexity, moderate complexity and high
complexity). Medical decision making refers to the complexity of
establishing a diagnosis and/or selecting a management option as measured
by:

- the number of possible diagnoses and/or the number of management
  options that must be considered;

- the amount and/or complexity of medical records, diagnostic tests,
  and/or other information that must be obtained, reviewed and
  analyzed; and

- the risk of significant complications, morbidity and/or mortality, as
  well as comorbidities, associated with the patient's presenting
  problem(s), the diagnostic procedure(s) and/or the possible
  management options.

The chart below shows the progression of the elements required for each level
of medical decision making. To qualify for a given type of decision making,
two of the three elements in the table must be either met or exceeded.

Number of diagnoses or management options	Amount and/or complexity of data to be reviewed	Risk of complications and/or morbidity or mortality	Type of decision making
Minimal	Minimal or None	Minimal	*Straightforward*
Limited	Limited	Limited	*Low Complexity*
Multiple	Moderate	Moderate	*Moderate Complexity*
Extensive	Extensive	High	*High Complexity*

Each of the elements of medical decision making is described below.

Excerpted from *1997 Documentation Guidelines for Evaluation and Management
Services*, published by the U.S. Health Care Financing Administration.

Figure 10.2 E&M Regulations (excerpt *continued*)

NUMBER OF DIAGNOSES OR MANAGEMENT OPTIONS

The number of possible diagnoses and/or the number of management options that must be considered is based on the number and types of problems addressed during the encounter, the complexity of establishing a diagnosis and the management decisions that are made by the physician.

Generally, decision making with respect to a diagnosed problem is easier than that for an identified but undiagnosed problem. The number and type of diagnostic tests employed may be an indicator of the number of possible diagnoses. Problems which are improving or resolving are less complex than those which are worsening or failing to change as expected. The need to seek advice from others is another indicator of complexity of diagnostic or management problems.

> •*DG: For each encounter, an assessment, clinical impression, or diagnosis should be documented. It may be explicitly stated or implied in documented decisions regarding management plans and/or further evaluation.*
>
> > • *For a presenting problem with an established diagnosis the record should reflect whether the problem is: a) improved, well controlled, resolving or resolved; or, b) inadequately controlled, worsening, or failing to change as expected.*
> >
> > • *For a presenting problem without an established diagnosis, the assessment or clinical impression may be stated in the form of differential diagnoses or as a "possible", "probable", or "rule out" (R/O) diagnosis.*
>
> •*DG: The initiation of, or changes in, treatment should be documented. Treatment includes a wide range of management options including patient instructions, nursing instructions, therapies, and medications.*
>
> •*DG: If referrals are made, consultations requested or advice sought, the record should indicate to whom or where the referral or consultation is made or from whom the advice is requested.*

•*DG = Documentation Guideline*

Current information can be obtained at HCFA's website, http://www.hcfa.gov

Legal Climate

In the current climate of concern about laws and litigation, an interesting caution has been expressed: "Be careful that what you put into a comment (in the medical record) is not in conflict with what you checked off with a pick list[5] — an internal conflict in a record is very hazardous if the insurance claim is challenged or you are in court." This atmosphere is another factor working against getting truthful information into the medical record.

The Impact on Physician — and Patient

Instead of starting with the patient's chart, and paying for what was done, payers are requiring physicians to jump through their hoops to obtain payment. This builds up to a bureaucratic quagmire of paperwork and struggle for the physician. The effect is micromanagement of physicians — and the *process* of patient care — by those whose concern should be the *outcome* — the health of the population and its cost.

Payers, both governmental and private, should focus instead on the big picture. Patterns of health status, healthcare, and cost can be viewed at the macro level — across the nation and by region, state, providers, and so forth as appropriate. When the pattern falls outside the "norm" (which can be measured by "usual" outcomes or by "best practice benchmarks" established by providers and payers), then the providers can be examined more closely to determine quality of care and possible fraud or abuse of the payment system. Or the "aberrant" pattern may represent better practice and outcomes — it may become the new benchmark. In the meantime, the great majority of physicians and other providers can be free to give their patients their best, unhindered by unnecessary "paperwork."

---

5.   Pick lists are often used as input devices in electronic medical records. For more, see ""Click and Enter" Technologies," page 238.

It has not been proven that such "micromanagement" improves care or lowers cost (in fact, the opposite has been shown).[6] But it does:

- take enormous amounts of time away from patient care
- actually interfere with that care
- discourage physicians, some to the point of leaving the profession.

Remember, the purpose of the medical record is to assist in patient care by serving as the memory of the physician, and communication among providers. Using it for reimbursement is only secondary, and should not drive its creation. Medical students are not taught to chart for the convenience of payers. They don't sit with a prescriptive book of "guidelines" telling them what to be sure to document.

Physicians learn *how to care for patients*, and what has to be documented in the record to ensure the best care. Physicians are taught how to observe and think about problems, and to write down their "train of thought." The record should show how the patient's problems were approached.

There is no reason to document every part of every system review and every negative finding. Such documentation, even if done religiously, would:

- Clutter up the record tremendously, making it harder to find the most important information.
- Put a terrible burden on providers, and waste of lot of their time.
- Interfere with the thought process essential for good medical judgment.
- Distract from the essentials.

The only way, in reality, to create such a "perfect" record is to *generate* it by computer. At that point, it becomes artificial, and meaningless.

The physician's viewpoint was expressed eloquently in the graphic description of a chart "audit" reprinted on the following pages.

---

6.   UnitedHealth Group, the second largest health insurer in the U.S., recently changed the policy of its HMO which required approval of expensive healthcare procedures and hospital stays. United Healthcare found it had been spending $100 million a year just for the approval process — and ended up approving 99% of the care, anyway. The change will allow physicians to make the final decisions on patient care. Kaiser Permanente, a pioneer health insurer and services provider in California, has had the physician-decision policy in place for over 50 years.

The Coding Audit

"You need two out of three components to code a 99213. Understand, this has nothing to do with the quality of medical care. The reality is that HCFA [the Health Care Financing Administration] will reclaim fees paid for inaccurate coding."

A pile of my audited charts was arranged in front of the coding consultant. Next to her sat our billing specialist. It was 8:30 on a Thursday morning, in the middle of the half hour that I usually reserve to think, dictate letters, read about my difficult cases, and perform the myriad tasks that pile up by the end of the week. I understood that our group had actually requested this review. The mastery of evaluation and management codes was as much a requirement for medicine in the 1990s as board certification. I had mentally prepared myself (or so I had thought) to handle this critique of my billing practices.

What I didn't expect was the unbidden escalation of my annoyance as we began the scripted process. The coding consultant started with my raw data. Twelve of 22 charts were coded properly; just 55% correct. My scalp started to prickle. The consultant explained that the inconsistencies were errors of either upcoding or downcoding. Since I had always thought that upcoding (charging more than supported by documentation) was the egregious error, my chief concern was the two charts that apparently did not pass muster in this category.

The consultant leveled me with her look. "Any error in coding can potentially cause penalty," she said. "Those five cases that you undercoded are a red flag to HCFA. They signal that you don't know how to code, and that can prompt a full audit. And then payments can be reclaimed ... " She droned on in her imperious tone. And I started to smolder.

I was angry that billing issues could even evoke in me that kind of emotion. With all of the ups and downs of training and clinical practice, I had gained a wider perspective and a cooler temperament than I had had in medical school days. Control of feelings was an element of my job. This sense of aggravation was, frankly, silly. But it was there! The spark ignited and I felt the fire flare.

"This doesn't take into account the time I spent explaining the issues to the patient, calling the family, calling the specialist, and making special

Sumkin, Joan, M.D. "The Coding Audit." *On Being a Doctor, Annals of Internal Medicine* 1998; 128:502. Reprinted with permission. A "99213" is a 15-minute office visit ("99214" is 25 minutes). See page 186.

arrangements, or the time spent thinking, feeling, caring ... " The consultant stopped me halfway through my diatribe.

"What you do doesn't matter," she said patiently. "If you don't document it correctly, you don't get reimbursed and you could get fined."

There it was. Bureaucratic arrogance was the crux of my frustration. The dissection of the medical encounter had become so detailed that actual patient interaction was now secondary to fleshing out the chart for HCFA.

I wanted to say all this, but instead I kept silent. Emotional pyrotechnics would be wasted on them while consuming me. The coding consultant and the billing specialist were getting uncomfortable. They truly had no context for understanding.

By the time the meeting ended, I was 10 minutes late for my 9:00 patient. I found it difficult to concentrate during the consultation. The elements of coding hounded me. Did I get enough review of systems for a 99214? How about pertinent PFSH (past, family, and social history)? How complex was her problem, anyway? Was it moderately complex or highly complex? By whose standards?

Later that day, between appointments, I checked messages and mail. There was a letter addressed to me with PERSONAL stamped on the front. I opened it and found a notecard decorated with flowers and headlined "Thinking of You." It was carefully typed.

> Dear Dr. Sumkin,
>
> How are you? I hope you don't mind me writing you a note. It was very good to see you in the parking lot a week ago. I miss you sometimes. We have been through a lot together. You were always there for me. I know I can't waste your time and the state's money but sometimes I would just like to set and talk a bit. I could always tell you how I was feeling inside and out and you never put me down. You never made me feel like I was worthless or dumb. Thank you.

As the letter went on, the heat dissipated. I entered the next exam room ... a doctor.

Physicians know how to communicate using the medical record. They record their thoughts and findings, especially the "important negatives" (not *every* negative). Just as importantly, physicians *look for* this information when reviewing the file of another physician, as is necessary for consultation. It's a proven method whose goal is — as it should be — high quality patient care. Prescribing how and what physicians should record is bureaucratic meddling.

Imagine the cumulative effect — the stress — of this kind of bureaucracy on the physician and the physician-patient relationship.

The "System" Should Back Off

There appears to be no mobilization against the factors — some discussed above — which are hard at work to degrade the truthfulness of medical records. The only forces working to keep medical record content what it should be are the conscientious efforts of the individual physician to maintain in the record the information vitally important in the care of the patient, and that same physician's understanding that a full, complete, and truthful record is the prime protection in case of a charge of malpractice. That physician should not be standing alone.

The healing profession and healing institutions of our society should support people doing the right thing — not reward those who may "follow the rules" but go against conscience. Healthcare providers want to provide high quality care, and the "system" should not interfere with this.

It's time to reexamine our values and goals. While we make plans on how to pay for health care, we need also to keep in mind how this will affect the honesty and accuracy of our health information. In the short run we *may* save dollars, but in the long run, the deterioration of our personal and national health — *and* the cost of its care — could be prohibitively expensive.

11

Optimizing the Electronic Medical Record

ONE CANNOT ARGUE with the fact that the electronic medical record (EMR) is a quantum leap forward in many respects. It picks up the patient's demographic data as a by-product of administrative processes. A single recording of a physician's order can not only record the order but also set in process its fulfillment. Recording a laboratory value puts the data in the record and also arranges for its billing. A drug order can write the prescription, send the order to the pharmacy, instruct the nursing staff, and initiate monitoring of its fulfillment — and also check for drug interactions.

Images of X-rays, MRIs, holographic documents, audio recording of the patient's speech, and even motion pictures of the patient's mobility can be displayed. The physiological reactions of the patient can be graphed along with drug therapy, and relationships can be seen at a glance. The EMR can be carried in a hand-held computer to the bedside. Several people can see it at the same time. Perhaps best of all, every bit of it is legible. All these are tremendous improvements over paper-based records.

But there should be a real concern that expediency needed for short-term market advantages, which have driven current EMR development by vendors, will be incompatible with achieving the greater benefits that patient care has been promised and that evidence-based medicine offers. Being early into the market, with an apparently easier product, may help today's sales but foreclose a better system which could be introduced a bit later.

The electronic medical record, despite all its advantages and potential, stands as perhaps the greatest threat to getting truth — accurate, complete, vital information — into our medical records.

And if we never get it into the records in the first place, we're certainly never going to be able to get truthful information back out.

Getting the "Whole Truth"

The Achilles' heel in the EMR development is its unsolved problem of capturing the essential detail formerly found in the physician's and other caregiver's entries — especially the diagnoses. This "narrative" part of the record used to be handwritten, or dictated and transcribed, in plain old words. The narrative contained the patient's complaints and statements of problems from his or her point of view, the physician's interpretation of the situation, the diagnoses considered and established, consultants' and other caregivers contributions to the debate, the treatments (descriptions of surgery and other modalities) employed, the patients' response to treatment, a summary of the case, and plans for the future.

The EMR problem in coping with this issue is caused by two factors:

- lack of the technology for capturing the detail

- demand for a "user-friendly" product

The first problem is due to the fact that the system is *code-dependent*, and we haven't provided the appropriate codes (see "Capturing the Clinical Detail," page 257). The solution is to code the detail (clinical entities) first, before coding to *ICD-9-CM* or other classifications. This is called "entity coding," and is described fully beginning on page 277.

The second problem results from our assumption, probably true, that most caregivers will not be willing or able to slow down to enter their information by typing on a keyboard. Pen-based methods (handwritten data entry which results in digitized information) have so far not lived up to earlier promises. The turnaround time presently required for dictation and transcription does not permit the EMR envisioned by the caregiver, who would like to be able to look back instantly at what has been entered, just as handwritten entries in the paper record now permit.

"Click and Enter" Technologies

To deal with this need for speed, electronic system designers are looking for shortcuts for input. "Pick lists" seem to be the most popular. A pick list is displayed on the computer screen offering a selection of terms for use by the physician, nurse, other caregiver, or patient. The desired entries can simply be "checked off" by selecting and clicking on them with a mouse (thus the term "click and enter"). Often, the choices branch in "cascading" fashion — items, as chosen, bring up additional lists, offering greater and greater detail. Check lists have, of course, been used in the paper based record (PBR) system for years, both for eliciting information from patients and for recording the observations of the caregivers.[1]

With pick lists, a summary of a patient record can easily be developed starting with simple check marks. For example, if the physician checks "normal" for "eyes" in recording the physical examination, the computer could draw on its stored boilerplate and report: "Examination of the eyes reveals no abnormality. The pupils react normally to light and accommodation ... ," with the prefabricated note proceeding to complete a textbook description of eyes absolutely normal in every respect. The output of such an entry method can be so sophisticated that it is virtually undetectable (except that real humans are not usually so consistent in their phrasing[2]).

Check-off data entry works fine for some applications where the choices are limited and fixed: a hardware store inventory, for example. But in healthcare, the terminology used is rich and extensive, and it varies from place to place. It includes colloquialisms of both the patient and the caregiver, describing the presenting problems as well as the caregiver's observations and conclusions. It has abbreviations, initialisms, and acronyms, some of which are national in usage, while others are local.[3] Pick lists and word wheels have not yet been developed which can cope

---

1.   Another, less frequently used, shortcut is the "word wheel." Word wheels respond to typing in the desired entry by bringing up all entries with the same spelling. Typing "a" brings up the first "a" word in the alphabetic list. Typing "ab" narrows the search to all words or phrases beginning "ab," and so on. Typically, the characters typed in are highlighted with the rest of the word or phrase shown also. As soon as the characters typed bring up the desired entry, the user only needs to select that entry. Users of the financial program Quicken® are familiar with word wheels as lists used to keep track of payers.

2.   However, the senior author once encountered a lengthy series of absolutely identical handwritten operative reports for appendectomies which read, in part, "the cecum was palpated for 23 cm. and no abnormalities were found." Interestingly, the handwriting for this entry was the same in every record, although different surgeons had operated.

3.   For more about abbreviations and acronyms and the problems they create, see "Standardizing the Meanings of Terms," page 81.

with all of the terminology in daily use, and they may never be able to do it.[4] (For more about the language of healthcare, see page 71.)

We have come to the gap in the medical record system which was the stimulus for this book — the failure of the information system to provide a way to capture and permanently record this diagnostic and other narrative information at the detail level. This problem is treated in depth beginning on page 257.

As a result of these difficulties, the pick lists today typically are lists of "category labels" ("rubrics") of the various classifications into which the payment system wants the information to find its way — e.g., *ICD-9-CM, CPT, HCPCS*. Thus, *many are really lists of insurance terminology rather than medical terminology.* And, of course, it is almost inevitable that EMR vendors will in fact "sanitize" the list so that users are not even offered codes which may give trouble in the payment system (whether they would be useful in describing the patient or not).

In some instances, there may also be lists of phrases which will help produce a narrative report from the record, better suited for output from the medical record than they are for its input. Neither approach allows accurate, unbiased, input.

Because of the influence of insurance billing, this problem is very serious. If the diagnosis or finding or treatment which the doctor or nurse really wants to record isn't on the list, the only option is to check off the "closest thing," and misinformation is the result. This is a problem which already exists with the present, non-electronic medical record system — whenever check-off forms are offered for input.

Of course, if something on a pick list provided by the insurance company (or other payer) is selected, the record will "go through" the system without challenge, and the demands of the greatest driving force — the reimbursement system — will be satisfied. But this method subverts the original purpose of the medical record — to provide the information essential to high quality patient care — and it seriously interferes with the possibility of some day adding to a vast pool of useful knowledge. These

---

4.   Note that such a check-off is a form of transformation of information, a subject discussed earlier (see "Modular Languages," page 83). Only occasionally will the transformed information be exactly the same as the user would have recorded, had "free recording" been easy to do.

purposes can only be served if the patient's problems and the caregiver's findings are accurately described.

"Improving" Pick Lists

Most vendors do, of course, provide options to expand on the pick lists furnished initially with the systems. There are usually two such options:

Adding Items

Local users can add items to the pick lists which come from the vendor. They can supplement and customize the pick lists for departmental and individual physician preferences, local jargon and abbreviations, local diagnostic and treatment options, special studies, and more. This is useful to conform with local practices, and to give additional information for care of the specific patient. However, such local changes don't lead to a standardized record, even within a single institution or enterprise. Nor is there usually any control over the local modifications — this would require carefully maintained documentation, such as a database giving meanings of the "local" pick list entries or "tailored" pick lists, the dates when terms are introduced, when modified, when taken out of service, etc. Nor does the vendor's system "learn" from one user's experience, gained in modifying the pick list locally, for the benefit of other users.

Adding Comments

A section of the EMR typically is provided in which the physician and others can enter free-text information and notes. Each patient is indeed unique, and the physician and patient need to be able to personalize the information. Such "extra" information may be entered through a keyboard, either by the caregiver personally or by dictating the entry for transcription, or even with voice recognition technology (see below). In some systems, it may be handwritten and result in storage of an image of the handwriting.

In more sophisticated systems, the physician and others, including the patient, can put notes into the record by speaking to the computer and having an audio recording made of their voices as an integral part of the EMR. (This entry can only be retrieved by "playing it back" locally through a loudspeaker or headset; it does not, without a conscious indexing step, get into the data system as a modification of the checked entry. A written copy would require a transcription step added to the process.)

Similarly, multimedia systems permit making video recordings in the course of the care, also right within the EMR. A motion picture of range of motion of a shoulder can, with today's technology, become a part of the "local" EMR at each visit, and be played back for the orthopedist and physical therapist to determine progress. But it must be emphasized that these niceties are added on to the basic record; they are not in such a form that they are computer accessible except in the individual EMR.

These methods for supplementing the pick lists for data entry are attractive from the standpoint of the "local" user, but even with them the system is not foolproof. With manually kept records, it was far easier to express the diagnoses and problems exactly as the physician wished. The patient's own words could be used. One could describe exactly what was found in surgery, and how the surgical procedure went, since these could simply be dictated. The physician himself or herself, the colleagues on review committees, the consultant, and other caregivers always had the full record, undistorted by the "efficiencies" of the computer, to fall back on. A record in which the information is truncated, distorted, or transformed under the influence of the computer loses these important attributes. So there are potentially serious problems even when one has the full electronic record available at the computer terminal.

Voice Recognition Technology

One emerging method for data entry is voice recognition technology (VRT). With VRT, the computer understands the human's speech and turns the words into digital representations, just as though the words had been typed at the keyboard. For a number of years VRT technology required the speaker to space her words, letting the computer understand each one separately. This has worked to give single-word commands to the computer, but its slowness has made it intolerable as a replacement for normal dictation.

Now, however, VRT products are coming on the consumer market, at street prices unthinkable just a few years ago, which offer continuous-speech recording on personal computers. The reported accuracy, i.e., the ability to put exactly what was said into digital form on the screen and in the computer file, is in the range of 95-98% . This is a tremendous step forward, but it still means that for about one word in twenty to one word in fifty will be wrong, with potentially dire consequences. So to ensure accuracy, either the dictator or an expert in medical terminology will have to review the document and make any necessary corrections.

To attain even 95% accuracy, however, the recording conditions must be favorable. First, the computer (software) must be trained to recognize the voice and speech pattern of the individual doing the dictating. This may not take more than an hour or two (vendors now say fifteen minutes), but it does mean that not just anyone can immediately dictate into the medical record. Favorable conditions also require a virtual absence of ambient noises, lack of interruptions, and the individual's normal voice. These conditions can be obtained in a dictating room, and it is not surprising that the early successes have been with radiology and pathology transcription, where the dictators are few and the settings for the dictation are controlled. But these controlled conditions are not present in the typical examining room or nurses' station. Also, the patient's medical record contains contributions from many different caregivers (and the patient herself), and the software needs "personal training" for each individual. VRT may some day become the usual mode of data entry, and replace the human transcriptionist, but that appears to be some time in the future.

Patient Involvement

Medical records are no longer strictly under the control of healthcare providers. More and more, patients themselves are putting information into the record. In an environment that supports informed shared decision making (ISDM), patients join with their physicians in the construction of their medical records, review them together, and often are given copies for reference.[5]

In such a setting the accuracy and completeness of the medical record is of prime importance – any distortions introduced by biasing influences and the inadequacy of the coded information are apparent to both the physician and the patient. ISDM simply can't work without adequate medical records.

---

5.   See "Informed Shared Decision Making," page 50.

Designing the EMR to Improve Patient Care

Both the design adopted for the EMR and the path taken to achieve that design are critical to its ultimate success. There are two "sine qua nons":

- The EMR must help in patient care.
- The EMR must not interfere with patient care.

The first consideration is to make sure that the EMR can fulfill the primary purpose of the medical record — providing help in the care of the patient. That is to say, the EMR must not be compromised by being an add-on to administrative procedures (as are some of the EMR systems being developed). This point is well stated in a report by a team of researchers in The Netherlands and the United States who developed a working electronic medical record system in a hospital intensive care unit. The practitioners — physicians, nurses, others using the system — were essential to the design. The report states:

> Much of the impetus for the development of [EMRs] has come from "second level" users (hospital management, governments, insurance agencies, researchers), who hope to be able to "tap" information directly from the ongoing primary care process. However, care providers will never use the system unless it is useful to them.

> First and foremost, an [EMR] should be conceptualized as a health professional's tool; secondary usages should also be secondary in design ...

✓ " ... We should ask questions like, 'When a doctor starts her working day, what information should be at her disposal?'; 'In the ongoing work of nurses, what are the tasks that computers can support?'"

> The system should be just as much healthcare worker-centered as it is patient-centered ... These functionalities are not "carrots" to get users to use the system; they should be seen as deriving from the fundamental prerequisite that systems should support work, not generate it.[6]

---

6.   Berg, Marc, MD, PhD, Chris Langenberg, MD, Ignas van de Berg, RN, Jan Kwakkernaat, RN. "Experiences with an Electronic Patient Record in a Clinical Context: Considerations for Design." Paper submitted to MIE '97, Fourteenth International Congress of the European Federation for Medical Informatics, May 25-29, 1997, Porto Carras, Sithonia, Greece.

In addition to supporting patient care, the EMR must also not impede care. The format must not interfere with its adoption by caregivers.

Work Habits Users should not be forced to change their work habits. Technology which does not require changes in work habits is more readily adopted than technology which does, even though the latter technology may offer distinct advances overall.[7]

Work Load The EMR should not require more work on the part of the physician (and other care providers) to get information in or out (the EMR simply won't be adopted if it takes more effort unless, of course, some irresistible reward or punishment can be invented).

Perhaps the most serious problem for the future of the EMR as the nucleus for a truly "paperless" system for the physician, and for its use as a source for epidemiological and other studies, is going to be any element of the system which slows down or impedes the process of care. The majority of users, regardless of the EMR's many advantages, don't want to spend any more time or effort using the system (read "putting the information in or getting the information out") than they did with its paper-based predecessor.

This resistance is reinforced by the managed care movement, which puts on constant pressure for patients to be seen more efficiently (read "rapidly"). Time required for learning the system adds to the "ease of use" barrier. Thus the electronic record must be extremely "user-friendly." The trick is to make the EMR quick and easy, and at the same time allow the level of clinical detail required for high quality patient care.

Increasing Security

The medical record currently exists in two formats:

- The full, permanent, patient record, including confidential, private information.

- The computer abstract, designed for billing and for regional data banks.

---

7. Weaver, Robert R. *Computers and Medical Knowledge*, Westview, Boulder, CO, 1991.

The Electronic "Surrogate" Record

We propose a new, intermediate form of the medical record, which could meet many of today's unmet needs, yet maintain — even increase — patient confidentiality. This is the *Electronic Surrogate Medical Record (ESMR)*.

The ESMR is an electronic mini-record which can be thought of as an adjunct to the original medical record or as a "semi-public" set of information within the medical record. It excludes the private, confidential information. The ESMR is created automatically as the EMR is created, by a filtering process which identifies the components of the ESMR in a standard, coded, sanitized data set containing the information required to provide:

- Security for confidential information in the EMR, by excluding it from the ESMR. A "firewall" is built between the total electronic medical record and the "surrogate."

- An electronic data source for users other than those directly caring for the patient. "External" users would have access only to the ESMR; and could not reach the private information in the EMR. In fact, there would be different levels of access for various users.

The original medical record, whether maintained as a paper-based patient record (PPR) or as an EMR or CPR (or a hybrid), should retain the complete, unadulterated detail of the traditional paper-based record, including both the original natural language and the corresponding electronic codes (see "Entity Coding," page 277). It should also contain any codes required for billing or other purposes.[8]

Although the required information content of the EMR has not been established (it awaits, among other things, agreement on a number of standards; see below), its delay in no way minimizes the importance of working toward the ESMR. The ESMR would make possible, for the first time, extensive and timely scientific investigations using actual

---

8.   It is critical that these codings be kept available for each case for future reference. These codes would be for the categories of *ICD-9-CM* or its successor, *CPT*, HCPCS (Health Care Financing Administration Common Procedure Coding System), and others which may be used in the future when additional classifications become feasible.

clinical experience. Previous attempts to use the information which is currently in electronic form have been thwarted by:

- its lack of detail and specificity (see "Capturing the Clinical Detail," page 257), and

- ambiguity of the codes (see "Living Successfully with Code-Dependency," page 291).

Obtaining the necessary detail has been impractical in the past because the information has been locked up in the original records and kept at local sites, from which its extraction has been prohibitively expensive. This cost barrier would finally be broken by the ESMR.

Standards for Health Information

The electronic medical record — and other potential uses of technology in healthcare — cannot move forward without standards. Standards are required to ensure compatibility within, between, and among various systems, both hardware and software.

In this context, a standard describes very specific criteria for something — e.g., that a specific peg will be shaped to fit in a specific hole. A "standard" electrical plug will fit into a "standard" outlet. A "nonstandard" plug will be left dangling from your hand.

Standards abound in a technological society such as ours. If the credit card in your pocket meets the relevant standard, for instance, it will physically fit into the slot of any cash machine anywhere in the world. Whether or not the machine will dispense cash at your request depends on myriad other factors, including more standards (and whether you have any money left in your account). Without a common consensus about the size of credit cards, though, we'd have to forego the convenience of being able to go nearly anywhere in the world today without significant amounts of cash or their substitutes in our pockets.

The Challenge of Health Information Standards

While the healthcare industry as a whole, much like other industries, depends on standards in most of its operations, it is in the area of information management and access ("informatics") that standards development seems to be lagging. Not that there aren't significant resources being applied to the effort — it's just that the challenges are so great. This is largely due to the fact that "knowledge" — the primary goal for informatics — is ultimately a distillation of information from a vast variety of sources, and is packaged in a vast variety of formats — including no format at all.

Computers in healthcare can't be fully utilized until they can all talk to each other. All sorts of "messages" must travel among a variety of machines. The computer that keeps track of the patient's billing and insurance information, for example, needs to be able to receive and send messages as well. For this to work, every item of information needs to be in a standard form.

With any form of communication, whether between humans or between machines, a message only "works" if the recipient knows what the sender meant. Humans have gotten fairly sophisticated over time in understanding messages, to the point that sometimes a simple look between two individuals speaks volumes. Machines, on the other hand, especially computers, need to have things "spelled out" for them. Standards govern how things are spelled out.

Currently, standards for messages (data in structured "containers") are the most highly developed. There are at least six groups working in this area: ASTM, HL7, X12N, NCPDP, ACR-NEMA, and IEEE. Their efforts are being coordinated by ANSI/HISPP.[9] However, standards related to the less-structured data elements found in healthcare (such as the "free-text" information found in diagnoses), remain elusive.

What makes the situation frustrating is that healthcare, which has clearly benefitted from so many recent advancements in its tools and technology, has largely failed to realize the potential of building collective knowledge. The reasons for this, and what can be done about it, are in fact part of what this book is all about. While healthcare providers continue to get better hammers and screwdrivers, they're getting a lot less help in deciding when to use which.

---

9.   See "Current Standards," page 252.

Who Sets the Standards?

Standards come about in two ways: officially and unofficially.

Official Standards

An official standard has a label, typically a description or number, issued by an accredited "standards development organization" (SDO).

Background   **Standards Development Organization (SDO)**

A standards development organization (SDO) is a formally accredited organization whose members work to create and refine standards in an area where the lack of any standards hampers progress towards a universally desired goal. An SDO, most often a nonprofit organization, typically includes members from the relevant industries (stakeholders), interested individuals from academic institutions, and representatives from various governmental units.

A distinction should be made between SDOs and other organizations which take initiatives and promote the development of standards, such as the Healthcare Informatics Standards Planning Panel (HISPP) and the Computer-based Patient Record Institute (CPRI) (discussed below), but which are not officially SDOs.

Primary among SDOs in the United States is the American National Standards Institute (ANSI).[10] It is a nonprofit, privately funded organization whose mission is the development of U.S. national standards on a voluntary basis. ANSI also represents the U.S. to non-treaty international standards organizations, such as the International Organization for Standardization (ISO), of which it was a founding member.

---

10. Founded in 1918, ANSI has a diverse membership consisting of private companies, professional, labor, and consumer organizations, and government agencies. ANSI also audits and provides accreditation for other standards development organizations (SDOs). ANSI has several components specifically concerned with healthcare, including ANSI IISP (Information Infrastructure Standards Panel), ANSI HISB (Healthcare Informatics Standards Board), and ANSI HISSP (Healthcare Informatics Standards Planning Panel). ANSI's web site is at http://www.ansi.org.

Background

ISO (International Organization for Standardization)

ISO is a worldwide, private federation of national standards groups from over 100 countries, one from each country. Established in 1947, its mission is to promote the development of standardization and related activities in the world with a view to facilitating the international exchange of goods and services, and to developing cooperation in the spheres of intellectual, scientific, technological, and economic activity. Each member in ISO is the national body most representative of standardization in its country.

ISO's work results in international agreements which are published as International Standards (the first was published in 1951). For example, the format of the common credit card is derived from an ISO International Standard. Adherence to the standard, which defines such features as an optimal thickness (0.76 mm), permits the card to be used worldwide.

Officially named the International Organization for Standardization, ISO is frequently (but incorrectly) referred to as the International Standards Organization. The mismatching sequence of letters is explained by the fact that ISO is not here an acronym, but rather a word derived from the Greek "isos," meaning "equal." Used as a prefix, iso- occurs in such words as isometric, meaning of equal measure or dimensions. This meaning led to the choice of ISO as the name of the organization. Also, the name ISO is valid in each of the organization's three official languages (English, French, and Russian), and thereby avoids the confusion that would arise through the use of an acronym.

ISO is headquartered in Geneva, Switzerland. It maintains a very informative and comprehensive web site at http://www.iso.ch.

ANSI develops standards in a variety of fields, including healthcare, occupational safety, medical devices, and medical informatics. These are referred to as "American National Standards". Since the members who agree on these standards are typically the major players in the area involved, approval by ANSI gives any standard the virtual effect of law. However, compliance with even an official standard is very often just voluntary.

Unofficial Standards

An unofficial standard is any standard not issued by an SDO. There are often several different formats or technologies competing to become the standard, often using the marketplace as their arena.

Probably the most common way we come face to face with unofficial standards is when a particular vendor manages to outsell enough of the competition so that this vendor's method or technology is dominant in the marketplace. Had vendor Sony been able to outsell its competition with Beta format VCRs, Beta would be today's unofficial standard in VCR technology instead of the prevailing VHS format. The marketplace ultimately determines the success or failure of any standard, but with unofficial standards it has a much more direct effect on the setting of a standard. Everyone agreed that Beta was a superior technology, but it lost out, anyway.

At some point — not always clear — there is enough agreement and consensus about a method or technology for it to be referred to (and treated as) the standard. Forward motion in technology (and many other areas) often is impeded — or comes to a stand still — for lack of the essential standards.

Oftentimes the market does not even come into being for a given technology or product until consensus is reached on a standard, official or not. The popularity of today's video rental stores is largely based on the fact that rental is so cheap and practical that most people would rather rent a movie than bothering to tape it or buy it. Part of the cheapness is based on the fact that rental stores only have to carry in their inventory a single video tape format, VHS. If they also had to carry Beta, it would double their inventory and space requirements, obviously increasing the price per rental. This is just one example where an unofficial standard has created opportunities for vendors and consumers alike.

In most cases, the consumer or user (who is the "voter" in the standards popularity contest) is not served by having multiple standards. When the consumer is served by multiple options, several standards may easily (or uneasily) coexist. An example of this from the world of small computers is the long-term coexistence of the PC (IBM compatible) and Apple computers.

The parties involved in the creation of unofficial standards are typically those with an interest in the outcome of the process. These parties are referred to as "stakeholders," and include such diverse groups as professional societies, trade associations, vendors (or an "alliance" of vendors) of manufactured items or services, interested individuals, scholars, and government agencies (in their non-legislative or non-rulemaking role).[11] Frequently these groups include some of the world's most motivated and knowledgeable experts in the relevant field — often volunteering their time for a cause they deeply believe in.

Current Standards

There are many today working toward official and unofficial health information standards, for the U.S. and for international use. Complicating the process is the relatively high rate of change in information technology: if it takes two years to develop a standard, but technology goes through a massive cycle of change in eighteen months, standards are obsolete before they become finalized.

Following are some of the major "players."

ANSI The American National Standards Institute (ANSI), described above (), is the primary standards development organization for healthcare in the United States.

HL7 One of the best known efforts is "Health Level Seven" (HL7), a nonprofit SDO developing standards for the electronic interchange of clinical, financial, and administrative information among differing computer systems and applications in the healthcare industry.[12]

---

11. The reaching of consensus on unofficial standards can be volatile and unpredictable, since sometimes the parties involved (at least when their incentive is economical) don't even pretend to be working towards a common standard. There is a great economic incentive to "own" the rights to an unofficial standard, since it assures a competitive advantage in the marketplace. However, until it becomes an unofficial standard, it is like a hand of cards that has been dealt — it must be played, without any assurance of winning, and a great risk of losing.

12. "Level Seven" is a reference to the "application level," the highest of the seven levels of the Open Systems Interconnection reference model ("OSI") of the International Organization for Standardization (ISO).

Founded in 1987 and based in Ann Arbor, Michigan, HL7 has gained wide acceptance both in the U.S. and abroad. Members include users, hospitals, vendors, consultants, and others. ANSI accredited HL7 as an SDO in 1994. In 1995, ANSI approved the fourth version of the HL7 standard (version 2.2), thereby making it the first American National Standard for the exchange of clinical data. Version 2.3 became an American National Standard in May of 1997. While there are other healthcare standards development efforts underway that deal with particular departments, HL7 was formed to focus on the interface requirements of the entire healthcare organization.

Often, "HL7" is used to refer to the standard itself. HL7 is a messaging standard in which certain "trigger" events in the healthcare arena cause the transmission of a specific message relating to the trigger event. HL7 defines the format of the messages according to the standard, allowing healthcare data to be interchanged among a variety of information systems in which the data themselves may be in a proprietary format internally.

Background	**Trigger events**
	A "trigger event " is one which forces another event to happen, usually automatically. For example, if the gas company doesn't receive your payment by the due date, this event (i.e., "payment = 0") triggers a reminder letter to be produced and mailed to you.
	This mechanism can be immensely helpful when used in health information systems. In the electronic medical record, a physician's order could serve as a "trigger event" for the computer.
	For example, the record might automatically remind (alert) the physician to switch a patient from a non-oral (NPO) to oral (PO) medication when the physician changes that patient's diet from "nothing by mouth" to "regular diet." System software could do this by continuously monitoring the patient's electronic medical record (EMR) using the following rule:
	• If diet order = "nothing by mouth", then "order the (specified) medication to be given intravenously (IV)."

> When the diet order changes, a different rule is applied:
>
> • If diet order = "regular diet", then give the (specified) medication by mouth.
>
> The computer system would automatically print out a new medication alert suggesting the use of the more cost-effective oral route of administration.

ASTM The world's largest source of voluntary consensus standards is the American Society for Testing and Materials (ASTM), founded in 1898 as a scientific and technical organization for the development of standards on characteristics and performance of materials, products, systems, and services, and the promotion of related knowledge. ASTM originally concerned itself with industrial materials, but its scope has broadened to include, for example, medical devices and services, standardized investigation of sexual assault, ambulance driving standards, civilian search and rescue operations, and the computer-based patient record (CPR).

There are a number of ASTM standards dealing with health information. One is ASTM Standard E 1384 - 96: "Content and Structure of the Computer-Based Patient Record." Another area being developed is "Medical Knowledge Representation." This subject is typically referred to as "Arden Syntax" or "ASTM E31.15" by those working on it.[13] In 1998, ASTM agreed that HL7 would publish future editions of this standard.

MEDIX MEDIX is another standards project in health information. This is an effort by the Institute of Electrical and Electronic Engineers (IEEE) Engineering in Medicine and Biology Society to develop standards for the exchange of data between hospital computer systems. It is formally known as IEEE P1157 Medical Data Interchange.[14]

---

13. The label E31.15 refers to a specific subcommittee of ASTM. E31 is the committee on Healthcare Informatics, while E31.15 is the subcommittee dealing with Medical Knowledge Representation.

14. The MEDIX effort is based on the standards for all seven levels of the OSI reference model, and is being promoted as a joint working group under the ANSI Healthcare Information Standards Planning Panel (HISPP)'s Message Standards Developers Subcommittee (MSDS).

DICOM DICOM is an acronym for "Digital Imaging and Communications in Medicine". It is a standard for the transmission of medical images and other medical information. In development since 1985 by the American College of Radiology (ACR) in conjunction with the National Electrical Manufacturers Association (NEMA), this standard is designed so that all of the programs and hardware which conform to it will communicate accurately with each other. This standard is of particular importance in radiology due the variety of digital imaging technologies used there, including CT scanners, MRI, ultrasound, and nuclear medicine. The standard includes the definition of a "header" which is sent with the actual images and provides the necessary context for the image, such as how the image was made. DICOM is an open (non-proprietary) standard.[15]

Standards for the EMR

For the electronic medical record (EMR) to be truly useful, it must solve more problems than it creates. It is a barrier to usefulness if a human is required to be an "interpreter" between the machine that takes the patient's blood pressure and the machine that holds the medical record. If a human has to write down the blood pressure reading, then take that paper message to another human who enters the information into the patient's electronic medical record, there is actually more work involved than when the paper message was simply filed in the paper medical record.

An EMR limited in this way falls far short of its potential. For example, if the blood pressure machine could transmit the reading in a message understood by the EMR, the blood pressure could be sent directly to the electronic medical record and have it be instantly and accurately recorded. The writing down and keyboarding steps would be eliminated (saving time), along with the corresponding room for error. To get to this level of sophistication and usefulness, we first need standards.

While standards such as HL7 and DICOM dictate how information is communicated electronically between machines, other standards such as *ICD-9-CM* and *CPT*, discussed elsewhere in this book, dictate how

---

15. More information can be found at http://www.rsna.org (click on "DICOM" under "Practice Resources").

information is communicated among healthcare consumers, providers, payors, and other interested parties. Some of these standards will be virtually invisible, while others will be household words in the world of healthcare. The electronic medical record must accommodate all these standards and facilitate their use. It's a big job, but it will eventually be mastered.[16]

16. The National Committee on Vital and Health Statistics (NCVHS) was mandated, under Section 263 of the Health Insurance Portability and Accountability Act of 1996 (HIPAA), to recommend to congress health information standards, including clinical terminologies, for electronic medical records by August, 2000. The NCVHS Computer-based Patient Record Workgroup is pursuing this charge. For current information, go to http://www.ncvhs.hhs.gov.

12

Capturing the Clinical Detail

WE HAVE BEEN STRUGGLING for years — mostly unsuccessfully — to get our successive healthcare *classifications* to serve all of our patient care information needs.[1] *Our primary problem is not with classification or classifications.* It is that we do not insist on *also* keeping our information accessible at the most elementary, entity level in which it is originally available.

Once aggregated, data can never be disaggregated. When we only code directly to a classification — as we do now with category coding — we aggregate our health information at the outset, and lose forever the clinical detail.

We Aren't Getting Enough Information

Category codes — the only kind of information currently available in our electronic system — don't tell us, in most cases, what disease(s) the patient *actually had*. There are lots of other things, of course, that the system doesn't tell us, but the problem is most acute with the matter of *diagnoses*.

Finding exact diagnoses usually requires going back to the hospital or office to look at the original medical record. To carry out this task from a research center is extremely difficult and costly — and thus rarely, if ever, done. The problem this presents to the "outside" investigator is illustrated by the following incident.

---

1. See also "Expanding Classification Possibilities," page 317, for more about a single classification trying to meet multiple needs.

Example

Tracking down a drug reaction

In the 1960s, a drug company was challenged that one of its products, enteric-coated potassium chloride, was causing a particular intestinal ulceration. Unfortunately, this diagnosis fell into a wastebasket category in the coding system. A "wastebasket" category is one that means "other" — all diagnoses which don't fit anywhere else can find a home in a wastebasket category (a classification must have a place to put everything in its universe).

To determine the accuracy of the challenge, the drug company went to enormous lengths:

• The company first approached the Commission on Professional and Hospital Activities (CPHA) for information. CPHA's Professional Activity Study (PAS) was at that time the only source for the required amounts of medical record data.[a]

• To come up with the hospitals where there were (possibly) relevant cases, CPHA needed to make special tabulations of several million hospitalizations.

• The drug company had to obtain *from each hospital* authorization for:

    • CPHA to perform the special tabulations.

    • CPHA to release to the drug company the identity of the hospitals which had any cases falling into that particular wastebasket category.

• The drug company had to send a representative to visit the hospital and, after getting additional permission on site, have the medical record librarian examine all the records in the category to see if the particular ulceration was involved.

• The drug company *then* had to, in each case, get the *attending physician's permission* to find out whether or not the particular drug had been used.[b]

This was a truly formidable and costly bit of investigation.

a. See "Hospital Discharge Abstract Systems," page 103, for more about CPHA and PAS.

b. Today, it would be the patient's permission which was required, rather than the physician's.

Research using only category-coded data has often been crippled by our inability to know just what diagnoses went into a given "pigeonhole." For example, at the time that one cause of Guillain-Barré Syndrome (GBS) appeared to be the swine flu vaccinations, the diagnosis, GBS, had been buried in a category of miscellaneous neurological problems entitled "354: Polyneuritis and polyradiculitis." Had it been specifically coded (received its own, unique code) in the computerized data banks which even then covered a substantial proportion of the nation's hospitalizations, investigation of the association of the vaccination and GBS would have been enormously facilitated.[2]

Still today, cases generally are not retrievable on the basis of specific diagnoses (AIDS has posed an especially difficult problem; see "Coding AIDS," page 263, and "The Definition of AIDS," page 271). In *ICD-9-CM*, over 100 categories contain over 100 diagnoses each. This means that over 10,000 diagnoses are forced into about 100 pigeonholes.[3] Less than 8% of the terms in the Alphabetic Index to *ICD-9-CM* are in reasonably approximate one-to-one correspondence with categories in the classification.

Lack of sufficient detail can actually endanger patient care, as well. Recall the earlier warnings that a number of the electronic medical records (EMR) under development are recording the diagnoses and procedures only as category codes. In such systems, the patient and physician are deprived of the information necessary for understanding the case, recalling the details, and communicating with other caregivers. *The fundamental detail has been forever lost* — sometimes neither the attending physician nor the researcher can find out essential information even by going back to the original medical record.

Our use of a coding system with inadequate specificity is surprising, an aberration from the detail we demand elsewhere in medical records. For example, when we record drug administration, we capture:

- specific drug (rather than a group, such as "antibiotics")

- dosage

---

2. For more about this, see page 16 and page 20.

3. See "ICD-9-CM Classification of the Circulatory System," page 515, for a dramatic demonstration of this complexity.

- route of administration

- schedule of administration

- duration of treatment

Patient age is recorded in years, not decades. We also record the exact date of birth. For newborns, we capture the minute of birth. We can thereafter measure age, as needed, by minutes, hours, days, weeks, months, and only considerably later, by years.

But when we code *diagnoses* to go into our health information system, we record only the *group* the diagnosis belongs to, not the diagnosis itself — let alone details related to the diagnosis which might be important.

With category coding, the movement of information is one-way. Once a diagnosis receives its category code, the original diagnosis is almost always lost forever. Since the primary purpose of the medical record is to aid in patient care, this loss can be disastrous.[4] It is also a great hindrance to expanding our medical knowledge.

Introducing "Entity Codes"

So, we need more codes — codes to identify the unique diagnoses. Since retrieval of clinical information (and an increasing amount of the data input) is now almost exclusively via codes, it should be clear that, *if clinical entities are ever to be retrieved, the clinical entities must be coded,* as well as their appropriate categories.

✓ We need to code *what it is*, as well as *where it goes*.

The term given to "what it is" coding is "entity coding" — what it *is* is the *entity* (where it *goes* is the *category*). Entities are the "things" that are put into the categories of classifications. Entity codes represent *individual* entities (terms) rather than *groups* (categories) of entities. Entities, once coded, can be put into any groups — and grouped in other ways later, if needed.

---

4.   See "To Err is Human," page 342.

The next chapter discusses entity coding in detail. Here we'll discuss how clinical detail is necessary for accurate classification and for our understanding, prevention, and treatment of disease.

The Path to Coding

Let's back up and look at how diseases get assigned to category codes in the first place — understanding that, with our present system, a disease must have such an assignment before it can be coded — and input — into our health information system.

To simplify, the sequence of events is this:

1. *Recognition.* A new illness, condition, or clue is recognized.

2. *Research.* Medical scientists study it and give it a name.

3. *Definition.* Criteria are established for the diagnosis.

4. *Classification.* Nosologists decide where the diagnosis fits in the relevant classification.

5. *Coding.* The diagnosis can now be given the code of the category where it fits, and thereby enter the health information system.

This sequence shows up several things:

- A diagnosis cannot be coded — now — until all of these steps have been completed.

- It cannot even be put in a "wastebasket" category until pretty far along the sequence.

- Our study and research of the disease is hindered by the difficulty of obtaining information on a disease not yet officially recognized and coded (a "Catch-22").

- We can't easily detect its incidence or location in the population.

- Even after it's coded, we can't go back and study its development and course.

- Our "early warning system" for threatening epidemics is severely crippled. It often depends on anecdotal revelation of disease symptoms, then pursuit by epidemiologists who are handicapped by lack of information.

Example

The Fen-Phen Story

Pam Ruff, an echocardiogram sonographer with a BS in biology, worked at MeritCare Medical Center in Fargo, North Dakota. On a day in 1994, she saw two women with heart valve deformities different from any she'd ever seen. This struck her as unusual, and she asked the women some questions. One thing they had in common was that both were taking a fairly new, popular drug combination for weight loss. Fenfluramine and phentermine, commonly called "fen-phen," had been prescribed in the U.S. since 1990. Both drugs had been approved by the FDA, but separately — using them in combination had not been an issue.

The sonographer kept seeing patients with similar deformities, and all were using fen-phen. She approached the cardiologists, but they were skeptical. Up until that point, these deformities had been observed only in patients with tumors in their intestinal tracts or cases of ergot (wheat/rye fungus) poisoning. After two years of record keeping, however, the number of such patients was up to two dozen. At this point, the doctors at MeritCare were 95% convinced of a connection, and took the matter to the Mayo Clinic, which studied the 24 patients. Meanwhile, in 1996 alone, 18 million prescriptions were filled for fen-phen.

In July 1997, the Mayo Clinic publicly reported its clinical observation of unusual valvular heart disease in the 24 patients who had been taking fen-phen. Mayo concluded, "These cases arouse concern that fenfluramine-phentermine therapy may be associated with valvular heart disease. Candidates for fenfluramine-phentermine therapy should be informed about serious potential adverse effects, including pulmonary hypertension and valvular heart disease."[a]

a. Connolly, H. M., J. L. Crary, M. D. McGoon, D. D. Hensrud, B. S. Edwards, W. D. Edwards, and Schaff. H. V. "Valvular Heart Disease Associated With Fenfluramine-Phentermine." *New England Journal of Medicine (NEJM)* 337, no. 9 (1997): 581-88.

Our present information system could not have picked up the "Fen-Phen" pattern, because we don't gather enough clinical detail.

Codes are not readily or quickly available for new terms (e.g., syndromes, diseases) in our category coding system because a classifying decision is required in order to determine where the terms belong, either in an existing or a new category. There is no speedily responsive system in place for making such determinations; they invariably must await the convening of (and consensus of) bodies of experts.

As a result, the only recourse is to code new terms into "wastebasket" categories — hoping to get into at least the right "chapter" of the classification; AIDS first got put into the "immune" diseases and later switched to the "infections" section (see below) — until an authoritative decision is made as to their proper allocation. And when authoritative decisions *are* finally made and published, there is no procedure for learning about prior "coding" decisions, nor for going back to the wastebasket categories where the cases were to reside (presumably temporarily, in a "holding area"), retrieving the cases, and finally changing the records to the correct classification.

The coding difficulties we've had with AIDS illustrate the problems in studying this disease over a period of time under the constraints of being confined to the *category codes* for information retrieval.

Example

Coding AIDS

AIDS was first described in the literature in 1981. The term began showing up in medical records, and the records had to be coded. Within the next five years, and within a single edition of the classification (*ICD-9-CM*), the disease was approached in the following ways:

- Phase 1, pre-1982: Put It Anywhere.

There was no rapidly responding agency to which coders could turn in order to find where to classify AIDS so, in order to keep the paper work flowing and reimbursement coming in, they simply made their own decisions — and we don't know *where* they put it.

- Phase 2, 1982: Put It in Three Places.

In October 1982, an official coding decision was published in the *Journal of the American Medical Record Association* (of course, we don't know how many coders read this issue). The Journal gave, as preferred, code 279.19, "Other deficiencies of cell-mediated immunity," and thus AIDS was put into a "waste-basket category" (not a classification specific to AIDS). *Alternative* codes were also given: 279.10, "Immunodeficiency with predominant T-cell defect, unspecified," and 279.3, "Unspecified immunity deficiency."

- Phase 3, 1986: Put It in Three *Different* Places.

"Unique" coding for AIDS did not begin until late in 1986, when an addendum to *ICD-9-CM* was issued assigning the unused codes 042, 043, and 044 to AIDS — a jump to an entirely different Chapter in the classification. This addendum contained nearly *five pages* of instructions as to how to classify AIDS cases, AIDS-like syndromes, and HTLV-III/LAV infections, taking into consideration various symptoms and "with" and "due to" relationships with other conditions. Note that this also changed AIDS from an *immune* disease to an *infectious* disease. (The definition of AIDS is discussed more fully on .)

Some further changes occurred two years later when the *nomenclature* of (diagnostic criteria for) HIV infection was revised.

The delay in uniquely identifying AIDS in the data system was due not only to debate over just how to classify it (the issue was always, "which pigeonhole?"), but also to administrative and bureaucratic factors.

Problems in retrieval of data still remain, primarily because of the rules as to labeling of the "principal diagnosis" in HIV cases (a "political/ resource consumption quagmire," in the words of one nosologist).[5]

Diagnoses Are Concepts, Not Things

Diagnoses are scientific propositions or conclusions. They are concepts, not concrete things, because we don't know everything about health and disease yet. We use them as "working hypotheses." As concepts, diagnoses are not static — they change with new information, greater experience, and new thinking.

For example, the diagnoses in the field of mental health change and are refined over time, as new knowledge is gained. The *Diagnostic and Statistical Manual of Mental Disorders (DSM)*, published by the American Psychiatric Association, is an ever-evolving discussion and diagnostic description of the concepts in the field of mental disorders.

Ideally, specific, unique codes should be assigned to each new definition ("generation") of a concept. Even better would be to acknowledge the

---

5.   Another recent example of such coding delays is the "Gulf War syndrome." See page 17.

fact that these symptoms and other criteria are entities themselves and provide entity codes for them.

The *DSM* does not, however, provide any of its own codes for the concepts defined. For the convenience of the physician, *DSM* gives the *ICD-9-CM* category into which that concept would be coded. So because we currently rely on category codes, mental illnesses are coded to the categories of *ICD*, rather than individually identified. The codes match quite closely because of the intense involvement of the American Psychiatric Association (APA) in the modification of *ICD-9* to create *ICD-9-CM*.

APA also worked with WHO in the preparation of *ICD-10*, and a good deal of correlation has been achieved. *DSM-IV* provides a table for placing its concepts into the categories of *ICD-10* for reporting purposes, along with a strong admonition that the codes are one-way, i.e., that the category codes do not necessarily retrieve the actual diagnoses placed into the categories.

The trouble is, even with a close correlation between the *DSM* concept and the *ICD* category, the code changes along with the concepts, *without leaving a trail* to the old concept. Part of the solution would be to tag (identify) each code as to which revision of *ICD and DSM* it belongs, so that it can be traced back to a former concept. For more about this, see "Living Successfully with Code-Dependency," page 291.

Also, a concept doesn't necessarily represent just one entity. Each concept may represent a single entity or a constellation or pattern of entities (subconcepts), each with its own terms and their variants. A change in a concept's definition is likely to mean a change in the particular entities which are used to form the pattern or constellation. If we were to retain the clinical entity information (not just the composite diagnosis) in the form of entity codes, we could assign patients to concepts under varying definitions simply by going back to the entities and allocating them to the different definition of the concepts.[6]

---

6.   See "The 'Labelling' of Dementia," page 274.

The Concept of AD/HD

Attention-Deficit/Hyperactivity Disorder (AD/HD) is a case in point. For the most part, in 1994 patients had pretty much the same problems as they had in 1979. But during the years between 1979 and 1994 — and between *DSM III* and *DSM IV* — new information and new thinking became available about causes and relationships.

The tables below compares the diagnostic criteria for Attention-Deficit/Hyperactivity Disorder (AD/HD) in 1979 and 1994. This diagnosis is determined from a pattern of symptoms and other criteria (entities) in the individual. The symptoms and other findings fall into groups which themselves are expressed as entity terms. The table shows that the patterns of entities are somewhat different under the thinking of 1979 and 1994. Note that the detailed list of symptoms under "inattention," "impulsivity," and "hyperactivity" is different in the two volumes, and that the disorder has been divided into several subtypes in *DSM-IV*. It is also recognized as an adult — not just childhood — disorder.

The first table compares the codes and labels given the disorder by *ICD-9-CM*, *DSM-III*, and *DSM-IV*. Note that in *DSM-IV*, two different subtypes — AD/HD, Predominantly Hyperactive-Impulsive Type, and AD/HD, Combined Type — receive the same *ICD-9-CM* code. The second table shows the specific criteria for the diagnosis.

Figure 12.1 Concepts and Codes for AD/HD, 1979 & 1994

Concepts for AD/HD as stated in		ICD-9-CM Category Assignments	
DSM III – 1979 Attention Deficit Disorder (ADD)	**DSM IV – 1994 Attention-Deficit/ Hyperactivity Disorder (AD/HD)**	**Code**	**Category Title – term retrieved from category code**
		314	Hyperkinetic syndrome of childhood

		314.0	Attention deficit disorder
			    Adult
			    Child

ADD with hyperactivity (ADD-H)	AD/HD, predominantly hyperactive-impulsive type	314.01	Attention deficit disorder with hyperactivity
ADD without hyperactivity (ADD)	AD/HD, predominantly inattentive type	314.00	Attention deficit disorder without mention of hyperactivity
ADD, residual type		314.80	Other specified manifestations of hyperkinetic syndrome of childhood
	AD/HD, combined type	314.01	Attention deficit disorder with hyperactivity
	AD/HD, not otherwise specified	314.9	Unspecified hyperkinetic syndrome of childhood

Correspondence between the ICD-9-CM code used for attention deficit/hyperactivity disorder and the DSM criteria in 1979 and 1994. Information is from ICD-9-CM and the *Diagnostic and Statistical Manual of Mental Disorders (DSM)* editions III and IV, published by the American Psychiatric Association.

Figure 12.2 Criteria for AD/HD, 1979 & 1994

	DSM-III - 1979 (ADD-H)	DSM-IV - 1994 (AD/HD)
Generally	The child displays, for his or her mental and chronological age, signs of developmentally inappropriate inattention, impulsivity, and hyperactivity.	Either inattention or hyperactivity-impulsivity symptoms have persisted to a degree that is maladaptive and inconsistent with developmental level.
Inattention	At least three of the following: (1) often fails to finish things he or she starts (2) often doesn't seem to listen (3) easily distracted (4) has difficulty concentrating on schoolwork or other tasks requiring sustained attention (5) has difficulty sticking to a play activity	At least six of the following: (a) often fails to give close attention to details or makes careless mistakes in schoolwork, work, or other activities (b) often has difficulty sustaining attention in tasks or play activities (c) often does not seem to listen when spoken to directly (d) often does not follow through on instructions and fails to finish schoolwork, chores, or duties in the workplace (not due to oppositional behavior or failure to understand instructions) (e) often has difficulties organizing tasks and activities (f) often avoids, dislikes, or is reluctant to engage in tasks that require sustained mental effort (such as schoolwork or homework) (g) often loses things necessary for tasks or activities (e.g., toys, school assignments, pencils, books, or tools) (h) is often easily distracted by extraneous stimuli (i) is often forgetful in daily activities
		Hyperactivity-Impulsivity At least four of the following symptoms:

Figure 12.2 Criteria for AD/HD, 1979 & 1994 *(continued)*

	DSM-III - 1979 (ADD-H)	DSM-IV - 1994 (AD/HD)
Hyperactivity	At least 2 of the following: (1) runs about or climbs on things excessively (1) has difficulty sitting still or fidgets excessively (2) has difficulty staying seated (3) moves about excessively during sleep (4) is always "on the go" or acts as if "driven by a motor"	(a) often fidgets with hands or feet or squirms in seat (b) often leaves seat in classroom or in other situations in which remaining seated is expected (c) often runs about or climbs excessively in situations in which it is inappropriate (in adolescents or adults, may be limited to subjective feelings of restlessness) (d) often has difficulty playing or engaging in leisure activities quietly (e) is often "on the go" or often acts as if "driven by a motor" (f) often talks excessively
Impulsivity	At least 3 of the following: (1) often acts before thinking (2) shifts excessively from one activity to another (3) has difficulty organizing work (this not being due to cognitive impairment) (4) needs a lot of supervision (5) frequently calls out in class (6) has difficulty awaiting turn in games or group situations	(g) often blurts out answers to questions before the questions have been completed (h) often has difficulty awaiting turn (i) often interrupts or intrudes on others (e.g., butts into conversations or games)
Onset	Before age 7	Some hyperactive-impulsive or inattentive symptoms that caused impairment were present before age 7.
Duration	At least 6 months	At least 6 months
Situation	(No criteria)	Some impairment from the symptoms is present in two or more settings (e.g., at school [or work] and at home).

Figure 12.2 Criteria for AD/HD, 1979 & 1994 *(continued)*

	DSM-III - 1979 (ADD-H)	DSM-IV - 1994 (AD/HD)
Impairment	(No criteria)	There must be clear evidence of clinically significant impairment in social, academic, or occupational functioning.
Not Due To	Schizophrenia, affective disorder, or severe or profound mental retardation	The symptoms do not occur exclusively during the course of a Pervasive Developmental Disorder, Schizophrenia, or other Psychotic Disorder, and are not better accounted for by another mental disorder (e.g., Mood, Anxiety, Dissociative, or Personality Disorder.

Comparison of the criteria for the diagnosis of Attention Deficit/Hyperactivity Disorder between 1979 and 1994. Information is from the *Diagnostic and Statistical Manual of Mental Disorders (DSM)* editions III and IV, published by the American Psychiatric Association.

Each of the criteria, including each of the "listed symptoms," in itself is an entity (term) describing the patient. "Easily distracted" is one entity, and each of the groups of criteria is also expressed as an entity, e.g., "hyperactivity." At a higher level of aggregation, "ADD-H" and "AD/HD" are also entity terms in the vocabulary of clinical medicine.

If the data were kept in the most discrete level of terminology, such as "easily distracted," and so coded, it might well be that cases which had been allocated to ADD-H would not be allocated to AD/HD, and vice versa. This presents a powerful argument for adopting a record system in which the most discrete level of entity is preserved by giving each statement of a symptom or sign, e.g., "has difficulty sticking to a play activity," a unique, unalterable, entity code, thus permitting far more powerful, bidirectional (looking backward as well as forward) studies over time, as biomedical knowledge, thinking, and understanding advance.

In the comparison of concepts shown in the table, it appears that a patient with the same findings might have been diagnosed differently in 1994 than in 1979. Had the discrete terms supporting the diagnosis —

and not just the diagnosis — been recorded and coded as entities (in this case the symptoms, age at onset, duration, and so on), it would be possible to determine whether the same case would have fitted the criteria for one or the other or both of the definitions.

The Definition of AIDS

It often takes a while to discover and then understand a new disease. AIDS provides a good example of this process, and how knowledge of the disease has been slowed by the delay in classification. Before a diagnosis can be accurately *classified*, it must be reasonably well understood — and defined. But before it is classified, when we rely only on category coding, we lose track of the disease. The defining of AIDS shows the importance of capturing the clinical detail.

AIDS was first described in 1981, but was not officially "defined" until 1985. To be diagnosed with AIDS, at that time a person had to:

1. be infected with the HIV virus, *and*

2. have any one of several dozen specified opportunistic infections[7] associated with the HIV infection.

This definition was modified in 1987 to add a number of opportunistic infections to the list of associated infections.[8]

In 1992, the definition was changed dramatically: any person with a blood count revealing fewer than 200 CD4 lymphocytes (also known as helper T cells) per cubic millimeter (mm^3) was considered to have AIDS.

The 1992 definition also *removed* the requirement of an accompanying opportunistic infection for a diagnosis of AIDS. This change was stimulated by two things:

---

7. An "opportunistic infection" is one caused by an organism which is unable to cause disease (to infect) in an individual (the host) unless the host's resistance has been lowered, usually by drugs or by another infection. Such lowered resistance provides a special "opportunity" for the infection.

8. In 1997, the important AIDS-related opportunistic infections included pneumocystis carinii pneumonia, cytomegalovirus retinitis and systemic disease, disseminated mycobacterium avium-intracellulare infection, mycobacterium tuberculosis infection, mucosal candidiasis, and herpes simplex virus infections.

First, the treatments for the opportunistic infections have become increasingly effective. Newer drug therapies have either eliminated or delayed the development of opportunistic infections in HIV+ individuals. This made the incidence of AIDS appear to be decreasing or slowing down as long as the 1987 definition was being applied. HIV infections themselves, however, were clearly still increasing in numbers. The old definition was giving us a "false negative."[9]

The second event behind the 1992 change was that the natural history of AIDS had become better known, and other studies confirmed that the CD4 cell count is a change which can be attributed to AIDS during a latent period between infection of the patient and the development of other symptoms and effects.

Changes in the definition of AIDS are important for several reasons:

• The statistics on AIDS are changed, but not the true incidence.

The best estimates are that the 1985 definition resulted in an increase in the reported incidence of AIDS of 3% to 4% over the period when there was no official definition. The 1987 definition, by adding a number of diagnoses to the list of specified opportunistic infections, increased the reported incidence by 19% to 24%. The 1992 definition increased the reported incidence by nearly another 50%. These changes were due solely to changes in the definition, not to the incidence or prevalence of the disease.

✓ Whole groups of individuals went into and out of being labeled as having AIDS.

Before 1992, patients who had the HIV infection but not the accompanying secondary, opportunistic infections did not have to be classified as having AIDS, and thus could honestly believe that they did not have AIDS. Furthermore, they did not have to be reported and thus could avoid certain economic and social problems, such as those

---

9.   Changes in definition of the disease affect morbidity statistics (dealing with the incidence and prevalence of the disease in the population) but not the mortality statistics, since deaths from AIDS occur in those individuals who have acquired the opportunistic infections, and this will be true after the definition changes as well as before.

connected with employment and benefits. When the 1992 definition removed the opportunistic infection requirement, these additional patients were instantly turned into actual, "labeled" AIDS patients. This, of course, had serious consequences for both patients and community.

Over the years, we have had to rely on information based on conclusions — the definition and corresponding coding of a disease — rather than on raw evidence (information upon which no conclusion had been made). We have as a result been at a disadvantage, from the start, in our war against AIDS.

Our health information system would not permit going back to the original records of all AIDS (or suspected AIDS) patients, in which were available not only immunological evidence of the HIV infection (an entity itself), but also information on the accompanying entities, that is, the opportunistic infections and the blood counts. Instead, the lowest available level of information was that of the coded diagnosis, "AIDS" (and that only after the term had been coined and applied to patients with the necessary constellation of entities leading — at that time — to the AIDS diagnosis). Had the details in the original record — other infections and the blood counts — been treated (and coded) as discrete entities, and had the information system permitted going into the records to that level of detail, we would now have a much truer picture of the progress of AIDS and of our efforts to combat it.

The Criteria for Diabetes Mellitus

More and more, a specific objective finding may be crucial in defining a diagnosis. For example, the Expert Committee on the Diagnosis and Classification of Diabetes Mellitus in late 1997 recommended that the diagnosis of diabetes mellitus should be made when a patient's fasting glucose level (FPG) exceeds 110 milligrams per deciliter (mg/dl), the proposed new upper limit of normal, which is lower than the old. If this recommendation is accepted, the FPG would become a key clinical entity in the definition of diabetes, i.e., the FPG would be taken into account in deciding whether or not the diagnosis would be considered valid.

Using the FPG as an entity would permit a longitudinal comparison of diabetes over time, a comparison impossible if only the term "diabetes mellitus" is used (and retrievable). One could determine at which FPG threshold the diagnosis was made. The source article for this information, a news story in the September/October 1997 issue of *Public*

Health Reports, points out that this new criterion could add 2,000,000 patients to the nation's "diabetes roster" with the stroke of a pen — a striking similarity to the AIDS story.

The "Labelling" of Dementia

The definitions of diagnoses don't just change over *time*. At any given time, the criteria for a diagnosis may differ from one *classification* to another.

The effects of the array of entities which go into a category with the same label in different classifications is well illustrated by a 1998 study of "The Effect of Different Diagnostic Criteria on the Prevalence of Dementia."[10] The authors studied the records of 1,879 subjects in the Canadian Study of Health and Aging and allocated to each the diagnosis of dementia under six classifications: The American Psychiatric Association's *Diagnostic and Statistical Manual of Mental Disorders, 3rd edition (DSM-III);* the 3rd edition revised *(DSM-III-R)*, the 4th edition *(DSM-IV)*, the *International Classification of Diseases*, 9th and 10th Revisions *(ICD-9* and *ICD-10)*, and the *Cambridge Examination for Mental Disorders of the Elderly (CAMDEX)*. The subjects were also evaluated in a clinical consensus meeting at which each expert clinician simply stated, for each patient, whether or not he or she believed that that patient had dementia, without reference to a published classification.

When classified under *ICD-10*, 3.1 percent of the study group would have been classified as having dementia; with *DSM-III*, 29.1 percent would have been labeled as having dementia, an astonishing 10-fold difference.

A portion of the findings is presented in the figure below. Clinical consensus diagnosed the largest group in the illustration. Only *CAMDEX* captured a complete subset of the cases identified by clinical consensus. Both *ICD-10* and *DSM-IV* diagnosed some patients as having dementia, even though the clinical consensus group had not given them that diagnosis.

---

10. Erkinjuntti, Timo, Truls ÿstbye, Runa Steenhuis, and Vladimir Hachinski. *New England Journal of Medicine (NEJM)* 337, no. 23 (1998): 1667-74.

Figure 12.3 Classification of "Dementia"

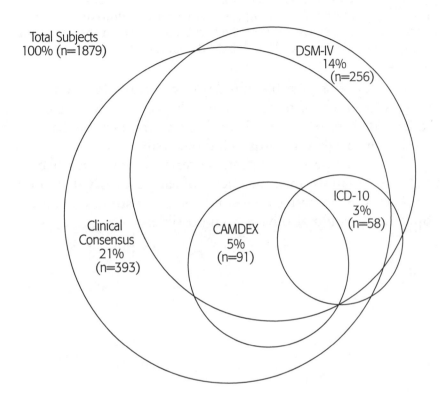

Redrawn from a diagram in "The Effect of Different Diagnostic Criteria on the Prevalence of Dementia." Erkinjuntti, Timo, Truls ÿstbye, Runa Steenhuis, and Vladimir Hachinski. *New England Journal of Medicine (NEJM)* 337, no. 23 (1998): 1667-74. Results not shown in the diagram were DSM-III 17% (n=546), DSM-III-R 17% (n=326), and ICD-9 5% (n=94).

The dementia study illustrates the impossibility of understanding and properly interpreting data which have been placed in a category of a classification unless the entities to be placed in that category (in the paper such entities are called "diagnostic criteria") are known. The researchers proposed that:

> All investigators should use the same minimal set of standardized, validated measures and record key demographics characteristics, so that patients can be reclassified and the findings interpreted in the light of emerging knowledge. The validity (construct, content, and criterion) of diagnostic classifications is essential for studies of the

epidemiology, risk factors, prevention, and treatment of any disorder. This use of standardized measures is critical, especially at the early stages of disease, when early detection of pathologic processes is essential if any intervention is to prevent or retard cognitive impairment. One proposal is that the focus should be on the spectrum of cognitive impairment, and the label "dementia" may even be abandoned.[11]

This study would not be possible in today's healthcare data system if the investigators were confined to the data which had already been category coded. It depended entirely on the investigators' ability to get back to the detail found in the original records. Had the system been such that the necessary entities (attributes, diagnostic criteria) were separately coded and available for analysis, then the effects of each category definition could have been studied with ease — and computer studies on much larger populations would also have been possible.

---

11. See "The label of dementia," page 338, for more about the effects of these varying diagnoses.

13

Entity Coding

WE NEED TO introduce a "front end" into our health information system to permit capturing the clinical entities. This front end is called "entity coding." Implementing it would require us to:

- Create a list of entities and their codes.

- Modify our medical records to carry entity codes in addition to category codes.

- Train coders to identify and capture clinical entities.

What Are Clinical Entities?

An "entity" is the smallest (most "granular") meaningful unit of information available in a given universe.[1] In this context, the universe is the clinical information in the medical record. "Clinical information" is all the information of whatever kind used in describing a person's illness and wellness, including description of the patient, behavior, occupation, problems presented, diagnoses made and suspected, procedures performed, response to treatments, places where that patient receives care, how the illness was contracted or injury sustained, caregivers, physical findings such as blood pressure, height, and weight, significant elements of personal and family history, laboratory values, drugs and other treatments, sources of the information, and more — i.e., everything needed to understand the case. These items comprise the medical record (and other health records).

---

1. "Universe" in this sense is the totality of information (things known) within a specific field; a "body of knowledge." A universe may be, for example, all species of birds in the world, or all we know about the human mind. For more about universes, see "Classifications & Classifying," page 133.

This sounds like the list in the patient data set, described earlier (page 140). In fact, everything in a patient data set is a clinical entity, plus there are many more potential clinical entities in the medical record.

Each of the items of clinical information listed above — patient's age, problem, blood pressure, etc. — are clinical entities.

✓ A "clinical entity" is the smallest *meaningful* unit of information *available* in a patient's medical record.

- "Meaningful" in the definition is used to eliminate terms which have no significance, at least not when standing alone — the word "blood," for example, is not by itself, in most contexts, a clinical entity. It must have a context and a unique identity.

- The word "available" is also significant. If the physician, for example, has recorded only "myocardial infarction," that is the clinical entity. If the term were "anterior myocardial infarction," giving greater detail, that would be the diagnosis clinical entity for that medical record (for that problem; there may be other diagnoses within the record).

The entities in the clinical record which can be most elusive are those which are expressed in words in the narrative portion of the record, such as the patient's statement of her problems, the physician's diagnoses (established and suspected), the surgeon's procedures, and nursing diagnoses.[2]

These "narrative" entities are the primary subject of this book, although occasionally today, and more so in the future, other entities from the record will be used in classifying patients. For example, blood glucose levels (FPGs) have become central to the diagnosis of diabetes mellitus;[3] blood counts of CD4 lymphocytes (also known as helper T cells) are important to the diagnosis of AIDS.[4]

---

2. Troubles arise mostly due to language issues; see "Expression of Clinical Concepts," page 71.

3. See "The Criteria for Diabetes Mellitus," page 273.

4. See "The Definition of AIDS," page 271.

Entity Codes

An entity code is a unique code which is:

- permanently assigned
- to a single, unique entity
- never reused

A "clinical entity code" is a code given to a specific clinical entity; the code permanently represents this smallest available unit of meaningful information.

To put entity coding in the context of this book, let's look again at the examples of various codes shown earlier on page 119. Here's that same list.

Figure 13.1 Entity Code Examples

Kind of Code	What It Represents	Example of Code
Social security number	Identity of a specific, unique individual	355-34-3222

The social security number is a true entity code — it is permanent, and identifies a single, unique individual, and is never reused.

Emergency information	A specific kind of emergency, to notify those who must take immediate action	Code Blue

This kind of code is a signal to action, rather than identification of information. It's not an entity code, but then, it doesn't need to be.

Telephone number	Electronic pathway to a specific telephone	651-699-0666

Telephone numbers *would* be entity codes if they stuck with a single thing (an address or a person) and didn't change periodically! Look at the trouble the phone people have to go through when they change area codes.

URL (Uniform Resource Locator)	Electronic pathway to a specific page (file) on the World Wide Web (WWW)	http://www.tringa.com/hccc.htm

The URL may be an entity code if it is permanent and never changes. However, very often the information at that site changes, so that the *page* is not unique. This defeats the URL as an entity code.

Catalog number	A specific item of merchandise	HQ47588

If the seller never changes the coding, and "retires" the code when the product is no longer available, this is a true entity code. Often this kind of code is "tagged" with additional identifying information. In the above example, HQ might mean the "Fall 1999 catalog." A key used with the code for "fan belt" might indicate that it's an "engine" part.

Healthcare classification code	A specific category within a specific classification	473.1

A classification code is not an entity code: it is not permanent, the category is not usually unique (the contents of the category periodically change), and the code itself often changes over time. It is a category code. However, it could become unique if it was tagged to identify exactly where and when it came from. (See "Making Meaning Precise," page 318.)

Entity code	A specific, unique item — code is assigned to the smallest available relevant item of information	ISBN 0-9615255-2-5

An ISBN is an entity code: it is permanent, identifies a single book, and is never reused. Note, however, that its *meaning* is known only if it has the key "ISBN" in front of it to identify it as such.

> ## An entity code is a unique code which is:
> - **permanently assigned**
> - **to a single, unique entity**
> - **never reused**

Entity Codes in Real Life: MICAR

For thirty years, the United States National Center for Health Statistics (NCHS) has been developing and using a program called the Mortality Medical Data System (MMDS) for mortality statistics. MICAR (Mortality Medical Indexing, Classification, and Retrieval System) was created to automate the entry, classification, and retrieval of cause of death information reported on death certificates.

MICAR uses, as its input, diagnoses in natural language, much as does a coder in the clinical world. The product of its data entry components are codes (numeric entity reference numbers (ERNs)) which replace that language. The ENRs assigned to the death certificates are permanently retained in the files of one component of the system, MICAR 100, and thus it would be possible, using that file, to return to the individual cases in which a given ENR was recorded. This use of the file is not common, however, because the system's purpose, its end product, is to allocate each case to the *ICD-9* and *ICD-10* in a uniform manner, following the cause-of-death coding rules prescribed by WHO. Nor would the original ERNs lead necessarily to the clinician's initial terms. MICAR is explained more fully in the appendices; see page 491.

Diagnoses as Entities

Although entity coding may be applied to a wide range of information, we'll focus here on *diagnoses*. We need to know specific details about diagnoses in order to render proper medical care. And diagnoses provide the basis for payment for healthcare services, and for most quality management assessments and epidemiological studies. We are using "diagnoses" as a broad term to also include such data as abnormal physical findings, symptoms, signs, problems, etc., as are classified in *ICD-9* and *ICD-10*.

✓ If diagnostic and procedure terms in the medical record are first identified as clinical entities and "captured" by being given unique entity codes, they can thereafter be allocated to their proper classification niche for whatever purpose — payment, research, etc. — and yet still retain their original, unique identities.

Introduction of an entity coding "front end" to the health information system would clearly be a tremendous step forward, permitting, for the first time, precise detail within the medical record — necessary for the care of the individual patient — even after the electronic medical record (EMR) has completely replaced the paper-based patient record.

How to Implement Entity Coding

Entity coding would not require any change in the "classification system" as such; we would still use the same classifications (i.e., *ICD-9-CM, CPT*) until new ones are introduced. The new front end in the medical record will capture and keep entity codes, while category coding continues, as now, with putting the case into *ICD-9-CM*. The reimbursement system and other current information needs would not be interrupted. But we would finally have the critical detail, wherever and whenever we need it.[5]

---

5. There will probably be a change, one day, in the route information follows in getting from the medical record to the pigeonhole in *ICD* or any other classification. Having the entity codes may well lead to "entity code classifying" in which, after the medical record information gets its entity codes, a computer algorithm will place the case into the appropriate category for each classification in use. See "Entity Code Classifying," page 320.

"Ground Rules"

The entity coding system for diagnoses must have the following essential features:

- The database must contain all "diagnoses," no matter how long the list.[6]

- There must be only one master database (list) of entity terms and entity codes for each type of information. Competing lists would defeat the entire purpose.[7]

- Each diagnostic entity must have its own permanent, unalterable, never-to-be-reused code.

- Entity codes must be instantly available to any coder.

- The system, once begun, must remain permanently available.

Creating the Master List

The starting place is developing the master list(s) of clinical entities. Although the term "entity" includes numerous kinds of information, it makes sense to begin with what we need the most: diagnoses. There must of course be "someone" responsible for holding and managing the master list and dissemination of codes; we'll call that someone here the "secretariat."

The Master List for Diagnoses could be initially defined as all the terms to be classified to *ICD-9-CM* or *ICD-10-CM*. The first step in its creation would be to glean the clinical entity terms from the alphabetic indices to *ICD-9-CM* (which already contains roughly 100,000 entries) and *ICD-10-CM*.

Terms can then be added from other sources:

- Other classifications, such as *SNOMED*, NHS Codes (Read Codes), other sources consulted by the U. S. National Library of Medicine in developing the Unified Medical Language System (UMLS).[8]

---

6. We are using "diagnoses" in a broad sense; see "Diagnoses as Entities," page 282.

7. We might entitle the master list for diagnoses, for example, "International Health Entity Codes" (IHEC). "IHEC" could identify each "official" entity code. See "Making Meaning Precise," page 318.

8. For more on UMLS, see the appendices, page 425.

- Textbook indexes, publications of the National Library of Medicine, and others.

- Response to inquiries from coders for entities not found in the growing database. Each new entity would be added to the Master List.

Once initially populated, the Master Database would simply grow by acquisition of new terms as they appear in the literature and as they are presented to the secretariat by coders requesting entity codes. Each diagnostic term encountered would automatically be an "entity," with no argument. It would be entered in the master entity database, and it would be given its own unique, permanent "entity code." No effort would be made to decide whether or not the term was the preferred term, a synonym (or even an alternate spelling), a new entity, or even whether it is a "legitimate" term at all. All the secretariat would do is assign codes to terms actually used in medical records, not make judgments about them.

Obviously, the database would accumulate a certain amount of "trash," such as entities encountered only once, misspellings, and so forth. But once assigned a code number, that code number would remain with the trash entity, doing no harm to the system, and could never be reused. A corollary is that the Master List database could never be purged (have entries deleted). If, over time, certain entities prove to be true synonyms for other entities, the database would include "pointers" to the other entities. The same would be true of "cross reference" entities.

By agreement, a published copy of the Master List might contain only those entities used during a specified preceding period of time, perhaps five years (one good reason for dating the entries). If the day comes that entity code classifying becomes prevalent, a feature of the computer program "downstream" would be to maintain a count of the frequency of usage of the various entity codes.[9] Periodically, perhaps annually, this "used" list could be compared with the full Master List database in preparation for the publication, similar in concept to a list of books in print. Remember that out-of-print books do not give up their ISBN numbers for other books to use. As a matter of fact, there are some ISBN numbers for books never even published; these cannot be reused, either.

---

9.   For more about entity code classifying, see page 319.

Background

> ## Why do we need codes at all?
>
> If we want to keep the most discrete detail possible — and the actual words used by the physician — why do we need any codes? Why not just use the words, themselves, since computers are so powerful? Aren't words and phrases (simply combinations of alphabetic letters and spaces) already "codes" in their own right?
>
> These are good questions. There are two basic reasons:
>
> 1. We want to capture relevant information, not everything. We want words and phrases which have been given meaning by humans. For example, we could capture "bed" and "sore" with the computer, but those words take on a special meaning together: "bed sore."
>
> 2. Computers do much better with code. They can learn things, and can manipulate data in many more ways.
>
> Serious efforts have been underway for years to develop computer logic which can take a clinical narrative and, without human intervention, tease from that narrative its meaning — its diagnostic terms, for example. None have reached the ability to do as good a job as a human reading the text and designating the diagnoses it contains. None are ready for "prime time."[a]

a. For more on this subject, see Gabrieli, Elmer R. "Aspects of a Computer-Based Patient Record." Journal of AHIMA 64, no. 7 (1993): 70-82.

Where Do We Get the Actual Codes?

Codes need to be assigned to identify each entity. Each code must be:

- permanent
- unalterable
- never to be reused

In addition, there are two critical "specifications" for the codes themselves:

- they must have no intrinsic meaning (so no one can make up or manufacture their own entity code)
- they must be identified as entity codes[10]

---

10. For more about identifying codes, see "Making Meaning Precise," page 318.

The entity code is essentially an accession number — each new entity receives the next code on the list. The codes may be simply consecutive numbers (or number-letter combinations), or random unique codes generated by a computer.

One source of nonrepeating numbers is the *time*. Time can be an absolute reference, expressed in relation to something such as Greenwich Mean Time (GMT). Most computers have an internal clock that measures time, typically to the nanosecond. As entities come in, the code they receive could represent the exact nanosecond they arrive. This would "date stamp" the entity, providing that much more information about it, as well as assigning a unique code. For the intitial list, we could simply count backwards from the year 2000 (or any date selected as "ground zero") until we reach one million "units," and then use those units as the first codes. After that, we can count forward and use the actual "timestamp" of issuance to identify each entity.

With whatever method is ultimately used, the availability of entity codes will be practically infinite — we don't need to worry about "leaving room" for yet-to-be discovered entities.

The Entity Coding Process

All system resources — medical record departments, professionals, trainers, libraries, computers, publishers — are already in place to handle the entity coding process.

Initially, at least, there would be two coding processes — the present, familiar coding to *ICD-9-CM* in order to keep reimbursement flowing, and the newer "look-up" and recording of entity codes.

Training for entity coding will be a one-time effort. When the information system is ready to put the classifying into the hands of the computer using entity codes and the necessary adjunct information as input, it will *never again* be necessary to train all the nation's coders with a new system.

When entity coding is implemented, the health information professional's coding duties would be to:

1.   Identify clinical entities.

Most of the diagnostic and procedure entities are readily visible in the traditional paper-based medical record because they have been listed by the physician, nurse, or other caregiver. But as all health information professionals know, some clinical entities will be noted in the body of the record but not listed, and these will need to be sought and teased out.

2.   Assign entity codes.

This should be the easiest part of the task. It involves looking up each clinical entity in the "coding book" (or within a computer-assisted coding product, such as are now in widespread use), finding there its code number, and assigning that code to the entity. Entity terms would be searchable alphabetically. They would also be available by phone, over the Internet, and online. Coding assistance would also be available, 24 hours a day, by the same routes. Entities without codes would be reported and immediately assigned a unique number.

Example

New codes handed out — a million times a day

Yes! Already, millions of unique codes are provided to users, electronically (and as "instantly" as traffic will allow), every day. Whenever a credit card transaction takes place, the merchant must obtain an "authorization number" from a centralized source before the transaction can go through.

This is often done electronically, by sliding the card through a machine which automatically calls in the needed numbers, and picks up the authorization code. Other times, a human makes a phone call, gives the credit card number, expiration date, and purchase amount and then within moments receives the authorization code.

A similar system can be set up to provide entity codes, as needed and on demand.

The entity coding process is illustrated by the flow chart below. Compare its simplicity with the diagram, "Coding Diagnoses with 'Category Coding'," page 214. Note also that the category coding process gives you the name of a category, and nothing else; entity coding preserves forever the identity of the diagnosis.

Figure 13.2 Coding Diagnoses with 'Entity Coding'

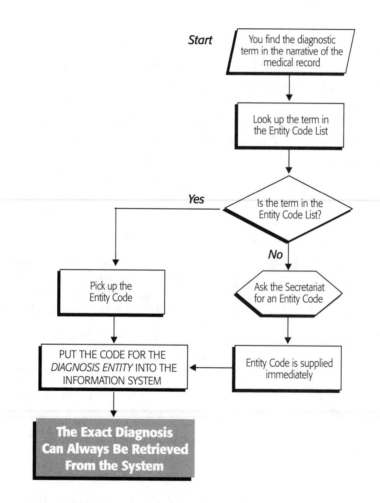

A flow chart showing the "Entity Coding" process (by the authors).

Features of Entity Coding

Entity coding has a number of attractive features:

It's Easy to Learn Learning to use an entity coding system is far simpler than learning a new classification. The coder is trained to recognize a word or string of words as a "clinical entity" and to find its code.

Coding is More Accurate Category coding — what we do today — is really a classifying, rather than coding, process. Entity coding is a simple "look up" process, and so much less prone to error; there should be no variations in coding. Also, there can be no codes "synthethized" by the coder, as is possible with some other methods, such as modular language coding.

Coding is Prompt Codes are immediately available for new terms, so diagnoses can be coded immediately and permanently, even though their classification may take awhile. Entity coding does not require a decision on the *classification* of an entity before it can be coded and placed in the information system.

The System is Auditable Each entity code must, by definition, be an exact exchange for the entity term coded. Thus entity coding is perfectly auditable, because the records of original entry retain the terms in natural language along with their codes.

Coding Need Never Change Again If classifying using the entity codes is implemented, subsequent classification changes need not impinge on the coder *at all*.[11] New classifications would only affect the computer systems which do the actual classifying, systems which can be part of electronic medical record (EMR) systems, institutional and enterprise computer systems, and systems elsewhere, such as with insurance companies and managed care organizations.

Data Quality Can Improve Data quality slumps each time we change from one classification to another. If entity coding is established to the point where the classifying can be turned over to the computer, the new classification can be used immediately, and the entity-coded data will not change at all. In addition, audits can be done to check the data quality.

---

11. See "Entity Code Classifying," page 320.

14

Living Successfully with Code-Dependency

IN THIS CHAPTER, we look again at codes, this time as "containers" for messages. We'll explore the framework in which codes exist, and what can be done to make them better at carrying and revealing their messages. We examine how we can design our information systems to help us, by taking advantage of everything that coding has to offer. First, we'll examine some of the present problems we have with healthcare codes, by looking at how we decode — and understand — them.

Decoding Healthcare Codes

The decoding challenge can reveal a whole complex of coding and classification problems. It seems like a simple enough task — you are given a code, you look it up in the list, and it tells you what the code means. Perhaps. But do you know which list?

You are shown the number "A560.1" and told that it is a code. How do you find out what it means? You first try to find out what universe it belongs to. Is it a catalog number? Probably not — it looks too short. Is it a telephone phone number? No — telephone numbers do not have decimal points, and North American telephone numbers are usually 4 digits (nnnn) for extensions, 7 digits (nnn-nnnn) for local numbers, or 10 digits (nnn-nnn-nnnn) for long distance, with sometimes a "1" in front, making an 11-digit number. Your code doesn't fit any of these patterns.

Suppose someone helps out, and gives the clue that the code is used in healthcare. That narrows it down. In some instances, the structure of the code will help to identify which code system is in use. Presently, a diagnosis category code by itself, e.g., "510.0," is not self-identifying. From just the code, we can't know which classification it's from, nor the year or revision of that classification.

Several of the commonly used healthcare code systems today are structured as shown in the table below.

Figure 14.1 Common Healthcare Code Structures

Classification	Content	Code Structure[a]
ICD-9	Diagnoses	nnn.n *or* Ann.n
ICD-9-CM	Diagnoses Procedures	nnn.nn nn.nn
ICD-10	Diagnoses	Ann.n *or* Ann.nn
ICD-10-CM	Diagnoses	Ann.nnn *maximum, but may be as short as* Ann
CPT	Procedures	nnnnn
ICD-10-PCS	Procedures	ccccccc *(except letters I and O) — must be exactly 7 characters long*
HCPCS National	Supplies, Services, Procedures	Annnn
IRD	Radiological Diagnoses	Not kept consistent
SNOMED III	Terminology used in human and veterinary medicine	A-n… *or* AA-n… (see page 429)
NHS Codes (Read Codes)	Health Care, Great Britain	5-Byte (alphabetic or numeric in any of 5 positions)

> a. n = numeric character
>   A = alphabetic character (not case sensitive)
>   c = character — either alphabetic or numeric

This information allows you to rule out several classifications, but that still leaves several possibilities. Several of the classifications — *ICD-9, ICD-9-CM, ICD-10,* HCPCS National, and *SNOMED III* — use codes which start with an alphabetic character, like yours.[1] So you have to know more. In *ICD-9* and *ICD-9-CM,* the only alpha characters used to start codes are the letters "E," "V," and "Y." In *ICD-10,* any letter of the alphabet (including "I" and "O," which are omitted in many codes because of confusion with the numerals "1" and "0") is a valid lead

---

1. These classifications are described in more detail in "Diagnosis Classifications," page 149.

character (except "U"). So it could be *ICD-10* — except for the fact that in *ICD-10*, there are only two numeric characters after the alpha before the decimal point (Ann.n).

In *SNOMED*, the "A" could be a lead character (as could all letters "A" through "F"), but it would be followed by a hyphen and 5 digits (A-nnnnn). NHS Codes (Read Codes) could start with an "A," but are 5 characters long without a decimal. Thus the code doesn't belong to *any* of these code systems.

The process of decoding — determining the meaning of a code (retrieving the information carried by the code) — is one which is usually taken for granted. Designers of coding systems seem to forget that a main reason for coding is so that the information can be *retrieved*, and that the users of the output deserve consideration along with those providing input. Far too much effort has gone into making the systems easy for the coder (although some designers have omitted even that consideration), and far too little for the retriever.

What You Need to Know to Decode

Decoding can only be done with assurance if you know the following about the code:

- *Context.* What universe the code pertains to (here, healthcare).
  - *Subcontext.* For example, if in healthcare, is the code a diagnosis or procedure code?
- *Coding System.* What coding system, e.g., entity coding, *ICD-9-CM*, *ICD-10*, is being used.
  - *Generation.* Which "generation" of the coding system was used, since the same code may have a different meaning from time to time.
- *Period in Use.* When a given code (or generation) went into use and when its meaning changed.

Context

Concerning healthcare codes, it would be natural to assume, since they are typically found only in healthcare data systems, that the universe is "health." Increasingly, however, health information systems also carry such information as occupation, residence, educational level, lifestyle, and so forth. So context alone (i.e., that the code is in a health information system) may not provide the needed information. Thus some method must be used to find out exactly what the code is talking about. Usually the easiest way today, and sometimes the only way, is to ask — and hope you can find someone who can give you the answer.

Generation of the Coding System

Assuming you can discover which coding system is being used, you need to know what generation or version of the code it represents. Mail order merchants often identify the date by prefixing every catalog item number with a key telling in which catalog the item was listed; for example, 99A, 99B, etc. Or the person taking the order asks which catalog you are using. Healthcare coding systems, however, have not yet devised a way to designate the exact source of a code used in a particular instance.

In fact, the generation problem in healthcare today is a serious one because the coding systems employed so often change the meanings of their codes. For example:

- In *ICD-7*, code 395 is "Ménière's disease," while in *ICD-8*, code 395 is "Diseases of aortic valve" (Ménière's disease had migrated to code 385).

- Several of the commonly used coding systems delete codes from time to time, yet there is no way to keep coders and others from using deleted codes. Unless this interferes with payment, or someone tries to look the code up in a book which no longer contains it, no one is likely to know. The user may fail to check a different generation of the code and, as a result, consider the code which can't be found merely a transposition or other error.

- Some systems move the terms they represent from one place to another. *SNOMED II* had the appendix (body part) as code T-66000, while in *SNOMED III* it is T-59200 (there is no code T-66000 in *SNOMED III*, and unless one had *SNOMED II* at hand, the code T-66000 would be a complete mystery).

- *Current Procedural Terminology* (*CPT*) also offers illustrations. In 1987, code 15350 denoted the application of a free skin graft, either from a donor (allograft) or from the same individual (homograft). In 1993, code 15350 denoted only an allograft. In 1987, code 10140 was restricted to the incision and drainage of a hematoma; in 1993, it was expanded to include also "seroma or fluid collection." Granted, *CPT* carries Appendix C, some 26 pages long in 1993, which lists the changes made from the previous edition. But this doesn't help the user trying to decode unless he can be absolutely sure from which edition of *CPT* the code was taken.

You must know which generation of the classification is being used, *and* have access to the coding references, to accurately decode.

Period in Use

But beware — knowing the date the code was assigned does not necessarily tell you what generation of what classification was *actually used*. It is natural to assume that data and tabulations covering the same time period, and therefore presumed to be based on the same classification, are compiled using the same code source. "T'ain't necessarily so."

Example

Not everyone gets on board

The senior author was a member of the United States delegation to the 1975 World Health Organization Conference on the *International Classification (ICD)*, which was convened to make decisions regarding the 9th Revision of *ICD*. It had been assumed that all the nations which had been parties to the agreement to use *ICD* in the international exchange of health data were using the 8th Revision, which was published by WHO in 1967. It was discovered that one major nation was still using the 7th Revision, published in 1957. Inspection of the coded data had not yielded this information. The implications of this fact for the quality of international health statistics are quite astonishing.

The changes between these two classifications was substantial. Individual categories changed in both their code numbers and their contents, a double source of confusion. For example, in *ICD-7*, "diseases of the adrenal glands" was code 274 with no subdivisions, while in *ICD-8*, it was code 255, with four decimal subdivisions. In *ICD-7* there were 33 categories for "congenital malformations," while in *ICD-8* there were 130 categories for "congenital anomalies." Within this chapter, code 753 in *ICD-7* was "other congenital malformations of nervous system and sense organs," while in *ICD-8*, code 743 was "other congenital anomalies of the nervous system," and the eye and the ear had their own three-digit codes. Obviously, meaningful comparisons between data compiled under these two classifications would be difficult, if not impossible.

In the 1960s, the assumption was made that all providers who submitted bills and all carriers who paid them would convert to the new (8th) Revision of *ICD* at the same time. This later proved to be a bad assumption. Some carriers didn't get their computer systems changed for a year or more. Some providers didn't get started at the same time as others. Even when a decision was made within an institution submitting data that it would convert to the new coding, there were many instances when the coding was indeed changed on a given date, but no control was made to be sure that the old coding applied to old data and the new coding to new data; all data, old and new, were coded to the new system.

Example

It seemed like a good idea at the time

In the mid-sixties, when insurance companies set up their computer systems to handle the new coding system, based on *ICD-8*, some companies used *only the first three digits* of *ICD*, on the assumption that all fourth digits were merely subdivisions of the 3-digit rubric and that the detail was irrelevant for purposes of payment (and setting up a larger field was very expensive). When it turned out that 4th digits were actually modifications as well as subdivisions, this fact was simply ignored (if it was known to the carrier at all), and the fourth digit was dropped (i.e., the code was truncated).

The resulting distortion of information was not visible, and was discovered only by accident. Its implications for payment and other uses of the information have not, to the authors' knowledge, ever been investigated.

It is virtually impossible to detect whether the correct classification was used or not. There is nothing inherent and visible in the code numbers themselves to indicate which classification is their source.

✓ All numbers look alike, and if no "clues" are present, the code cannot be decoded with any certainty.

The Missing Link in Our Medical Knowledge

Interhospital comparisons and research, especially "longitudinal studies" (studies over a period of years), which were key incentives for the establishment of multi-hospital information systems, have been severely hampered by the lack of specificity available from the codes. Even more, by the incompatibility between the category labels and codes, and also the category contents, in succeeding generations of the classification itself. The unsatisfactory compromises required by the use of already-grouped data greatly reduced the potential value of the studies, often to the degree that it was futile to even attempt them. The coding of AIDS, discussed above (page 263), presents an example of the problem of longitudinal studies even within a single generation of *ICD*.

Longitudinal studies have often been impossible because diagnoses moved from one category to another as later generations of the classification were substituted for earlier ones. Sometimes investigators will develop a "concordance" to code the diagnoses of interest to their categories in each of the series of successive classifications, in order to estimate the effects of the modifications on event rates and thus to smooth the transition. A perfect fit is rarely if ever possible, so the results can only be approximate.

When the category shift is from a broad category to a finer category, hidden diagnoses may become visible for the first time. Acute myocardial infarction (AMI) is an example:

Example   **Acute myocardial infarction (AMI)**

As biomedical knowledge grows over time, diagnoses are often found to be made up of smaller and smaller parts. For example, in the mid-50s in the United States, physicians often recorded simply "coronary thrombosis" or "coronary artery occlusion" as sufficient. As diagnostic resources improved, experts in cardiology pointed out that the specific artery occluded was important in diagnosis, treatment, and prognosis. The diagnoses then became more specific, and the resulting diagnostic entities more discrete.

Until *ICD-8* was put in use in 1965, AMI was included in a category labeled "Heart diseases specified as involving coronary arteries." Thus no estimates as to morbidity or mortality of AMI can be made from hospital data or death certificates recorded prior to 1965, when AMI was given its own pigeonhole, even though the medical records (and death certificates) themselves contained the information. Returning to the original medical records is so impractical that no studies requiring greater detail prior to the provision of the needed categories can be mounted.

A further problem arose when, in response to clinicians' demands, the modification of *ICD-8* by the Commission on Professional and Hospital Activities (CPHA), H-ICDA, added a refinement by designating the anatomical site, e.g., "anterior," and subdivided the category accordingly. The "official" modification produced by the United States government (ICDA-8), which was in use simultaneously with H-ICDA for about half the nation's hospitalizations, used a different schema, subdividing AMI as to whether or not it was accompanied by hypertension. Currently, *ICD-9-CM*, but not *ICD-9*, its parent volume, has the anatomical subdivisions.

So data which have already been category coded to different classifications in which the categories have different definitions cannot be accurately compared or aggregated. Under these circumstances, studies which need to count the same things (apples and apples) over time often have to be ruled out. While getting back to the original medical records (if they can be located) may reveal the essential detail, this is often impossible, or at least prohibitively expensive. A compromise sometimes is to water down the study by making the grouping so broad that the cases are sure to be included, whatever the classification. For example, "heart disease" is sure to include AMI.

This inability to carry out essential longitudinal studies may be shrugged off as an academic problem, just an annoyance in the cloisters. But the fact is that we need to know what is going on in health and in healthcare over periods longer than the nominal decade between revisions of *ICD*. Are genetic defects really increasing or declining? We might be able to judge a question that broad if we could aggregate all the kinds of genetic defects. But we may be completely thwarted if we wish to pinpoint the specific kinds of defect which are increasing or declining. The explosion in knowledge in this field compounds the issue. We need to add the "missing link" in our medical knowledge by making sure we retain enough discrete, unambiguous information that we can confidently compare data over time. This means not only coding clinical entities, but also permanently identifying each entity and category code so that it becomes unique in its meaning.

"Crosswalks" Don't Solve the Problem

"Crosswalks" or "conversion tables" are often proposed as solutions to the problems of changing category contents and shifts in the placement of entities within categories. Crosswalks are tables attempting to show that what was, say, category 200 in one classification is category 210 in another. Of course, in a few instances, a given category has no changes between classifications, either in its label or its content, and 200 really is the same as 210. Most of the time, however, this is not true, and footnotes or disclaimers appear in the crosswalks.

Example

Crosswalk to ICD-10-CM

When the United States National Center for Health Statistics (NCHS) undertook the construction of *ICD-10-CM*, they also commissioned ZKC Associates Ltd. to produce a crosswalk, entitled *"ICD-9-CM* to *ICD-10-CM* Conversion."

The table is prefaced with a note that the "pound sign (#) following an *ICD-10-CM* code indicates the best match of one to many matches." There are 4 modifiers for the pound sign. These modifiers, labeled "Best-Match Mechanics," pertain to what the analysts did with NOS (Not Otherwise Specified) and NEC (Not Elsewhere Classified) codes, and apparent discrepancies between codes and index entries. The fourth modifier, "d," is especially revealing: "Some of the designations are mostly intuitive." Overall, over 13% of the "matches" have one of the cautions appended (4648 out of 35082). The rates range from 10% to 19% among the chapters of *ICD-9-CM*.

It should be further noted that the table carries the English labels for the categories in truncated form. Truncation is used to make sure that the label can fit into a designated space on a printed form or a limited-length field in a database (common length is about 25 characters, including spaces). Both *ICD-9-CM* and *ICD-10-CM* truncate labels to 24 characters, a constriction which, of course, changes the original term and often interferes with understanding, i.e., one would have to refer to the original classifications to understand exactly what the label of the category really was.

Sample pages of the *ICD-9-CM* to *ICD-10-CM Conversion* follow this page.

Figure 14.2 ICD-9-CM-to-ICD-10-CM Conversion
Infectious and Parasitic Diseases

Infectious and Parasitic Diseases				Page 55 of 56	
ICD-9-CM Code	**ICD-9-CM Abbreviated Title**	**ICD-10-CM Code**	**Best Match**	**ICD-10-CM Abbreviated Title**	
136.5	SARCOSPORIDIOSIS	A07.8		PROTOZOAL GI DIS NEC	
136.8	INFECT/PARASITIC DIS NEC	B60.0		BABESIOSIS	
136.8	INFECT/PARASITIC DIS NEC	B60.8		PROTOZOAL DISEASE NEC	
136.8	INFECT/PARASITIC DIS NEC	B64		PROTOZOAL DISEASE NOS	
136.8	INFECT/PARASITIC DIS NEC	B99	#a	INFECTIOUS DIS NEC/NOS	
136.9	INFECT/PARASITIC DIS NOS	B89		PARASITIC DISEASE NOS	
137	LATE EFFECT-TUBERCULOSIS				
137.0	LATE EFFECTS-RESP TB/NOS	B90.9		SEQUELAE OF RESP TB	
137.1	LATE EFFECTS OF CNS TB	B90.0		SEQUELAE OF CNS TB	
137.2	LATE EFFCT-GENITOURIN TB	B90.1		SEQUELAE OF GU TB	
137.3	LATE EFFCT-BONE/JOINT TB	B90.2		SEQUELAE OF BONE TB	
137.4	LATE EFFECTS OF TB NEC	B90.8		SEQUELAE OF TB NEC	
138	LATE EFFECTS OF AC POLIO	B91		SEQUELAE OF POLIO	
139	LATE EFF-OTH INF/PARASIT				
139.0	LATE EFFECT-VIRAL ENCEPH	B94.1		SEQUELAE OF VIRAL ENCEPH	
139.1	LATE EFFECTS OF TRACHOMA	B94.0		SEQUELAE OF TRACHOMA	
139.8	LATE EFF-INF/PARASIT NEC	B92		SEQUELAE OF LEPROSY	
139.8	LATE EFF-INF/PARASIT NEC	B94.2		SEQUELAE OF VIRAL HEPATI	
139.8	LATE EFF-INF/PARASIT NEC	B94.8		SEQUELAE INFEC/PARA NEC	
139.8	LATE EFF-INF/PARASIT NEC	B94.9	#a	SEQUELAE INFEC/PARA NOS	

BEST-MATCH MECHANICS

1. IF THE ICD-9-CM CODE INCLUDES ALL ENTITIES CONTAINED IN THE ICD-10-CM CODES AND THE LIST OF ICD-10-CM CODES INCLUDES ONE WHICH IS DESIGNATED NOS, THAT IS CONSIDERED BEST-MATCH. SEE #a

2. IF THE ICD-9-CM CODE INCLUDES ALL ENTITIES CONTAINED IN THE ICD-10-CM CODES AND THE LIST OF ICD-10-CM CODES DOES NOT INCLUDE ONE WHICH IS DESIGNATED NOS BUT DOES INCLUDE ONE THAT IS DESIGNATED NEC, THAT IS CONSIDERED BEST-MATCH. SEE #b

3. IF THE ICD-9-CM CODE CAN BE MATCHED TO AN ICD-10-CM CODE BY INSPECTION ALONE, BUT STUDY OF THE CONCATENATED FILE REVEALS INDEX ENTRIES TO THAT ICD-9-CM CODE FROM OTHER ICD-10-CM CODES, THE BEST-MATCH IS THE OBVIOUS ONE. SEE #c

4. SOME OF THE DESIGNATIONS ARE MOSTLY INTUITIVE. SEE #d

Sample page from Chapter 1 of *ICD-9-CM to ICD-10-CM Conversion*, showing key to "Best Match Mechanics." © 1997 ZKC Associates Ltd.

Figure 14.3 ICD-9-CM to ICD-10-CM Conversion
Congenital Anomalies

Congenital Anomalies

ICD-9-CM Code	ICD-9-CM Abbreviated Title	ICD-10-CM Code	Best Match	ICD-10-CM Abbreviated Title
750.9	CONG UPPR GI ANOMALY NOS	Q38.8		PHARYNX ANOMALY NEC/NOS
750.9	CONG UPPR GI ANOMALY NOS	Q39.9		ESOPHAGEAL ANOMALY NOS
750.9	CONG UPPR GI ANOMALY NOS	Q40.3		STOMACH ANOMALY NOS
750.9	CONG UPPR GI ANOMALY NOS	Q40.9	#a	UPPER ALIMENT ANOMAL NOS
751	OTH CONG ANOM DIGEST SYS			
751.0	MECKEL'S DIVERTICULUM	Q43.0		MECKEL'S DIVERTICULUM
751.1	CNG ATRES/STEN SM INTEST	Q41.0		DUOD ABSENC/ATRES/STENOS
751.1	CNG ATRES/STEN SM INTEST	Q41.1		JEJ ABSENCE/ATRES/STENOS
751.1	CNG ATRES/STEN SM INTEST	Q41.2		ILEUM ABSEN/ATRES/STENOS
751.1	CNG ATRES/STEN SM INTEST	Q41.8		ABSEN/ATRES SM BOWEL NEC
751.1	CNG ATRES/STEN SM INTEST	Q41.9	#a	ABSEN/ATRES SM BOWEL NOS
751.2	CNG ATRES/STEN LG INTEST	Q42.0		RECT ABSEN/ATRES/STN&FST
751.2	CNG ATRES/STEN LG INTEST	Q42.1		RECT ATRES/STEN-NO FISTU
751.2	CNG ATRES/STEN LG INTEST	Q42.2		ANUS ABSEN/ATRES/STN&FST
751.2	CNG ATRES/STEN LG INTEST	Q42.3		ANUS ATRES/STEN-NO FISTU
751.2	CNG ATRES/STEN LG INTEST	Q42.8		ABSEN/ATRES LG BOWEL NEC
751.2	CNG ATRES/STEN LG INTEST	Q42.9	#a	ABSEN/ATRES LG BOWEL NOS
751.3	HIRSCHSPRUNG'S DISEASE	Q43.1	#c	HIRSCHSPRUNG'S DISEASE
751.3	HIRSCHSPRUNG'S DISEASE	Q43.2		COLON DYSFUNCTION NEC
751.4	CONG ANOM INTESTN FIXATN	Q43.3		INTESTINE FIXATION ANOM
751.5	CONG ANOM INTESTINES NEC	Q43.4		INTESTINAL DUPLICATION
751.5	CONG ANOM INTESTINES NEC	Q43.5		ECTOPIC ANUS
751.5	CONG ANOM INTESTINES NEC	Q43.6		CONG RECTUM/ANUS FISTUL
751.5	CONG ANOM INTESTINES NEC	Q43.7		PERSISTENT CLOACA
751.5	CONG ANOM INTESTINES NEC	Q43.8	#b	INTESTINE/ANUS ANOM NEC
751.6	ANOMALY-GB/BILE DCT/LIVR			
751.60	CNG ANOM-GB/DUCT/LVR NOS	Q44.1		GALLBLADDER ANOM NEC/NOS
751.60	CNG ANOM-GB/DUCT/LVR NOS	Q44.5	#d	BILE DUCT ANOMAL NEC/NOS
751.60	CNG ANOM-GB/DUCT/LVR NOS	Q44.7		LIVER ANOMALY NEC/NOS
751.61	CONGENIT BILIARY ATRESIA	P61.0		TRANS NEONAT THROMBOCYTO
751.61	CONGENIT BILIARY ATRESIA	Q44.2	#c	ATRESIA OF BILE DUCT(S)
751.61	CONGENIT BILIARY ATRESIA	Q44.3		BILE DUCT STENOS/STRICT
751.62	CONGEN CYSTIC LIVER DIS	Q44.6		CYSTIC LIVER DISEASE
751.69	CNG ANOM-GB/DUCT/LVR NEC	Q44.0		GALLBLAD AGENES/HYPOPLAS
751.69	CNG ANOM-GB/DUCT/LVR NEC	Q44.1		GALLBLADDER ANOM NEC/NOS
751.69	CNG ANOM-GB/DUCT/LVR NEC	Q44.4		CHOLEDOCHAL CYST

Page 12

Sample page from Chapter 14 of *ICD-9-CM to ICD-10-CM Conversion*, showing increased degree of detail in diagnoses. © 1997 ZKC Associates Ltd.

Figure 14.4 ICD-9-CM to ICD-10-CM Conversion
Injury and Poisoning

Injury and Poisoning

ICD-9-CM Code	ICD-9-CM Abbreviated Title	ICD-10-CM Code	Best Match	ICD-10-CM Abbreviated Title
800.2	CL SKULL VLT FX/HEMORRHG			
800.20	CL SK VLT FX/HEM-CNS NOS	S02.029	#c	C VL SK FX-DHEM/COMA NOS
800.20	CL SK VLT FX/HEM-CNS NOS	S07.1		CRUSHING INJURY OF SKULL
800.21	CL SK VLT FX/HEM-NO LOSS	S02.020	#c	CL VAULT SK FX DURAL HEM
800.21	CL SK VLT FX/HEM-NO LOSS	S07.1		CRUSHING INJURY OF SKULL
800.22	CL SK VLT FX/HEM-BRF LOS	S02.021	#c	C V SK FX-DHEM/<1 HR COM
800.22	CL SK VLT FX/HEM-BRF LOS	S07.1		CRUSHING INJURY OF SKULL
800.23	CL SK VLT FX/HEM-MOD LOS	S02.022	#c	C V SK FX-DH/1-24HR COMA
800.23	CL SK VLT FX/HEM-MOD LOS	S07.1		CRUSHING INJURY OF SKULL
800.24	CL SK VLT FX/HEM-LNG LOS	S02.023	#c	C V SK FX-DH/>24 COM&RTN
800.24	CL SK VLT FX/HEM-LNG LOS	S07.1		CRUSHING INJURY OF SKULL
800.25	CL SK VLT FX/HM-LS/NO RT	S02.024	#c	C V SK FX-DHEM/>24HR COM
800.25	CL SK VLT FX/HM-LS/NO RT	S07.1		CRUSHING INJURY OF SKULL
800.26	CL SK VLT FX/HEM-LOS NOS	S02.029	#c	C VL SK FX-DHEM/COMA NOS
800.26	CL SK VLT FX/HEM-LOS NOS	S07.1		CRUSHING INJURY OF SKULL
800.29	CL SK VLT FX/HEM-CONCUSS	S02.029	#c	C VL SK FX-DHEM/COMA NOS
800.29	CL SK VLT FX/HEM-CONCUSS	S07.1		CRUSHING INJURY OF SKULL
800.3	CL SK VLT FX/CRN HEM NEC			
800.30	CL VLT FX/HM NEC-CNS NOS	S02.039	#c	CL VL SK FX-HEM/COMA NOS
800.30	CL VLT FX/HM NEC-CNS NOS	S07.1		CRUSHING INJURY OF SKULL
800.31	CL VLT FX/HEM NEC-NO LOS	S02.030	#c	CL VAULT SK FX HEMOR NOS
800.31	CL VLT FX/HEM NEC-NO LOS	S07.1		CRUSHING INJURY OF SKULL
800.32	CL VLT FX/HEM NEC-BR LOS	S02.031	#c	C VL SK FX-HEM/<1 HR COM
800.32	CL VLT FX/HEM NEC-BR LOS	S07.1		CRUSHING INJURY OF SKULL
800.33	CL VLT FX/HEM NEC-MD LOS	S02.032	#c	C V SK FX-HM/1-24HR COMA
800.33	CL VLT FX/HEM NEC-MD LOS	S07.1		CRUSHING INJURY OF SKULL
800.34	CL VLT FX/HEM NEC-LG LOS	S02.033	#c	C V SK FX-HM/>24 COM&RTN
800.34	CL VLT FX/HEM NEC-LG LOS	S07.1		CRUSHING INJURY OF SKULL
800.35	CL SK VLT FX/HM-LS/NO RT	S02.034	#c	C V SK FX-HEM/>24HR COMA
800.35	CL SK VLT FX/HM-LS/NO RT	S07.1		CRUSHING INJURY OF SKULL
800.36	CL VLT FX/HM NEC-LOS NOS	S02.039	#c	CL VL SK FX-HEM/COMA NOS
800.36	CL VLT FX/HM NEC-LOS NOS	S07.1		CRUSHING INJURY OF SKULL
800.39	CL S VLT FX/HEM NEC-CONC	S02.039	#c	CL VL SK FX-HEM/COMA NOS
800.39	CL S VLT FX/HEM NEC-CONC	S07.1		CRUSHING INJURY OF SKULL

Sample page from Chapter 17 of *ICD-9-CM to ICD-10-CM Conversion*. Note the variety of combination codes in ICD-10-CM. © 1997 ZKC Associates Ltd.

Making Meaning Precise

By this time it should be clear that we need a better, foolproof way to handle the coding/decoding problem. There are ways — if we put our powerful technological tools together with what we've learned over the years.

How We Understand Information

First, let's examine how we understand information, starting with language. A word, like a code, is a unit of information. But words can have a number of different meanings, depending upon their language of origin and the context in which they stand. For most words, there is no unambiguous meaning — meaning comes from language, culture, context (this is why we can't just use words as codes).

"Art", for example, can mean an "asthetic object" in English, but in German it may mean "kind" or "species." Within a language, the reader still must know the context to determine the meaning of a single instance of usage of the word. Consider the following usages of the word "art":

> Life is short and the art long.
>
> Hippocrates

> The most beautiful thing we can experience is the mysterious. It is the source of all true art and all science. He to whom this emotion is a stranger, who can no longer pause to wonder and stand rapt in awe, is as good as dead: his eyes are closed.
>
> Albert Einstein

And words change their meanings over time. Translators of the Bible respond to this, because they are driven, in part, by fear that the words used centuries ago will not be understood properly by today's readers. Either the words are no longer in use and will not carry any meaning, or usage has changed their meanings, and the modern reader will be misled.

So just as it is important to know a word's context, the time of its use must also be known. Consider *this* usage of the word "art":

> Tell me thy company, and I will tell thee what thou art.
>
> Miguel de Cervantes, *Don Quixote*

Just so, the context of any bit of information is essential to understanding its meaning. Where did it come from? When? Depending on the type of code, other essential information may include subject of the code, unit of measure, and so forth.

So to understand information — or to receive and decode messages — we usually need "supporting information." We need the code, plus identification to place it in the proper context. A parallel can be found in international commerce, where goods are sent — in a standard format and with clear identification — all over the world.

The Secrets of Commerce

During the mid-1950s (about the same time the senior author began harnessing computers to healthcare information), the international shipping of goods went through a major revolution — *containerization*. This method allowed many and varied goods to be securely packaged and labeled in one container at the point of origin, and shipped great distances via ship, train, and truck — all without needing to be unpacked and repacked along the route. This method worked so well that by the mid-1960s our language had a new word: "containership" (sometimes "container ship" is used). By 1970, containerships were loading and unloading in special "containerports." The hallmark of this cargo "container" is that it is a worldwide standard, and commerce now depends on it.[2] For all practical purposes it has become an international standard volume measurement as well, as manufacturers buy and sell items in "container" quantities.

---

2.   For more about standards, see "Standards for Health Information," page 247.

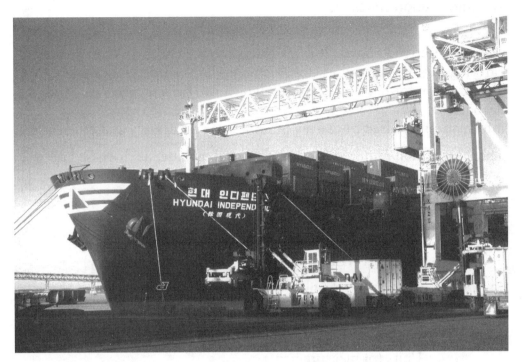

Containership and loading crane. Photo by David Wasserman for Artville.

Approximately 20 years after the shipping industry agreed on its containers, the information industry began to develop its own electronic version of these standard containers. Research begun in the mid-1970s (funded by the U.S. government, including the Department of Health and Human Services) resulted in a set of standards, known as "TCP/IP protocols." These protocols define how all electronic (digital) information can be packaged into containers called "datagrams" (sometimes more generally referred to as "packets"), which may then be shipped across the world or down the hall. Each datagram contains, among other things, the addresses of its source and destination, so that special computers known as "routers" can send the container along its way.

✓ Just as with containerized cargo, the world now enjoys the benefits of "information containerization," as vast amounts of information travel the shipping lanes of the Internet.

The Information "Package"

An effective coding system will have much in common with the two systems described above. It is instructive to see codes as "containers" carrying cargo — messages. Each time we code something, we are creating an information "package" which can be sent, received, and decoded to reveal a message. The "package" should include all information required to convey that message accurately and efficiently.

The information required for decoding will include, as discussed above, one or more of the following:

> Context
>> Domain (healthcare, retail goods, demographics)
>> Code list (ICD-9-CM, CPT, ISBN, Social Security)
>> Time (year of publication, date of use)
> Type of information
>> Language (English, Spanish, etc.)
>> Units (of measurement)
> Other essential information

Or, like a good news story, the code package must tell:

> Who
> What
> When
> Where
> Why

This essential information — what you need to decode — we're calling here the "key" for that code; it's what you need to unlock the meaning of the message. In a previous chapter we said that the actual characters making up the code itself were its "value" (see "Codes & Coding," page 117). If we view the code package as travelling like the ship container, the code's "value" is the cargo and the "key" is the labeled container.

✓ A *key* contains everything required to permit the code to be decoded.

Self-Identifying Codes

Every healthcare code should carry a "key" with it, permanently, to provide whatever is needed to determine the exact meaning of its value. Often, the key will quite simply provide the "code list" where that code originated. Knowing the list, the decoder can easily look up the code to find its meaning. Especially if the code list (coding system) is standardized and "registered" (see), the "key" need only identify the code list; then all other information needed (language, domain, etc.) can be looked up in the code list itself.

We'll call such codes here "self-identifying codes" ("SICs"):

value + key = self-identifying code

The ISBN Code Example

An example of such a code is "ISBN 0-9615255-2-5" — the code which uniquely and permanently identifies this very book to the rest of the world. Looking up the value "0961525525" in any ISBN database (that contains this number) will always yield the title of this book, plus whatever other fields of information have been linked to it (such as authors, price, publisher, etc.). It should be noted that in this example, while the letters "ISBN" are not actually a part of the ISBN code *value*, they are essential to give meaning to the ten digits. We refer to the letters "ISBN" as the "key" for this code.

In fact, when the ISBN number is encoded into a EAN-13 bar code symbol (the "zebra stripes"), as it is on the back cover of this book (and in the illustration below), it becomes a self-identifying code — it provides enough information, by itself, for decoding it precisely.

Figure 14.5 ISBN Bar Code Example

ISBN 0-9615255-2-5

Any bar code reader that "understands" the EAN-13 bar code system (and most do) will correctly interpret the bar code symbol to reveal both the code's value *and* the fact that it belongs to the master ISBN database. The EAN-13 system has the number "978" — for "Bookland," a fictitious land of books — precede the ISBN number itself, to identify the code as an ISBN number. This is why the bar code on a book is often called the "EAN Bookland" bar code.[3]

Background	EAN International

EAN International

In 1974, the "European Article Numbering Association" (EAN) was formed to develop a standard article numbering (coding) system for Europe, similar to the UPC (Uniform Product Code) developed by the Uniform Code Council (UCC) and used in the U.S. The successful system grew to be used outside Europe, and in 1992, EAN changed its name to EAN International.

The system — now called EAN-UCC — is most commonly known for its bar codes and Electronic Data Interchange (EDI) standards. It's managed by EAN International in 94 countries around the world, and in North America by the UCC in collaboration with the Electronic Commerce Council of Canada (ECCC).

---

3. The barcoded equivalent of an ISBN number uses the very last digit as a "check digit" to verify that the code was accurately read in the first place. This explains why the final digit of the human-readable number, often printed under the bar code stripes, frequently is different than the final digit of the original ISBN, which is itself a "check digit."

The EAN-UCC system consists of:

- A system for numbering items (consumer products and services, transport units, locations, etc.) which permits their unambiguous identification.

- A system for representing supplementary information (batch number, date, measurement, etc.).

- Standard bar codes to represent information which can be easily read by computers (scanned).

- A set of messages for EDI transactions (EANCOM messages).

Key to the success of the system are the "Numbering Organisations" (NOs), national associations that provide full EAN-UCC system implementation support, in the local language, to their member companies. The NOs:

- Allocate numbers.

- Provide training on numbering, bar coding, and EDI.

- Supply information on the standards and on the evolution of the system.

More information is available at the EAN website, http://www.ean.be.

Tagging Healthcare Codes

Making our healthcare codes self-identifying is essential to eliminate the ambiguity plaguing us today. We need to make sure that *every code*, whether entity or category, carries with it a key which tells the user exactly the source of the code:

- The name of the "code series" to which it belongs, e.g., *ICD-9-CM*, *ICD-10*, "International Health Entity Codes" (IHEC), etc., and

- The specific version of the classification, e.g., 1997 modification, and

- Any further correction or modification of the series, and

- Any other information found to be essential.

Entity codes Once an *entity code* is combined with its key, that "key + value" *combination* will become unique, and we will always be able to accurately decode it. It will be:

- permanently assigned

- to a single *unique entity* (the diagnosis entity as found in the master list)

Category codes Similarly, once a *category code* is combined with its key, that "key + value" *combination* will be:

- permanently assigned

- to a single *unique category* (the diagnosis category, as defined in a certain place, at a certain time)

- and we'll always be able to decode it accurately

For example, with the *ICD* series, the key should tell at least:

> ICD + Revision Number + "Edition" (e.g., U.S. Clinical Modification) +
> Version Number (e.g., "1998") + Errata (date or number)

Thus keys could have solved the swine flu vaccine incidence problem in the earlier example, in which the investigator was trying to find at least which *category* would contain the condition. The category in which to find Guillain-Barré syndrome might be given "key + value" combinations as follows:

Figure 14.6 Tagged Codes for Finding Guillain-Barré Syndrome (GBS)

Sample Key — Components				Code	Label of Category Containing GBS
Classifi-cation	Modifi-cation	Edition	Version		
ICD	7	W[a]	X[b]	357	Other diseases of spinal cord
ICD	8	W	X	354	Polyneuritis and polyradiculitis
ICD	9	CM[c]	X	357.0	Acute infective polyneuritis [d]
ICD	10	W	X	G61.0	Guillain Barré Syndrome (Acute (post-)infective polyneuritis

a. "W" standing for the international version published by WHO.

b. "X" meaning the original, without modification. Zero wouldn't be used, nor would 1, because of the possible confusion with the letters O and I.

c. "CM" meaning the clinical modification published by the United States.

d. This category represents *only* GBS.

So here is how these codes might look:

ICD7WX-357	=	Other diseases of spinal cord
ICD8WX-354	=	Polyneuritis and polyradiculitis
ICD9CMX-357.0	=	Acute infective polyneuritis
ICD10WX-G61.0	=	Guillain-Barré syndrome

And see what a difference a key would make with this *ICD* code, for example:

395

If we (1) *already know* that this is an *ICD* code, and (2) have the luxury of several editions of *ICD* on hand, we can narrow down its meaning to:

Ménière's disease (*ICD-6 & 7*)

Diseases of aortic valve (*ICD-8 & 9*)

Which of course leaves us nowhere; these aren't even in the same body system! But if the code was self-identifying, it might look like this:

ICD7WX-395, or

ICD8WX-395

And we'd know exactly where to look it up.

Example

Keys for clinical concepts

If there are to be serious studies of health and healthcare over time, it is also essential that a unique identification — key + code — be attached to clinical concepts. This has not, to the authors' knowledge, ever been a part of any information system. To illustrate how this would work, the authors of *DSM* could have attached their own "concept code," with its key, to each of the concepts they defined in the first edition (see "The Concept of AD/HD," page 266). Then with each refinement of the definition of the concept in succeeding editions, a new code + key would be assigned to the new definition.

As the old code appeared in records after the "changeover date," it would have been clear what definition was being used — the old concept code would have referred to the concept definition in effect during the time between its appearance, and the time it was supplanted by a newer definition.

The computer could easily relate the constellation of symptoms of the particular patient and diagnosis. The computer could also generate the list of subconcepts, working "backward" from the concept definition, and reaggregate them under different definitions.

For example, the "Tetralogy of Fallot" is a specific constellation of four congenital heart defects occurring together:

(1) ventricular septal defect
(2) pulmonic valve stenosis or infundibular stenosis
(3) dextroposition of the aorta
(4) right ventricular hypertrophy

The computer could generate the list of these four components — each of them could also be found separately.

The Luxury of Space

Some may view the "tagging" idea as "excessive" — taking up too many resources. That is almost an instinctive reaction for those of us who grew up in the "early days" of data processing (perhaps 10 or 15 years ago!). In those days, space for storing information was at a premium. Initially, hospital discharge abstract systems used punch cards: eighty columns per card, one card per case.[4] Data systems had to be cleverly designed to compact an entire case into that card. When we switched from *SNDO* to *ICD*, the mere shortening of the code was a great advance.

But there is such a thing as false economy, and this has been amply demonstrated by the cost of the Y2K problem. In earlier days, computers were slower and storage was limited. Many programmers dealt with the limitations by saving space in programs: the year could be represented by just two digits — why bother putting "19" at the beginning of each date? It worked for awhile, but then billions of dollars and hours had to be spent to remedy the shortsightedness, as we suddenly realized that to our computers, the year "2000" would be indistinguishable from "1900."

Now, thanks to continuing advances in informatics technology (and lessons learned from Y2K), we can start with what we want and need, and not be inhibited by "economy thinking." We can design our health information system to take full advantage of the vast storage capacity and sheer processing power available.

---

4.   For more about hospital discharge abstract systems, see page 103.

Standards for Keys

Imagine a tagged code as a shipping container fully loaded with its cargo. Just like the other "containers" discussed above, the structure and content of the key must be standardized. That way, anyone can understand where the container came from, what's in it, and where it's going. And it will "fit" in its place in the system.

Self-identifying codes are not a new idea. As we have seen, the book world depends on the ISBN number, which is always identified as such; the number never travels by itself (see page 307). And since the mid-1990s, we've all become familiar with codes like "http://www.tringa.com," in which the "http://" is essentially a "key" for the Uniform Resource Locator (URL) code value of "www.tringa.com".

What makes the above coding systems useful is that they can be depended on. Vast resources have been expended on systems that depend on these codes to yield precisely the same information each time. In 1999, someone spent 7.5 million dollars for the rights to use one code from the URL master list — the code's value was "business.com". This type of expenditure requires a great deal of confidence in the coding system.

In the above examples, there are one or more organizations who are responsible for maintaining the master code list for each system. Someone is ensuring that there are never any duplicate codes issued, and someone is ensuring that everyone who uses the codes follows the rules required to make the coding systems work. Both systems have much in common, even though the ISBN code decodes into a thing (book), and the URL code decodes into a place (website).

For healthcare codes to be as effective as the above two examples, there must also be a "keeper of the master list" for each coding system used. For diagnosis and other entity codes, we have elsewhere in this book suggested a secretariat for this function (see "Creating the Master List," page 283). It would also be useful to have a registry (a "list of lists") with which all code keys could be registered. Organizations like the American National Standards Institute (ANSI) already have programs in place to provide this type of service (see more at http://www.ansi.org/).

The key registration process would include (just as the current ISBN and URL registrations do) submitting information relevant to decoding the particular code involved. With this in place, a computer could be programmed so that whenever it was confronted with a code it didn't recognize, it would simply look up the code's key in the registry, and then proceed to decode the code with the information it had obtained from the registry.

Markup Language May Hold the "Key"

One possible tool for tagging "key" information onto diagnosis and other healthcare codes is "markup language."[5] Markup includes any method used to specify the meaning or interpretation of a quantity of free-form data, typically text. Markup adds instructions on how the data should appear, be structured, or otherwise enhanced. Marking a word to be **bolded**, for instance, is called an "appearance directive." Marking a phrase as "CHAPTER HEADING" is specifying a "structural" element. Marking a word or phrase to be a **hypertext link** creates a connection to other information (such links are plentiful on the Internet; clicking one takes you to another page or site). In electronic documents, including those produced by most wordprocessing programs, this is done by inserting special coded instructions into the text itself. These coded instructions, commonly referred to as "tags," are not usually visible on the computer display or in the printed document. Most of what you see with your Internet browser is controlled by markup language.

A markup language is a system that specifies which tags are required and which are optional (and under what circumstances), the syntax of the tags (how they're distinguished from the document content itself), and what the tags themselves mean. The most famous markup language in existence today is HTML (HyperText Markup Language), since it forms the basis for almost every web page on the Internet. Rapidly catching up is XML (eXtensible Markup Language), the markup language we'll discuss here. Like HTML, XML is derived from SGML (Standard

---

5.   The authors are not recommending or promoting any specific kind of markup language nor, for that matter, any markup language at all. This section is included to give some idea of the state of technology today (early 2000), and how that technology might be helpful in providing health information solutions.

Generalized Markup Language).[6] Like SGML, XML employs a type of coding often referred to as "semantic" coding because it focusses on the *meaning* of the data rather than simply its appearance.

Markup languages typically surround the subject text with starting and ending tags, often delimited by angled brackets (<xxxxx> and </xxxxx>). In XML, the capability of any start tag can be extended by adding additional information via its "attribute=value" structure. This feature of XML might be utilized to tag healthcare codes. For example, a diagnosis code (I21.1, acute transmural myocardial infarction of anterior wall) appearing in the medical record might be tagged as follows:

```
<DXCODE Type="ICD-10" Version="1.0" Lang="English">I21.1</DXCODE>
```

The attributes feature can *also be used to provide security and privacy information, as well as audit trail data.*

Markup languages may be either proprietary or based on (open) standards. If used for healthcare codes, it would be essential that the language was standardized, open, and universally available, so that codes could be easily interpreted and data readily exchanged.

Another strength of XML is that it allows text to be organized and structured, much like fields and records allow the data in databases to be organized and structured.[7] What makes XML "extensible" and so useful is its "Document Type Definition" (DTD) concept, inherited from SGML. The DTD is the master plan that governs how the information in the document will be structured and stored, much like the structure definition of a database. The DTD essentially defines information "containers" (similar to fields in a database) which users then assign text

---

6. A wonderfully concise overview of the possible contributions that SGML and its progeny might make to the electronic medical record (EMR) was written by British author Tim Benson in 1996. Our EMR compares to the British electronic *patient* record (EPR). Benson's work is entitled *SGML, HTML and EPR: Application of the Standard Generalized Markup Language (SGML) in Electronic Patient Records*, Version 2.0, 11 September 1996. It was commissioned by the British National Health Service (NHS) Executive's EPR Project Board. Benson's article is silent as to XML (since it hadn't been "invented" yet) but from his assessment of the technology then it follows that he would likely support the use of XML in electronic medical records today. The fact that his article is as relevant today as it was then shows just how much foresight Benson had at the time. The complete article was still available online in January of 2000, at http://www.mcis.duke.edu/ standards/HL7/committees/sgml/references/sgmlepr.htm.

7. See page 172 for a brief overview of database management.

The freedom to create DTDs to suit any purpose may well be XML's greatest advantage. It may also be the greatest challenge for its adoption and successful implementation by the healthcare informatics community. To enable the collection, exchange, and consumption of healthcare information, we would need to reach agreement on what DTDs would be defined and used, and under what circumstances. This is yet one more "standards" challenge that must be met, aside from all the challenges presented by the technology itself. (See "Standards for Health Information," page 247.)

Nonetheless, XML is in fact increasingly being accepted by the healthcare industry, including its use in EMRs. The standards challenge posed by XML is being met head-on by the Health Level 7 (HL7) Patient Record Architecture (PRA) effort, which is being proposed as an addition to HL7's existing standards. HL7 defines PRA as "an XML framework for document exchange, manipulation, portability and longevity for health care." Acceptance of XML here may make it easier to develop and implement standards for tagged healthcare codes.[8]

So as this is being written in the beginning of the year 2000, XML and related SGML technologies appear to hold great promise for helping us live more successfully with our healthcare "code-dependency." There is no reason to believe that XML-type technology can't be used as the "glue" language that helps us get all our other information applications communicating with each other. As we move forward, however, it's essential that we keep our information needs and goals in sight. However we end up working with healthcare codes, it's mandatory that each code be permanently accompanied by its key, so that it doesn't get "lost" in the shuffle.

---

8.   The first level of the PRA development already makes a provision for "containers" that can hold what PRA calls a "'healthcare.code' — an association between a piece of text and an HL7-recognized coded vocabulary such as SNOMED or LOINC or ICD-9 ... " The containers can be any paragraph, list item, table cell, or "chunk" (a paragraph component) containing clinical information and found in a document in the medical record itself. At this point, however, the necessity for unique identification of codes (self-identifying codes, as we have termed them) is not apparently a subject within the HL7 effort. For additional details, see "Introducing HL7's Patient Record Architecture" by Liora Alschuler, Co-Chair, HL7 XML SIG, in the January 2000 *HL7 News*. Also see additional references to PRA at http://www.hl7.org.

15

Expanding Classification Possibilities

EVERY CLASSIFICATION is developed for a specific purpose. Its use for other purposes is never optimal. *ICD-9-CM* is a multipurpose classification, attempting to serve many masters. *ICD* is most suitable for its original use, international comparisons of mortality and morbidity data. Yet it also "seeks to meet the needs of policymakers, statisticians, third-party payers, managers, clinicians, and investigators in a wide range of socio-economic and cultural settings around the world."[1]

When *ICD* was modified for "clinical" use in U. S. hospitals (i.e., for uses other than morbidity and mortality statistics, such as disease indexing and inter- and intrahospital comparisons of practice), additional demands were placed on it.

And by far, the most influential use of *ICD-9-CM* today is in the payment system, which stretches its uses even more. Any classification which tries to meet these competing demands must be a compromise, one which will never quite satisfy any user.

Karel Kupka, M.D., Secretary to the International Conference for the Ninth Revision of *ICD*,[2] has suggested that:

✓ "The fine art of compromise is making everyone equally unhappy."

---

1. Kerr L. White, *Historical Introduction to ICPC, International Classification of Primary Care*, Oxford University Press, 1987.

2. The International Conference for the Ninth Revision of the International Classification of Diseases was convened by the World Health Organization (WHO) in Geneva in 1975. Dr. Kupka was at that time the Chief Medical Officer for the International Classification of Diseases at WHO. The Conference was attended by delegations from 46 member nations. Participants also included representatives from the United Nations, the Organization for Economic Cooperation and Development, the International Labour Organisation, the International Agency for Research on Cancer, the Council for International Organizations of Medical Sciences and ten other international non-governmental organizations concerned with dental health, dermatology, gynecology and obstetrics, mental health, neurosurgery, ophthalmology, pediatrics, pathology, radiology, and rehabilitation of the disabled.

We can't have more than one classification in the system today, and thus satisfy the various constituencies, because, with the data already aggregated (into the *ICD-9-CM* categories), they can only be placed in broader, rather than different, groups. They can never be disaggregated so that one can start over and classify them another way.

Once data have been category coded, classifying those data for purposes other than the original one requires either:

1. "recoding" (a misnomer — it actually means "further grouping;" e.g., to DRGs, which compounds the problems of the original lack of specificity), or

2. going back to the original records to start over from the narrative.

Recoding, of course, usually makes the grouping less appropriate than the user would like. Going back to the original records on a large scale is prohibitively expensive, since the original medical records are the only place where the needed detail exists, and they are not yet in computer-accessible form. And they are likely to be in thousands of different settings from coast to coast.

We should work toward making the "system" more flexible, so that cases can be allocated to more than one classification — each tailored to a specific use. The key is to code smaller units of information, before the case is classified, so that those units can be retrieved and rearranged for other purposes. The entity coding "front end," discussed on page 277, would give us this flexibility. We would finally be able to build "custom" classifications.

Especially important would be classifications truly appropriate for billing under a variety of circumstances, e.g., inpatient vs. home care. Our acknowledged problems with DRGs are primarily due to the compromises which had to be made in DRG design because of the limitations of *ICD-9-CM*, the only available source of input at the time the DRGs were created.

The ability to have classifications tailored to different purposes is exciting. Each classification could obtain data directly from the detailed, entity-coded information rather than having to make do with already grouped data. Candidates for new classifications which come to mind include:

- Payment classifications correcting the perceived defects in DRGs for hospital care and APGs for outpatient care.
- Epidemiologic classifications focused at etiology, disability, or any other axis.
- Evidence-based medicine classifications.
- "Facilities-specific" groupings of patients.
- Groupings for public policy uses.

The list is limited only by the imagination of the user.

Opening the Door for Multiple Classifications

We need just three things in place to permit a virtually unlimited number of classifications:

- Entity-coded clinical information.
- Algorithms for allocating cases to each classification, using the entity-coded information as input.
- Moving the classification task to computers.

We're going inevitably in this direction, anyway, with the advances in technology and the overwhelming, growing volume of health information.

Let's assume that we have the entity coding "front end" in place, and are capturing a goodly portion of essential clinical information.

For each specific classification (such as *ICD-9-CM*), an expert "team" — nosologists (specialists in classification), clinicians, biomedical specialists, medical specialists, research scientists, computer experts, and whoever else is needed for the task — would create algorithms[3] to assign the entities (or groups of entities) to categories in that particular classification. This is exactly what the United States National Center for

---

3. An *algorithm* is a set of rules for carrying out a process, such as the care of a patient with a given set of problems, or the calculation of a statistic. The rules are such that a specific set of steps is required in sequence, with each step dependent on the preceding step.

Health Statistics (NCHS) did with MICAR for death certificate information, for both *ICD-9* and *ICD-10*.[4]

Then computer programs would be written, using the algorithms, to find the necessary entity coded information in the medical record and assign the case to the proper category, in whatever classification is being used. We'll call the process — using the computer to classify cases using diagnosis and other entity codes, as described below — "entity code classifying."

Entity Code Classifying

Of course, classifying starting with entity codes is not as simple as it looks. Because classifying in today's information system does not simply put diagnoses or procedures into groups, it puts *cases* (or *patients* or *episodes of illness*) into the groups. To do this grouping, the classifier, whether a person or a computer, must take into account information in addition to just the diagnosis or procedure. Guidance is provided by "classifying rules" in the classification itself. The task of algorithms is to turn these rules into explicit step-by-step procedures for actually doing the classifying.

For purposes of classifying cases, a diagnosis or procedure entity must usually be considered in the context of:

- the source of the information (institution, country)
- the patient's other attributes such as age, sex
- whether or not there was surgery
- any concomitant diagnoses (complications and comorbidity)
- laboratory values and other findings
- other factors

This means that placing a patient — a case — into either a diagnostic or procedure category can virtually never be done from one entity alone. The diagnosis or procedure is not the sole governing factor in classifying the case. The computer needs to know what other codes to pick up, and how to use them. Simple "mapping tables," which show where each

---

4.   See more about MICAR on page 491.

diagnosis or code belongs in the classification, are not adequate because they do not account for the rules and additional information needed.[5]

This challenge was tackled by the NCHS during the development of the Mortality Medical Data System (MMDS). The component known as the Automated Classification of Medical Entities (ACME) portion has a process to take the diagnoses on the death certificate and "automate the underlying cause-of-death coding rules." These rules are, of course, specific for both *ICD-9* and *ICD-10*.[6]

Entity Objects

We therefore need to capture from the record not only the diagnosis entity, but some other things as well.

✓ The "naked" diagnosis has to bring with it some clothes and luggage. We need a term to describe the traveler thus outfitted — we'll call it an "entity object."

For example, a *diagnosis entity object* would be a set of data containing the "diagnosis entity" plus the adjunct information needed to place the specific case in the proper category of a given classification (e.g., *ICD-9-CM*).

A given diagnosis entity will require different adjunct information for each classification into which it is to be placed. *ICD-9-CM*, for instance, requires different information in many categories than does *ICD-10-CM*. So the "diagnosis entity object" would always be "classification-specific." The objects would be defined by the specialists in that particular classification.

The following Venn diagram pictures the relationship of all the information about a patient, and that which is used in creating entity objects. The largest circle represents all of the information in the medical record. The smallest circle represents just the diagnosis entity (here, "Diagnosis Entity A"). The other two circles represent the complete diagnosis entity objects needed to classify the case to *ICD-9-CM* and to *ICD-10-CM*.

---

5.   One place where mapping tables are available is the Read Clinical Classification System (NHS Codes). See page 96.

6.   See more about MMDS in the appendices on page 491.

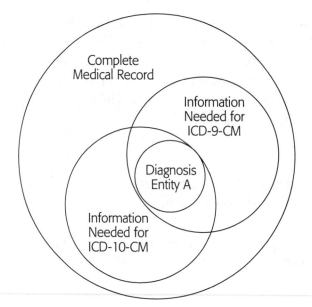

Illustration showing the relationship between all the information about a patient, and that which is used in creating entity objects for two different classifications, *ICD-9-CM* and *ICD-10-CM*.

The Adjunct Information

The attributes ("adjunct information") required for a given entity object might include demographic information, findings,[7] management, response, complications, comorbidity, and outcome. In fact, any item of information in the medical record may, for some classifications, be adjunct information necessary for proper categorization of the case. A great deal of this information is, in the electronic medical record, already in coded form and so accessible for carrying out the classifying process by computer. For example, patients' ages, laboratory values, drug

---

7.   "Findings" as used by Lawrence Weed in connection with Problem Knowledge Couplers means the items of information used to discriminate among possible causes or as factors used in guiding management. See Weed, L. *Knowledge Coupling: New Premises and New Tools for Medical Care and Education.* Springer-Verlag 1991.

identification, dosage, and treatment schedules (and more) are sent to the EMR automatically by the computer system which initially records them and submits charges for them. And more will be available in the future. The "Electronic Surrogate Medical Record" (ESMR; see page 246) can be designed and implemented with the adjunct information needs in mind, and supply the information readily in computer-readable form.

Entity Object Specification

The entity object specification provides the blueprint for allocating the case to the proper category in the relevant classification. From the coder's standpoint (i.e., the person transferring information from the original medical record, or the electronic system which picks up the data items from the Electronic Surrogate Medical Record[8]), the task is to find, and to provide the appropriate entity information for, each item in the entity object specification.[9] The classifier, whether human or computer, can take it from there.

The major problem which remains, before such a system can be a reality, is that of attaching codes to the entity terms which are in the narrative portions of the record: the physicians', nurses', and other caregivers' diagnoses and procedures, as well as problem statements and observations from the patient and family. Thus *the entity coding "front end" must be in place in the information system before the benefits of classifying by computer algorithms can be obtained.* Once that step is in place, the classifying system (which can be developed, to a large extent, in parallel to the coding system), can be implemented.

---

8.   See "The Electronic "Surrogate" Record," page 246.

9.   Much of the information is automatically in the record in electronic form. If appropriate standards for information transfer and content are in use (see "Standards for Health Information," page 247), part of each entity object would be already completed. The remainder — finding the entity codes for specific diagnoses and procedures — is a new and critical challenge for the human coder or for computer system design and programming.

The Joys of Entity Code Classifying

Algorithms — rules — must be written to classify a case using information from the medical record. And of course, a human can use these algorithms with great success.

But once the information is entity-coded, and so in electronic format where it can be searched and captured instantly by computer, it makes sense to let the computer now also do the classifying. The beauty of an algorithm is that it must be written so unambiguously that the computer can understand it. Imagine the speed — and flexibility — of a system which uses computers to "sort" entity-coded information into categories. The number of categories — and their corresponding classifications — is now virtually unlimited. The only limitation is the time and resources required to build the algorithms and write the computer programs, and this needn't be done all at once.

Entity code classifying has a number of attractive virtues, which will be discussed in more detail below:

- All classifying algorithms are created by *experts in that classification*. The computer has no choice but to apply the algorithms to all cases uniformly, "without fear or favor." Today classifying is in the hands of thousands of humans, dispersed throughout the nation, who apply less rigorous algorithms. Uniformity is impossible to determine or enforce.

- Coding is more consistent. Entity coding is very precise in its own right. Category coding achieves equal precision when it is done with a single set of algorithms based on the entity codes and their prescribed adjunct information.

- Accuracy can be audited.

- There need be no delays in category coding. The entities are coded immediately, and can be retained in the relevant *ICD* "wastebasket" categories until official classification decisions are made.

- Coded diagnoses may be *reclassified* and/or reallocated to more precise categories at a later time.

- Data quality stays high.

- We save money.

Expert Classifying

Today's coding system — category coding — is really a "distributed" classifying process.[10] There are several hundred thousand people today, in hospitals, doctors' offices, nursing homes, and so forth, making classifying decisions. Most have been trained, to varying degrees. Hardly any are clinicians, scientists, or experts in classification. In addition, almost all coding is done manually, notwithstanding "computer-assisted" coding.

Category coding, of course, uses the rules of the classification as "algorithms" for classifying the case. But when humans use the algorithms ("manually"), two things interfere with consistency:

- The algorithms are often not written as carefully as if they had to be programmed for a computer. Computers always do exactly what you tell them to — for better or for worse.

- Not all humans will use the algorithms properly. Studying each one through for proper application of the rules often would take far more time than can be committed.

Entity code classifying can help with consistency because:

- The algorithms will be written precisely — by specialists trained in the conventions of the classification being used, many of whom will have helped develop the classification itself — in enough detail so that the computer can follow the directions.

- The computers will apply the algorithms as written. Any problems, either with the algorithm or the computer appliction, can be dealt with immediately, in one location (where the program is created), and tested again on the computer.

Under the new system, the list of decisions — and resulting classifying algorithms — would grow in one central location, with each decision added to the library of decisions. There would be no opportunity for "creative classifying" or "algorithm invention" at myriad sites throughout the nation. In today's decentralized category coding, the decisions are made invisibly in hundreds of thousands of locations, with no aggregation of logic.

---

10. See "The Process of Classifying," page 144.

More Consistency

Classifying is now done in thousands of places across the U.S., and there is no way to assure consistency. For example, let's assume that we have two excellent, trained, experienced coders. We would probably assume that the same patient will get the same code from both coders, and that similar patients would receive similar codes. Unfortunately, this often is not the case.

The accuracy of coding is very low.[11] The studies which have been made of coding accuracy have involved having two (or more) expert "coders" code the same medical records. The rates of disagreement between the two have simply illustrated (1) the difficulty of going through the medical records to find the necessary information, and (2) the fact that there can be more than one right answer for many, perhaps the majority, of "coding" decisions.[12]

In other words, two coders may well come up with different answers, with both answers being correct. See some excellent examples of this in the real world beginning on page 216.

With computer classification, the consistency and accuracy of coding would greatly improve. The algrorithms would always take the same information down the same trail. Modifications to those algorithms can be made as unforeseen situations are encountered. And all the classifying would be done by one "master coder" — the computer.

Accuracy Can Be Audited

Today it is virtually impossible to audit the accuracy of coding. There is no unequivocal "audit trail." The "recoding" by computer from *ICD-9-CM* to DRGs is, in contrast, auditable because the grouping is done by

---

11. Hsia, D.S., Krushat, W. M., Fagan, A.B., et al. "Accuracy of diagnostic coding for Medicare patients under the prospective payment system." *NEJM*, 1988, 918, 352-55. Institute of Medicine. "Reliability of Medicare hospital discharge records." Washington, DC: National Academy of Sciences, 1977. Lloyd, S.S. & Rissing, J.P. "Physician and coding errors in patient records." *JAMA*, 1985, 254, 1330-36.

12. Thompson, B. J. and Slee, V. N. "Accuracy of Diagnosis and Operation Coding." *Medical Record News* 1978; 49: No. 5; Thompson, B. J. "Implications of an Interactive Encoding System for ICD-9-CM," *J Clin Computing* 1983, XII: No. 4.

computer, using agreed-upon rules, and then the audit trail simply reverses the direction, and leads back from DRGs to the original *ICD-9-CM* categories, where the trail ends. If we did all our classifying by computer, it would be completely auditable, category back to entity code, and we can check its accuracy. And of course the entity coding itself is absolutely auditable. Code and term have a one-to-one correspondence.

Cases Can Be *Reclassified*

When a diagnosis appears for which there is no category code, because the disease has not yet found its way into a classification category, it is now put in a "wastebasket" — that is, it gets a wastebasket code. This is a sort of "holding tank," except that the diagnosis can never move on to its legitimate classification. This is because once it has received the wastebasket code, it has permanently lost its individual identity. The proper category code for the case can only be applied to cases which come after that classification decision has been made.[13]

With computer classification, the computer will retain, along with the category code (even be it a "wastebasket" code), all of the diagnosis entity and adjunct information. Thus when the "final" category code becomes available, the computer can take cases out of the "holding area" and assign them to the appropriate category. The computer merely goes back to the original record information and starts over with the classifying process.

No Delays

Today, newly discovered diagnoses can't be coded until they have been officially classified; that is, assigned a category in the current classification. If we were to implement entity code classifying, using computers, from now on:

- The diagnoses themselves can be coded immediately, with entity codes.

- Each can be placed in a "relevant" holding category, e.g., respiratory, circulatory, and so on.

---

13. This process is discussed more fully in "The Path to Coding," page 261.

- Once a classification decision is made, the diagnoses can be reallocated to the proper category.

- We can even go *back* and pick up earlier cases from the date entity coding was instituted!

Data Quality Stays High

In our present system, which relies only on category coding, the process of changing from one classification to another diminishes data quality. There are hundreds of thousands of coders to be retrained, hundreds of computer programs to be rewritten, and, as a result, a period of several years during which the category-coded data lose much of their credibility. A new system must be learned while an old one is also in use. Coding under the new system is slower for awhile. Mistakes are common. Both providers and computer systems adopt the new codes at different times (often at dates which are not known to users of the data). Further modifications are not always incorporated.

With computer classification, change occurs in *only one place*. Coders need not be concerned with the classification, at all, because they are coding entities, not classifying cases.

We Save Money

With our existing system of coding, implementation of a new classification is complex, traumatic, and extremely costly. The category coding process must change *completely* along with the classification, including system development and installation, and training of all coders and users.

Once entity coding is in place, and coders have been trained for that, they will never have to be trained again. We would only have to pay for a *one-time* coding change. The costs would include development and installation of the entity coding system and training of the coders. There would never be another *coding* change, ever!

There are also the "immeasurable costs" incurred with our present system. While the costs in money to revamp the system are enormous, *those faulty decisions in the healthcare system which are the result of bad data may be much more expensive to society than we'll ever know.*

16

The Challenge of ICD-10

WE NOW FACE another — and significant — classification change. In 1992, the World Health Organization (WHO) published the tenth revision of *ICD*, *The International Classification of Diseases and Related Health Problems, Tenth Revision* (known as *ICD-10*).[1] By treaty, the United States is required to report its health statistics to WHO using the new revision (in 1998, the U.S. began reporting death statistics using *ICD-10*). In preparation to use *ICD-10* for the rest of our clinical data, it was modified for use in the U.S., just as *ICD-7*, *ICD-8*, and *ICD-9* were modified.[2]

At the same time, the Health Care Financing Administration (HCFA), which is responsible for *procedure* classification, developed the *ICD-10 Procedure Coding System (ICD-10-PCS)*.[3]

So there are now two new "coding" systems waiting to be implemented nationwide:

- *ICD-10-CM* for diagnoses
- *ICD-10-PCS* for procedures

Consequences of Change

With the way our present coding system is set up, a classification change is a major upheaval, and very costly. The anticipated change from *ICD-9-CM* to *ICD-10-CM* — in particular — is going to be a big one.

---

1. See "The Tenth Revision of ICD," page 166.

2. See "The Clinical Modification of ICD-10," page 168.

3. See "ICD-10-PCS — A New Coding System," page 191. The *ICD* series pertains only to "diseases." WHO has never promulgated an operation or procedure classification, except in an exploratory fashion in 1978.

ICD-10's clinical versions appear to represent far more substantial changes than might have been expected. The resulting impacts on the health information system, however, are not so much related to the *magnitude* of the changes in the classification as to the *fact* of the changes.

If we follow the same course as we have in the past, the next phase will be to publish the coding books (and training materials) for the required number of installations (places where the coding takes place — hospitals, doctors' offices, etc.), train the hundreds of thousands of coders, develop and install necessary software, and, generally:

- Incur enormous costs in dollars.

- Suffer a drop in data quality until the new system is stablized.

- Cause a potentially disastrous disruption of the payment system.

- Get ready to repeat the process in ten years or so.

Immediate Costs

The outright cost of making the coding change itself is huge. Some costs can be spread over the entire system. Others are internal to each site.

There are far-reaching effects for the coders themselves, who have to learn a whole new coding system. They must obtain the new code books (and perhaps computer-assisted coding products) and study the new system until familiar with it. What was the thinking of the authors? Are different principles involved in the groupings than in the current *ICD-9-CM*? Are there new rules to be followed? New things to be coded that didn't concern us before? (Yes.)

This preparation usually involves going somewhere and taking classes, time taken away from productive work during the educational process. Then there will be an inevitable decline in productivity as familiarity is being gained in actual coding. And there will be a temporary decline in coding quality, with the resuting necessity of "reworking" the coding for some of the cases. More coders may be required, in a transition period of months to years.

Outside the immediate healthcare setting — hospitals, clinics, physician's offices — there has grown up a sizeable industry for teaching and supporting healthcare coding. A new classification will require this industry to develop training materials and training facilities for the new classification, and prepare consultation and reference services. A tremendous amount of resources will go into this — raising the costs of coding and, therefore, of healthcare.

Example

The sheer magnitude of it

In the late 1980s, the cost of conversion to coding with *ICD-10* for the Health Care Financing Administration (HCFA) alone was estimated at $100,000,000.

A story in *American Medical News* quoted a 1989 study by Coopers and Lybrand to the effect that a change in the physician's office from one coding system to another, i.e., from *CPT* to something else, could mean $1 billion in "environmental costs" to physicians and other users.[a] The change from one generation of *ICD-CM* to another is a project of the same order of magnitude, and it involves the nation's hospitals as well as the physicians' offices.

a. Martin, Sean. "Revamp of AMA's Coding System Under Way." *American Medical News* (1998): 5-6.

Data Quality

Information, and therefore healthcare quality, suffer badly with the classification change. Delays (and differences of changeover times), coding errors, loss of continuity in the categories, and other factors contribute to this; see "Data Quality Stays High," page 328.

The Payment System

When we change to the next generation of the *ICD* clinical modification, we will then also most likely be using the new classification in the Medicare and other payment systems. If we try to change these systems prematurely, however, it could have disastrous consequences for reimbursement, including unprecedented disputes over payment between providers and payers.

Payment today is for the "package" of services "normally" required for patients in Diagnosis Related Groups (DRGs).[4] DRGs were constructed to meet two criteria:

1. patients in a given group would all consume essentially the same amount of resources, and

2. a given group would be constituted of patients with more or less the same clinical problem and management, so that the grouping would make clinical sense.

To construct such hospital payment groups, one must have data on a large series of cases. The data on each patient includes the patient's diagnoses, the type of treatment employed, certain demographic and other information, and each patient's hospital "costs." The series must be large enough so that the numbers distributed to each of the groups will provide statistically adequate samples.

Data for the original generation of DRGs were collected using a clinical or hospital version of *ICD-8* as the source of diagnosis and operation information, and each group's definition depended on the *ICD-8* codes. With the arrival of *ICD-9-CM*, the groups had to be redefined, which meant collecting the same information as before, but under the new classification, and then carrying out the analysis all over again. Since *ICD-9-CM* was put into use before DRGs became the key to the payment system, it was possible to carry out the necessary analysis for similar groups of patients classsified under both the *ICD-8* and *ICD-9* categories. Not only were the new DRGs "tested" in this fashion and recalibrated, but the analysis was carried out without disrupting the payments to hospitals.

With the changeover to *ICD-10-CM*, if DRGs will be used for payment, the same procedure will be required for their construction. A new series of cases must be accumulated, and the DRG groupings must be defined using the new category codes. Ideally the same cases would be classified to *ICD-9-CM* and also to the new *ICD-10-CM*, and the subsequent DRG assignment analyzed as to:

• its adequacy for describing the cases clinically, and

---

4.   See the appendices, page 421, for more about DRGs.

- its impact on payment to providers and to the payment system.

When significant differences are found as a result of the changes in the categories going into the DRGs, new DRG definitions will be required.

But the situation is entirely different than it was in 1978. Then the financial solvency of the healthcare system was not at stake. Today it is. With the implementation of *ICD-10-CM*, presumably the data will simply come in one day under *ICD-9-CM* and the next day (and thereafter) under *ICD-10-CM*. No one has had the temerity to suggest that for a considerable time data must be classified simultaneously to both systems in hospitals and physicians' offices. But no other method can tell us whether DRGs constructed from the categories of *ICD-10-CM* (even though they may appear similar to those of *ICD-9-CM*) will have the same actual clinical content and thus the same resource consumption. Not only may the categories that appear similar have subtle — or dramatic — differences, but there will be missing categories and new categories whose impact cannot be foretold.

The ideal course of action would be to study "off-line" the same series of cases (several hundred thousand of them in a properly collected sample) coded to both *ICD-9-CM* and to *ICD-10-CM*. With such data in hand, the transition to the new payment classification could be a reasonable one to both payers and providers, and thus it would be straightforward. (Of course, there would at the same time be an opportunity for any other changes desired in the payment groupings.)

Such a careful revision of payment groupings will require several years, for data collection, analysis, and establishment of prices. Time will be required to accumulate an appropriate series of cases, conduct the analysis, and carry out the other steps necessary to establish the prices for the new groupings. Yet such a study cannot even begin until the new codes are stabilized and made available. Meanwhile, payments must continue to be made to providers.

Example

> **Entity coding can help**
>
> If and when we install the entity coding "front end" to medical records, we could classify using the entity coded information. It would then be a relatively simple matter to classify the same cases to both *ICD-9-CM* and *ICD-10-CM*, as a parallel operation in the current reimbursement system, and thus be able to study the impact of the new classification on DRGs and other payment mechanisms. New payment groups could then be introduced that are fair to both payer and payee.

How to Buy Time

ICD-10-CM may be required in the billing system as early as 2001. This does not leave enough time to properly address the issues raised in this book, to "refine" our health information system, nor to carry out the critically important studies necessary to recalibrate the DRG and other prospective payment classifications.

The good new is, we don't *have* to rush into a change. There's a way to accomplish what's needed.

We need "breathing space" right now. We need to reinforce the bridge *before* the next train rolls over it.

The most immediate pressure to convert to *ICD-10-CM* is due to the United States' obligation to use *ICD-10* in reporting health data to WHO. So it's natural to think in terms of "switching" the national system to *ICD-10* (via *ICD-10-CM*). But it doesn't have to be done this way. There are alternatives.

In anticipation of changing to *ICD-10-CM*, the National Center for Health Statistics (NCHS) has had a "crosswalk" — a conversion table from *ICD-9-CM* to *ICD-10-CM* — prepared.[5] This is intended to assist in classifying cases to the new system. However, it could also provide the solution to the "time challenge."

The *ICD-9-CM* to *ICD-10-CM* crosswalk could, with minimal effort, be reworked to convert from *ICD-9-CM* *directly to ICD-10 itself*. The new crosswalk would be both simpler and more accurate — it's always easier

---

5.   See "Crosswalk to ICD-10-CM," page 299.

to move data into larger categories than into smaller. *ICD-10* has only 13,000 (larger) categories, about the same number as *ICD-9-CM*, while *ICD-10-CM* has much smaller categories (about 60,000 of them).

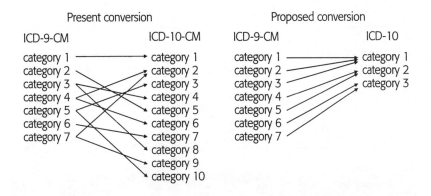

Thus when information coded to *ICD-10* is required, as to meet the United States obligations to the World Health Organization, the new crosswalk can be used to easily convert the data from *ICD-9-CM* (in which it is already coded) directly to *ICD-10*. And this conversion can be done at the federal level — so the 500,000 or so coders across the nation needn't be concerned with it.

The crosswalk approach would allow us to simply *continue with ICD-9-CM* for all billing and other reporting purposes — while we attend to the system. If we take this route,

- The equilibrium of the payment system will not be disturbed.

- The essential reimbursement studies can be done.

- The nation can get its statistics into *ICD-10* categories much sooner than if we had to wait to change the entire input across the healthcare system.

- We'll have time to deal with other important aspects of the system.

17

A New Beginning

The Power of Codes

THERE'S ONE ASPECT of our health information system which we may have "glossed over": the power of the codes, themselves.

Think of codes as "labels." We know about the potential consequences of labelling people. For example, label a child as "slow," and at least two things will happen:

- The child will think of herself as slow, and perhaps not try so hard.

- Others will also think of her as slow, and not expect as much from her.

And the label becomes a self-fulfilling prophecy. The label, by itself, can profoundly affect her whole life. The same is true in healthcare.

A patient's chart receives a code for a diagnosis (or group of diagnoses). This code will influence, among other things:

- the health and medical care the patient receives

- whether insurance will cover the care

- amount of reimbursement (if any)

- other and future diagnoses

- how that patient views himself, and how others view him

- qualification for disability or other benefits

- whether the case is included in studies of health and healthcare

We have an obligation to take utmost care when using codes.

Example

The label of dementia

The authors of the dementia study[a] noted the far-ranging ramifications of making a diagnosis — of "labelling" a patient's condition — beyond any research difficulties:

"From the viewpoint of research, a given person may or may not qualify for a therapeutic protocol, depending on the label applied to his or her condition."

"Clinically, it makes a great difference whether a patient is labeled as having dementia. The diagnosis often sets the threshold for investigation, treatment, and prognosis."

"Third-party reimbursement depends on the diagnosis, as does the patient's ability to obtain insurance."

"Legally, the diagnosis of dementia may deprive a person of the right to drive, manage personal affairs, and make a will."

"Diagnostic methods that generate prevalence figures that vary by a factor of 10 have important implications for healthcare planning. It makes a substantial difference whether 3 percent or 29 percent of the population over 65 years of age has dementia; the resources needed for prevention, treatment, and long-term care differ dramatically in these two cases."

"Our findings, and the prospect of the early diagnosis and treatment of dementia, point to the urgency of further debate and studies to redefine and refine the characterization of categories of cognitive impairment and dementia."

a. See "The 'Labelling' of Dementia," page 274.

Looking at Where We Are

There has been tremendous progress in healthcare information in the last century. We have gone from skeletal handwritten individual records to a nationwide system of computers which can collect and disseminate vast amounts of information. The potential is mind boggling. Imagine, for example, being able to utilize "neural networking" technology with health data. This technology teaches the computer to look at enormous amounts of information, and to find patterns and connections.

In the movie *Safe Passage*,[1] the father is having more and more frequent blind spells, and no one can figure out why. One son, a scientist, follows him around for a few days with pen and paper, making notes of *everything* he observes. He finally sees a pattern — the dad goes blind every time he drinks tea *and* the cat is in the room. This connection could not have been anticipated, but with enough data, it was eventually revealed.

Computers can do the same kind of observation, but can digest much more information. If all we have in the system is diagnoses, we have something, but all we have really is conclusions. If we also had suffecient details, we could learn so much more.

The tremendous growth in data, however, has led to problems, just as urban areas which grow too fast run into difficulties. Without time to plan ahead, and anticipate some of the effects of such growth, cities get overcrowded, too much traffic, pollution, and other problems. Moving people to the suburbs creates another set of problems.

Our health information system — coding and classification — has grown, to a large extent, in the same way. But solving the problems will be much, much easier. For one thing, we don't have to tear up a lot of concrete, or demolish buildings, or waste anything, or even reroute traffic. On the contrary, everything thing we've built, and everything we've learned, can be utilized to build a better system. We have nothing to lose, and everything to gain, by taking action now.

---

1.   1994, starring Susan Sarandon and Sam Shepard, directed by Robert Allan Ackerman. Based on the novel by Ellyn Bache.

The "Wish List"

The growing demands on our information system are putting increasing pressure on it for change. The "wish list" has been growing; almost everyone has something on it. The demands include:

- the move toward evidence-based medicine

- the desire for a better payment system

- the wish that there were a single set of codes for diagnoses and another single set for procedures

- the need for more appropriate statistics to guide our healthcare policies and planning

- the urgency of making sure that the electronic medical record carries the essential information for patient care

- the need to learn from our past — gain knowledge from our experience

This is a beautiful time to reexamine our system, and refine it to better meet our needs. If we grab the opportunity, we can finally attend to our collective wish list.

But we have to act now, resisting the pressure of a change to *ICD-10-CM* before we're ready, with potentially disastrous consequences. We are rapidly approaching a "fork in the road," and need to make a quick decision — and act on it.

> When you come to a fork in the road, take it.

> **Yogi Berra**

Most books end with a conclusion. This one ends with a challenge.

Saving the Medical Record

The medical record is the nucleus of our healthcare system, for the care of the individual patient, for reimbursing providers, and for providing intelligence for tasks ranging from the operation of individual facilities to developing national — in fact international — healthcare strategies. In addition, the wealth of biomedical information being captured in the 2.5 billion encounters per year could add enormously to the knowledgebase available to evidence-based medicine and disclose otherwise undetectable gaps in our understanding of both health and healthcare.

Now its integrity is being threatened, but there are at least four things we can do to save it:

1. Examine our priorities, and start doing all we can to support truth, completeness, and accuracy in the medical record.

    a. Get rid of pressures that distort information.

    b. Make sure payment covers necessary care.

    c. Don't punish people for doing the right thing.

    d. Maximize the potential of our technology.

2. Permanently capture in coded, computer-usable form, the clinical detail from our medical records: introduce entity coding.

3. "Tag" all codes used in healthcare to make them unambiguous. For this we need standards, just as in all other areas of modern technology.

4. Start using computers to do the classifying, using entity codes and expertly developed algorithms. This will let us put cases into different, tailored classifications as needed.

Example

To Err is Human

We have stressed repeatedly that while health information is critical for a number of purposes, nowhere is it more important than at the patient's bedside. This is corroborated by the story below.

Near the very end of the twentieth century, Americans received some very startling news via feature stories in the Washington Post, the New York Times, and on National Public Radio. We were told that medical errors in hospitals account for more deaths every year than those caused by motor vehicle accidents, breast cancer, or AIDS. The source of the news was a report issued by the Institute of Medicine (IOM), entitled "To Err Is Human," and subtitled "Building a Safer Health System".[a]

Dr. William Richardson, chair of the IOM committee that wrote the report,[b] said, "These stunningly high rates of medical errors — resulting in deaths, permanent disability, and unnecessary suffering — are simply unacceptable in a medical system that promises first to 'do no harm'."

The report noted that the majority of medical errors are caused by the way the nation's health system is organized, *not by individual negligence*. Included on the list of causes were illegible writing on both prescriptions and on medical records, a healthcare system that lacks coordination, and patients being treated by *multiple caregivers who lack complete information for the patients*.

According to the report's authors, part of the solution is that healthcare organizations need to create an overall culture of safety. The report also recommends improved data collection and analysis, and development of effective systems at the level of direct patient care.

a. The IOM is a body formed by the National Academy of Sciences (NAS) in 1970 to secure the services of eminent members of appointed professions for the examination of policy matters pertaining to the health of the public. While technically a private agency, most of the studies carried out by the IOM are requested and funded by government agencies.

b. Also president and CEO of the W. K. Kellogg Foundation of Battle Creek, Michigan.

The Bottom Line

We have two options:

1. The system can continue as is — with all the effort, expense, and problems that will entail at the time of the change from *ICD-9-CM* to *ICD-10-CM*. Then a similar upheaval will occur when *ICD-11* appears, and on into the future. And all of our information problems will persist. And we'll spend a *lot* of money.

2. The change to *ICD-10-CM* can be made painless, and the necessary improvements can be made to the information system at the same time, if we decide to take a different road — *before* changing to *ICD-10-CM*.

This new road will begin with several steps:

1. To buy time:

    a. Modify the existing NCHS crosswalk to convert data from *ICD-9-CM* directly to *ICD-10* to meet our international statistical obligations. This would be much faster than a system-wide change.

    b. Continue using *ICD-9-CM* for present purposes. This would avoid any disruption in the payment system.

2. To improve coding:

    a. Create the initial master database of entity terms and codes.

    b. Establish the communication system for dissemination of the entity codes.

    c. Prepare the medical record systems to carry the entity coded data.

    d. Implement entity coding.

    e. Establish standards for tagging *all* codes used in health and healthcare.

3. To be ready for the future:

    a. Study the whole health information system — its needs and how best to meet them, using our collective experience, our brightest minds, and our best technology.

    b. Prepare to initiate entity code classifying.

After all these years of experience with classifying and coding in our healthcare system, it's time to take the "lessons learned"[2] and move forward.

---

2. A favorite phrase of J. M. Juran, "quality guru."

Section 4: Coding Systems

A

International Classification of Diseases

THIS APPENDIX contains a number of references concerning the International Classification of Diseases. These are as follows:

- *The International Classification: Its Evolution and Implementation*, a reprint of a 1990 article by the senior author discussing the history of the *International Classification* and some reflections about its future.[1]

- Reproductions of the Introductions to the 6th and 9th Revisions of *ICD*; these are helpful in understanding the background, purposes, and thinking behind the classification.

The International Classification: Its Evolution & Implementation

The years since about 1940 have seen substantial changes in the *International Classification*, a series of "disease" classification volumes periodically revised and published by the World Health Organization (WHO) and in use throughout the world. For simplicity, the series is referred to here as "The Classification." This paper reviews its history briefly, examines the latest of the changes which are found in the forthcoming 10th Revision, *ICD-10*, and discusses some of the implications of implementing *ICD-10* in the United States healthcare system.

A Brief History of The Classification

The Classification started out in 1900 as *The International List of Causes of Death*, which was primarily a statistical tool for the international exchange of mortality data.[2] The *List* was later given the added task of accommodating morbidity statistics, that is, statistics on non-lethal as well as lethal conditions. Public health professionals turned to it for information on causes of

---

1. The Commission on Professional and Hospital Activities (CPHA) requested this paper for a symposium entitled "*ICD-10* — Will It Refocus Healthcare Information from Death to Health Status?" (Chicago, IL, 29 November 1990) and described as "an ... opportunity ... to discuss the issues involved in obtaining more comprehensive and qualitative patient data ... [and] ... guiding the direction of healthcare into the year 2000 by reviewing and recommending strategies for implementing ... *ICD-10*." The paper is reprinted here without change.

2. A brief history of the *International Classification* is given here; for a detailed history, see the Introductions to the Revisions, page 364.

injuries. The next significant usage was termed "clinical," when it was adopted for hospital disease indexing. In the eighties, through "recoding" into Diagnosis Related Groups (DRGs), it became the vehicle used in the United States payment system for telling payers why care was given. Tomorrow, with the 10th Revision, it is likely to become also the principal means of classifying additional reasons why people seek help from, and are affected by, both the public health programs and the healthcare systems of the world.

The evolution of The Classification has had two chief attributes. The first is that its purpose has changed, as just described. Once having only a single purpose, it has over the years attempted to serve a number of purposes. One reflection of this is the change in the titles of the actual volumes. The 1948 revision, the 6th, was called *The International Statistical Classification of Diseases, Injuries, and Causes of Death*. The 1955 Revision, the 7th, saw the name become *The International Classification of Diseases, Injuries, and Causes of Death*, a title which was retained through the 9th Revision. The title of the 10th Revision, *ICD-10*, seems to combine both previous ideas: *International Statistical Classification of Diseases and Related Health Problems*. It has remained a classification, however; it is not and never has been either a nomenclature or a taxonomy, as some have referred to it.[3]

The second attribute of the evolution of The Classification has been in the fineness of its pigeonholes. The world's exchange of vital statistics in 1900 was satisfied with 179 categories; *ICD-10* is reported to provide nearly 13,000.

The rate of change in the evolution of The Classification is demonstrated by the graph in Figure 1. The published steps in the evolution are shown in the table which is Figure 2. The newer uses, namely in payment for care, and in accommodating additional relationships with preventive and curative measures (such information as in the new Chapter XXI) have not been involved long enough to have their maximum impact: they may be expected to exert future demands for changes in classification systems.

---

3.   The distinction between a classification, a nomenclature (i.e., a system of approved terms), and a taxonomy (i.e., an orderly classification of the entities in the "disease" universe according to their logical relationships with respect to a particular viewpoint) is well discussed in the *Introduction* to *ICD-9*.

Figure A.1 Evolution of ICD Since 1945

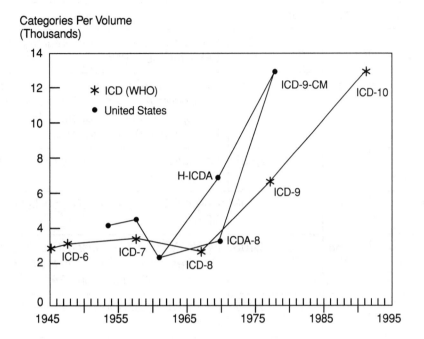

Categories Per Volume
(Thousands)

Some detail on the events between the accommodation of morbidity as well as mortality data in The Classification and the appearance of the 10th Revision may be useful:

Figure A.2 Evolution of the International Classification

Volume	Year	Categories[a]	Comments
ISC	1900	179	*International Statistical Classification,* primarily for mortality statistics
ISC	1920	205	International Statistical Classification
ISC-6	1948	3,248	*International Statistical Classification, 6th Revision*(WHO[b]); introduced morbidity categories
ISC-6 (*SMHC[c]*)	1955	3,720	Subdivisions and modifications introduced by SMHC for hospital use in PAS
ICD-7	1958	3,440	*International Classification of Diseases, 7th Revision* (WHO)

Figure A.2 Evolution of the International Classification *(continued)*

Volume	Year	Categories[a]	Comments
ICD-7 (*CPHA*[d])	1958	3,858	Subdivisions and modifications introduced by CPHA for use in PAS
ICDA	1959	2,616	"Disease Index" — *International Classification of Diseases Adapted for Hospital Records and Operation Classification*, USPHS[e] Publication 719, Revised 1962
ICD-8	1967	2,883	*International Classification of Diseases, 8th Revision* (WHO)
H-ICDA	1968	4,208	*Hospital Adaptation of ICDA*, published by CPHA
ICDA-8	1968	3,106	*Eighth Revision International Classification of Diseases, Adapted for Use in the United States*, USPHS Publication 1693
ICD-9	1977	7,023	*International Classification of Diseases, 9th Revision* (WHO)
ICD-9-CM	1978	11,992	*International Classification of Diseases, 9th Revision, Clinical Modification*, published by CPHA
ICD-10	1992	12,630	Current popular designation for *International Statistical Classification of Diseases and Related Health Problems* (WHO). Expected date of availability 1992.

a. Category counts were developed by counting the categories in the volumes and multiplying each category for which modifiers were stated to be required by the number of modifiers for the category (some modifiers are optional).

b. World Health Organization, Geneva.

c. Southwestern Michigan Hospital Council, Hastings, Michigan, where the Professional Activity Study (PAS) originated. See "Hospital Discharge Abstract Systems," page 103.

d. Commission on Professional and Hospital Activities, Ann Arbor, Michigan, which took over operation of PAS in 1956.

e. United States Public Health Service.

Introduction of Morbidity Classification

The desire for adding an internationally standardized classification for morbidity to that for mortality was reflected in the 6th Revision by two changes: (1) a significant expansion of The Classification by the addition of more categories for non-fatal conditions, and (2) responding to the public health concern, the introduction of a "dual classification" system in which the numbers 800-999 were given dual meanings, depending on whether they were prefixed by an "E" or by an "N." If the prefix was an "E," the number referred to an "external cause" of the injury, e.g., violence or neglect, while if the prefix was an "N," the number gave the "nature" of the injury, e.g., fracture or poisoning. For the most part, those charged with prevention of morbidity and mortality sought to control the external causes, while those giving care were interested in the resulting injuries. The term "dual classification" came from the idea that for each injury there were two possible categories.[4]

"Clinical Use" of The Classification

Then came the adoption of The Classification for clinical use. For decades, medical records in hospitals had been indexed according to diagnosis in the record departments. To accomplish this, they had been coded (that is, given numerical codes relating to the diagnoses). Coding had been done for three reasons: (1) to make the information more compact, (2) to increase specificity in communication (for example, one orders goods by catalog number rather than description), and (3) for economy in handling the information (even before the use of computers). Soon it became common to use the numerical codes instead of the diagnoses themselves for many purposes.

Prior to the mid-1950s, hospitals had, generally, coded the diagnoses to the *Standard Nomenclature of Diseases and Operations (SNDO)*,[5] published by the American Medical Association. *SNDO* presented some problems in the retrieval of series of cases, however, both because it was constructed in such a manner that more than one code could be devised for the same diagnosis, and also because there was no convenient way to retrieve clinical series of cases for the physician. It was virtually impossible to think of all the codes which might have been used for the diagnoses which should fall into the group of cases a physician might want

---

4. One of the basic principles behind a classification is that there must be a place (but only one place) for everything in the universe to which the classification pertains — here "diseases, injuries, and causes of death." This principle technically was not violated, because the "E codes" (for external causes of injuries) were in a "supplementary classification," and presumably optional, either as supplements to the code for the injury, or substitutes, depending on the user. With *ICD-10*, the "E codes" have been brought into Chapter XX, inside The Classification itself, and, for the first time, it seems "required" that trauma be given codes for both cause and nature of injury.

5. Thompson, E.T., and Hayden, A.C., editors, *Standard Nomenclature of Diseases and Operations*, 4th Ed., 1952, American Medical Association, Chicago. Last edition, 5th, published in 1961.

for a study, and *SNDO* provided no grouping method useful for this purpose. Consequently, cases essential to a given study were often not found.

Medical record librarians (the title then employed) sometimes used novel methods of handling the problem of giving codes to the diagnoses. Dr. Edwin Crosby, first the Director of the Joint Commission on Accreditation of Hospitals, and later Director of the American Hospital Association, had a favorite story about one librarian who always found the cases Dr. Crosby wanted, but the code numbers used for the retrieval were not in any coding system he knew. When Dr. Crosby asked the record librarian where she got the codes, he found they were simply the page numbers from *SNDO*.

Other medical record librarians solved the problem of retrieval of series of cases by another method. They used *SNDO* to find the diagnostic terms, i.e., the acceptable English expressions[6] and their *SNDO* codes. Then they indexed the cases by placing them in *ICD* categories, using a table found as an Appendix in the 4th edition of *SNDO*. This table showed which *SNDO* codes fell into each *ICD-6* category. This indexing with *ICD* proved so useful that the Professional Activity Study (PAS)[7] switched to having the participating hospitals code directly to *ICD* effective the first of January of 1955.

Indexing by *ICD* proved to be welcome to the physician, the chief user of the disease index. The physician wanted all the cases which might be relevant to a particular study. It was far more desirable to simply ignore some cases in the group that the medical record librarian had obtained than to fear that some needed cases had not been found; throwing aside a few extraneous charts was far preferable to missing some which should have been retrieved.

Some of the groupings of *ICD* did prove too broad for disease indexing, of course, and in the early days, PAS simply issued little pieces of paper, which were fastened into the *ICD* with scotch tape, in order to give the added specificity. PAS first adopted the modifications made by two pioneer medical record librarians[8] and then added some more as experience dictated. All the modifications represented primarily the subdivision of some categories to give more "clinical detail" (narrower groups) than was found in *ICD* itself.

---

6. *SNDO* was, after all, the "standard [coded] nomenclature," promulgated by the American Medical Association.

7. The Professional Activity Study (PAS) was the first hospital discharge abstract system. It was initiated under the aegis of the Southwestern Michigan Hospital Council with grant support from the W. K. Kellogg Foundation, and was transferred to the Commission on Professional and Hospital Activities (CPHA) in 1956 in order to give PAS a national presence. Participating hospitals (eventually over 2,000 of them) send coded case abstracts to PAS, where they are processed by computer in order to furnish the hospitals their own disease (and other) indexes and statistics, and to build a multihospital data bank for research purposes. PAS, like CPHA, was founded by the author.

8. Loyola Voelker, CRL, of the United States Public Health Service Hospital in Baltimore and Dorothy Kurtz, CRL, of the Columbia-Presbyterian Medical Center in New York.

Using hospital disease indexes which had been coded to the privately modified *ICD*, primarily in the Columbia-Presbyterian Medical Center in New York, in the Public Health Service Hospital in Baltimore, and in PAS hospitals, the American Hospital Association and the American Association of Medical Record Librarians were able to conduct a study[9] of the relative merits of *ICD* and *SNDO* for hospital disease indexing. *ICD* won, and the result was the publication in 1959, by the United States Public Health Service, of the *International Classification of Diseases Adapted for Indexing of Hospital Records and Operation Classification (ICDA)*.[10] This volume was derived from the 7th Revision of *ICD*, dated 1955. Note the addition of a "rudimentary" classification of operations which was added for hospital use; The Classification itself had never dealt with surgical procedures.

Meanwhile, the American Medical Association became aware of the need for grouping of cases for disease indexing, and the Fifth Edition of *SNDO* (1961) introduced as an appendix an "Abridged Statistical Classification for Clinical Indexing." This was a four-digit code which replaced the *ICD* Appendix which had been in the 4th Edition. But it was too late. The switch to *ICD* had already taken place; the 5th Edition was the last edition of *SNDO* published.

So hospitals for more than thirty years have coded their diagnoses for disease indexing using modifications of successive versions of The Classification.

With the publication of the 8th Revision of *ICD* in 1965 by the World Health Organization (WHO), a period of turmoil began in the United States. Hospitals in the Professional Activity Study were not satisfied with the clinical detail *ICD-8* provided. So the Commission on Professional and Hospital Activities in 1968 developed and published its *Hospital Adaptation of ICDA (H-ICDA)*. The United States Public Health Service then, also in 1968, issued its competing modification, Publication Number 1693, entitled *Eighth Revision International Classification of Diseases Adapted for Use in the United States*, which came to be known as *ICDA-8*. Roughly equal numbers of hospitals used *H-ICDA* and *ICDA-8*.

All agreed that this was an undesirable situation, and when preparations began for the *International Classification of Diseases, 9th Revision (ICD-9)*, the Commission on Professional and Hospital Activities (CPHA) was invited to participate in developing the United States position.

Creation of a Revision of The Classification

It may be of interest to recount the procedure by which a Revision of The Classification occurs. The Classification is in the hands of the World Health Organization, whose policy it is to examine it every ten years or so, creating a Revision if that seems indicated. In preparation for this effort, WHO member nations submit their input to regional "Centers" for The

---

9.   "Efficiency in Hospital Indexing of the Coding Systems of the *International Statistical Classification* and *Standard Nomenclature of Diseases and Operations*," *Journal of American Association of Medical Record Librarians*, Vol 30 No 3, June 1959.

10.   USPHS Publication 719 (Price $1.00). The volume was revised in 1962 and given an alphabetic index in a second volume (Price, for the set, $1.75).

Classification, which consolidate that input. An international conference is finally called, at which time the whole issue is studied, and decisions are made as to the new Revision. The author was a part of this process for the United States for the 9th Revision in 1975. A similar process accounts for *ICD-10*.

First came agreement on the United States input for the WHO Center for Classification of Diseases for North America in its preparation for *ICD-9*. The United States government spent several years developing its position. The basic *ICD-9* structure had been fixed by WHO as to number and length of "chapters" and the specific categories within them, and a decision that there could only be four digits in the codes. Working within this framework, the United States government sought to accommodate the demands of a number of users. First, there were vital and public health statistics, because the United States government is bound by treaty to use *ICD* in its international exchange of such data. Then, because of the United States history of using adaptations and modifications of *ICD* for hospital indexing and the grouping of cases for medical auditing, as well as for carrying out healthcare studies, the government gave the clinical specialties chances to state their wishes, that is, to recommend the degree of diagnosis detail felt to be essential in The Classification, as well as the groupings into which to place "their" various diagnoses. Some specialties, such as ophthalmology and psychiatry, had given far more attention to such matters than others, and thus were more assertive in their presentations and obtained some of the greater detail they wanted. But many compromises were required. Some compromises, for example, were over territory, i.e., which section of The Classification should contain certain diagnoses. The clinical interests sometimes competed with those of the vital statisticians, and the clinical interests were subordinated; after all, the basic purpose of The Classification is public health rather than clinical medicine. In the end, much detail desired in the United States had to be sacrificed.

Once consolidated, the North American input had to compete in Geneva with input from other countries (via the "Centers"), ranging from the developed nations with trained personnel and considerable computerization to the third world countries where virtually all input is in "nonmedical terms" from lay persons. *ICD-9* had to serve all. Nations also had to compete on a political level, e.g., there must be a balance among nations in how many suggestions from each could be accommodated. Unique national situations, such as osteopathy in the United States and Russian psychiatric theory, had to be considered. The resulting *ICD-9* was remarkably good, considering the compromises required to satisfy these competing interests.

United States Clinical Modification of The Classification

But even then, some of the attributes of *ICD-9* in psychiatry, obstetrics, and classification theory were so unacceptable to United States clinicians that they decided that, if *ICD-9* were to be the vehicle for hospital indexing and retrieval of case data for clinical studies (at that time, reimbursement was not in the picture), it must be modified, and the *International Classification of Diseases, 9th Revision, Clinical Modification (ICD-9-CM)* was created as a joint effort between the United States clinical community[11] and the National Center for Health Statistics. The cost of this adaptation in volunteer physician time alone was enormous.

ICD-9-CM was put into use in the United States in January 1979, replacing the adaptations and modifications of *ICD-8*. Of course, there was soon a demand for interpretations and for accommodations for additional terms. For a time answers were given by the various discharge abstract systems and by the American Hospital Association. None of these sources were "official." There was informal collaboration among them, but there was a clear need for one central voice. The American Hospital Association (AHA), the American Medical Record Association (AMRA) (now the American Health Information Management Association (AHIMA)), the Health Care Financing Administration (HCFA), and the National Center for Health Statistics (NCHS) joined together as "cooperating parties" in the establishment, in 1984, of a journal called *Coding Clinic for ICD-9-CM*. Coding Clinic is published by the AHA's Central Office on *ICD-9-CM* quarterly. A Coordination and Maintenance Committee for *ICD-9-CM*, whose official members are federal employees, meets periodically and considers possible revisions, which, after approval by HCFA (procedures) and NCHS (diagnoses), are disseminated in Coding Clinic. Official status was given to these pronouncements by a notice in the Federal Register (see Volume 54, No. 1339, Friday, July 21, 1989) designating Coding Clinic as the only publication endorsed by HCFA for this purpose.

Coding Clinic publishes such content as "Conversion Tables for New ICD-9-CM Codes" and "New and Revised Codes" and, for many of them, the rationale, clinical and theoretical for the changes. For example, a new procedure might have a description of the procedure along with the code to be used. Diagnoses are often discussed in some detail so that the coding implications are supported. The changes, in this form of publication, are given as "delete" and "insert" and so on, and to incorporate them in the published volumes is a major clerical undertaking. The volumes were not printed to encourage handwritten entries in either the Tabular List or the Alphabetic Index. And many settings in which coding is done will have a number of copies of the books.

The 1992 changes, for example, numbered several hundred for both diagnoses and procedures. The table showed current code assignments which were to replace previous code assignments. These were changes to be made in the Tabular List, but there was no companion table indicating the changes that should rightly have been made also in the Alphabet Index. As a result, a number of publishers offer annual new versions of *ICD-9-CM* revisions, with various competing enhancements. Some have anatomical diagrams. Some offer color-coding to indicate the influence of various codes on payment. A substantial industry has been spawned in this manner, since the revisions are now implemented annually (in October).

ICD-10

Unlike revisions of computer programs, preliminary versions of which are subjected to intensive "beta testing" in the real world, neither the exact features of, nor the "bugs" in, a revision of The Classification can be found until it goes into real life use. Physicians, public

---

11. A special organization, the Council on Clinical Classifications (CCC) (of which the senior author was president), was formed in order to carry out this task. Sponsors of CCC were the American Academy of Pediatrics, the American College of Obstetricians and Gynecologists, the American College of Physicians, the American College of Surgeons, the American Psychiatric Association, and the Commission on Professional and Hospital Activities (CPHA). CPHA was the initial publisher of *ICD-9-CM*.

health officials, statisticians, medical record professionals, systems engineers and programmers, writers of instruction manuals, providers, and payers—all must wait until the ink is dry in the final volumes before they can begin to get ready for the introduction of the new code. Nor can one tell until that time the degree to which *ICD-10* will satisfy all the interests in the United States which use The Classification, or whether a United States modification will be required, as it was with *ICD-9*. It is widely believed that such a modification will be needed (and rumor has it that one has been prepared and is under wraps).

The changes between *ICD-9* and *ICD-10* are substantial. Four of them bear special mention:

1. The codes have been changed from purely numeric (except for the "E" and "N" codes mentioned above) to alphanumeric codes. As shown in the table below, all codes are prefixed by a letter. The old "N" codes become "S" and "T" codes; the old "E" codes become "V" and "Y" codes. Alphanumeric codes will, of course, as stated, permit many more pigeonholes while using the same number of characters. And there will be no codes which will simply transfer from one book to the other.

2. The codes have been restricted to the format x99.9, i.e., one alphabetic character followed by two numeric, a decimal point, and a single numeric character. At various places in *ICD-10* supplementary digits are offered, e.g., "0 without open wound into cavity" and "1 with open wound into cavity," but with the admonition that such digits be placed in a separate "box."

3. The "dagger (†) and asterisk (*)" feature of *ICD-9*, which allowed the same diagnostic label in some instances to appear in two locations, under its etiology and also under its manifestation, was severely criticized. It has been replaced by some 82 "homogeneous 3- and 4-character categories" designed as asterisk categories, with the format "xnn.n*" which provides a supplementary code, e.g., H36.0* — Diabetic retinopathy (E10† - E14† ... with common fourth character .3)" and H36.8* — Other retinal disorders in diseases classified elsewhere." For the latter, H36.8* code, three other diseases with which it may be used are given. Despite the direction, as given above, that a supplementary code is to be put in a separate box, the use of the dagger and asterisk would require a 6-digit field in a computer record; a fifth digit is required for the decimal point and a sixth for the dagger or asterisk.

4. The number of chapters has been expanded from 17 to 21, although this is slightly misleading: *ICD-9* had two "non-chapters," the "E codes" and the "V codes," which were in "supplementary classifications." These are now in Chapters XX and XXI, respectively. Then two "new" chapters are the results of breaking out the eye and ear from their inclusion in the chapter on the nervous system. Further "internal" changes, moving entities between categories and chapters have, of course, taken place as well.

The basic structure, chapter headings, and code ranges are shown in the table below, to give some idea of the changes from *ICD-9*.

Figure A.3 Structure Comparison of ICD-9 & ICD-10

CH.	ICD-9	ICD-10	ICD-9 Chapter Title	ICD-10 Chapter Title
I	001- 139	A00- B99	Infectious and Parasitic Diseases	Certain Infectious and Parasitic Diseases
II	140- 239	C00- D49	Neoplasms	Neoplasms
III	240- 279		Endocrine, Nutritional and Metabolic Diseases and Immunity Disorders	
		D50- D99		Diseases of Blood and Blood-forming Organs and Certain Disorders Involving the Immune Mechanism
IV	280- 289		Diseases of Blood and Blood-forming Organs	
		E00- E99		Endocrine, Nutritional, and Metabolic Diseases
V	290- 319	F00- F99	Mental Disorders	Mental and Behavioral Disorders
VI	320- 389	G00- G99	Diseases of the Nervous System and Sense Organs	Diseases of the Nervous System
VII	390- 459		Diseases of the Circulatory System	
		H00- H59		Diseases of the Eye and Adnexa
VIII	460- 519		Diseases of the Respiratory System	
		H60- H99		Diseases of the Ear and Mastoid Process
IX	520- 579		Diseases of the Digestive System	
		I00- I99		Diseases of the Circulatory System

Figure A.3 Structure Comparison of ICD-9 & ICD-10 *(continued)*

CH.	*ICD-9*	*ICD-10*	*ICD-9* Chapter Title	*ICD-10* Chapter Title
X	580- 629		Diseases of the Genitourinary System	
		J00- J99		Diseases of the Respiratory System
XI	630- 676		Complications of Pregnancy, Childbirth, and the Puerperium	
		K00- K99		Diseases of the Digestive System
XII	680- 709	L00- L99	Diseases of the Skin and Subcutaneous Tissue	Diseases of the Skin and Subcutaneous Tissue
XIII	710- 739	M00- M99	Diseases of the Musculoskeletal System and Connective Tissue	Diseases of the Musculoskeletal System and Connective Tissue
XIV	740- 759		Congenital Anomalies	
		N00- N99		Diseases of the Genitourinary System
XV	760- 779		Certain Conditions Originating in the Perinatal Period	
		O00- O99		Pregnancy, Childbirth, and Puerperium
XVI	780- 799		Symptoms, Signs, and Ill-Defined Conditions	
		P00- P99		Certain Conditions Originating in the Perinatal Period

Figure A.3 Structure Comparison of ICD-9 & ICD-10 *(continued)*

CH.	ICD-9	ICD-10	ICD-9 Chapter Title	ICD-10 Chapter Title
XVII	800- 999		Injury and Poisoning	
		Q00- Q99		Congenital Malformations, Deformations, and Chromosomal Abnormalities
XVIII		R00- R99		Symptoms, Signs, and Abnormal Clinical and Laboratory Findings not Elsewhere Classified
XIX		S00- T99		Injury, Poisoning, and Certain Other Consequences of External Causes
XX		V01- Y99		External Causes of Morbidity and Mortality
XXI		Z00- Z99		Factors Influencing Health Status and Contact with Health Services
	E800- E999		Supplementary Classification of External Causes of Injury and Poisoning	
	V01- V82		Supplementary Classification of Factors Influencing Health Status and Contact with Health Services	

Implementation of ICD-10

Implementation of *ICD-10*, as of any classification change, will not be a trivial undertaking.[12] It will (1) present new opportunities, (2) result in a period of questionable data, (3) require hard work, (4) have a substantial price tag in dollars, and (5) have a profound effect on the payment system.

First, the opportunities: *ICD-10* should provide more and better information. As implied by the CPHA symposium title,[13] recording and coding of conditions and situations not previously carried in the data system, i.e., coding the conditions provided for by the new Chapter XXI (those formerly classified to the supplementary "V" codes, along with other factors), will provide a new source of information on why people encounter the healthcare system and what happens to them. Using these (computer) records which are more detailed, and which contain information about factors not recorded in the past, will permit new healthcare studies and statistics.

Second, there will be less trustworthy and sometimes confusing information during the transition period, a period which will likely span several years. Inevitably there will be a period when one must be very cautious in interpreting the data, and it will be extremely difficult to measure the errors present. There are several reasons for this:

Using any new code leads to errors. During a learning period one can always expect coding problems. Some may not be detected; those which are found will have to be corrected, thus delaying the data processing (and payment).

It will often be difficult to tell which codes were used in a given individual case.[14]

Based on experience with past classification changes, one cannot assume that the old classification will be abandoned and the new one adopted on the specified date (or the same date) by all involved: coders, intermediaries, insurers, and others. When *ICD-9-CM* was introduced, for example, not all state governments were able to accept it for Medicaid in the same year. Thus data for the same time period will be in different classifications.

To the extent that the plans of the federal government have been disclosed, it is likely that vital statistics agencies will use *ICD-10* at an earlier date than the Health Care Financing Administration (HCFA). This will result in the inability to correlate data from these two important segments of the government.

---

12. Implementation is presumably scheduled for the year 2001.

13. *"ICD-10* – Will It Refocus Healthcare Information from Death to Health Status?" (Chicago, IL, 29 Nov 1990).

14. In this regard, the change to alphanumeric codes may have one advantage. Except for those codes beginning with "E", which can mean either "External cause" or "Endocrine", "N", which can be either "Nature of Injury" or "Genito-urinary", or "V", which can be either "External causes" or "Factors ... ", codes with alphabetic prefixes are from *ICD-10*, those without are from *ICD-9* (see the "Structure" table above).

Third, a great deal of work is required in any coding change, and there is even more work when the coders also have to learn a new classification. Hundreds of thousands of persons[15] will have to learn the new classification system.[16] Furthermore, the problems of analyzing data under the new classification are formidable. First, computer programs will have to be rewritten to substitute the changed codes for the old and to accommodate the new codes and their categories. A great deal of effort will be required to be sure that longitudinal studies which cross over between the old and the new classifications are valid. Conscientious researchers will have to worry particularly about the accuracy of the data acquired in the transition period.

Fourth, the transition will be very costly in dollars. The following is a partial list of items which will require outright expenditures (the costs associated with "data problems," enumerated above, are not included): publishing "plain vanilla" copies of *ICD-10*; writing and publishing annotated versions of *ICD-10*; writing and publishing instruction manuals; establishing training programs for those who code manually; rewriting computer programs for computer-assisted coding aids; reprogramming the computer systems for handling data, both in the statistical and the payment systems; rewriting "DRG optimizing" programs.

Fifth, DRGs will have to be redefined (or new payment categories developed) using the data as coded in *ICD-10*. Unless this task is handled with great skill, one can expect, at the very least, unprecedented disputes over payment between providers and payers. A brief outline of what such a change in payment groupings entails is as follows:

> For the past several years, payment to United States hospitals from Medicare, and from other payers, has been via the Prospective Payment System (PPS). Payment has been for the "package" of services "normally" required for patients in Diagnosis Related Groups (DRGs). DRGs were constructed to meet two criteria: (1) patients in a given group would all consume essentially the same amount of resources, and (2) a given group would be constituted of patients with more or less the same clinical problem and management, so that the grouping would make clinical sense.

---

15. This number comes from estimating the number of individuals in hospitals, other health care organizations and agencies, and in physicians' offices who have to do the coding. To the extent that these persons use computer-assisted coding devices, the work and errors will, of course, be less.

16. It should be emphasized that *ICD* is neither a taxonomy nor a nomenclature; it is a classification. The education process is not simply being sure that the "coder" looks up the term in a different book. The person coding (actually, the person is "classifying") must (1) know the meaning of the diagnostic (or "problem") term, (2) know how The Classification "works," (3) look up each term in the alphabetic index to *ICD* (in a separate volume) in order to find out in which category of The Classification the user should look next, (4) go to that category (in the other volume) and find out if there are special considerations, such as "inclusions" or "exclusions," which must be taken into account, (5) often go to another category on the advice of the instructions under the first category, and (6), only after this exhaustive process, "code" the term to the category. This a complex process. See Thompson, B.J. and Slee, V.N., "Accuracy of Diagnosis and Operation Coding," *Medical Record News*, 1978; 49: No.5.

To construct such hospital payment groups, one must have data on a large series of cases, with the data on each patient including the patient's diagnoses, the type of treatment employed, certain demographic and other information, and each patient's hospital "costs." The series must be large enough so that the numbers distributed to each of the groups will provide statistically adequate samples.

Data for the original generation of DRGs were collected using a version of *ICD-8* as the source of diagnosis and operation information, and each group's definition depended on the *ICD-8* codes. With the arrival of *ICD-9-CM*, the groups had to be redefined, which meant collecting the same information as before, but under the new classification, and then carrying out the analysis all over again.

With adoption of *ICD-10*, the same procedure will be required. A new series of cases must be accumulated, and groupings must be defined using the new data source. A serious problem arises with the implementation of *ICD-10*, because presumably the data will simply come in one day under *ICD-9-CM* and the next (and thereafter) under *ICD-10*. Time will be required to accumulate an appropriate series of cases, conduct the analysis, and carry out the other steps necessary to establish the prices for the new groupings. Meanwhile, payments must continue to be made to providers.

The ideal course of action would be to study the same series of cases (several hundred thousand of them in a properly collected sample) coded to both *ICD-9-CM* and to *ICD-10*. With such data in hand, the transition to the new payment classification should be a reasonable one to both payers and providers, and thus it would be straightforward. (Of course, there would at the same time be an opportunity for any other changes desired in the payment groupings.)

Such a careful revision of payment groupings would require several years, for data collection, analysis, and establishment of prices. Yet such a study cannot even begin until the new codes are stabilized and made available, unless entity coding is introduced prior to the transition and an adequate sample of cases is coded both to entities and to *ICD-9-CM*, and also coded to *ICD-10*. This course of action would permit an orderly transition to the new classification in the payment system.

The cost of the transition from *ICD-9-CM* to *ICD-10* in dollars as well as in quality of information, as the present plans for its implementation are understood, will be enormous. One can only hope that the data will be sufficiently more useful (and used) to justify the change.

Implementation of ICD-10 as an Opportunity

The difficulties and costs involved in the forthcoming transition to *ICD-10* must not be underestimated. However, the fact that change is required for implementation of *ICD-10* provides a priceless opportunity to take advantage of the "disarray" and to implement at the same time (and even prior to) the transition a new approach to coding that will forever after simplify the implementation (and reduce the associated costs) of changes in classifications.

The information to be put into the categories of *ICD-10* is already at hand in the medical records of hospitals and other providers. It is the same diagnosis information (except for the greater range of conditions provided for in Chapter XXI of *ICD-10*) that is presently coded to the categories of *ICD-9-CM*. This same information will, of course, also be placed into the categories of any future revisions of The Classification.

The key to capitalizing on this opportunity is to insert a new step, now, of assigning "entity code" numbers to patient diagnosis information. Since the patient information stays the same, the entity code numbers can stay the same ad infinitum. In entity coding, the diagnosis terms are replaced with codes which are their exact counterparts, i.e., decoding gives the exact diagnosis, not the rubric (label) for a group of diagnoses, as is often the case in category coding.[17] The person coding the entities manually simply looks up the term to be coded in a "telephone directory" type of reference and copies the code number; there is no need to make a classification judgement. The person coding by computer would see no change, since assignment of entity codes (as well as to today's *ICD-9-CM* codes and DRGs) would be done via computer programming. The entity codes would be permanently recorded in the "patient's [computer] data set."

The Classification process, the actual placing of the data into the categories of *ICD-10* (or any classification, for that matter) would be carried out by computer. Such a system would permit changes in The Classification, and creation of any number of local or global classifications, without requiring corresponding changes throughout the entire coding system. Only The Classification itself, and the software required for assignment of entity codes to category codes, need be revised.

The one-time establishment of entity coding would be straightforward, it would be essentially painless to the coder, and it would avoid many of the costs, both in data quality and in dollars, inherent in the planned direct substitution of *ICD-10* for *ICD-9* as the vehicle for coding as well as classifying.[18] A nationwide change to entity coding could begin right now; it would not (and should not) have to wait for publication of *ICD-10* to get the process of change started. Control of the completeness and quality of the data could be retained through any number of classification changes. Indeed, efforts now spent on continuous change could instead be spent on refining the data quality to meet present and future needs.

In reviewing and recommending strategies for implementing *ICD-10*, one must keep in mind the goal: obtaining more comprehensive and qualitative patient data. That data already exists, in its most discrete form, in the patient's medical record. If the discrete data is permanently recorded in the patient's data set via entity coding, nothing will be lost by this and future changes in The Classification, but rather there will be great gains in the quality of medical data, which will help achieve the highest quality of medical care. And, in fact, this goal may be achieved at a much lower cost than that which will result from the direct conversion to *ICD-10* which is presently planned. It is a very good time to learn from past experiences, to put to work the tools never before available, and to build a more solid foundation of quality data for the future of world healthcare.

---

17. There are two basic ways to code information: (1) assigning to each individual term its own unique code (number), and (2) assigning to each term a code which represents a class, which class may include one or more individual terms. The first technique is called "entity coding;" the second is "category coding." *See* Slee, *Health Care Terms*, 2d ed., St. Paul: Tringa Press, forthcoming. Further details on entity coding are available from the author.

18. As an example of one immediate advantage of the entity coding alternative: prior to the universal implementation of *ICD-10*, a sample of cases with entity codes could be classified to both *ICD-9-CM* and to *ICD-10* and the resulting data file could be used for redefining DRGs.

Introductions to ICD-6 & ICD-9

The "Introductions" to *ICD-6* (1955) and *ICD-9* (1977), documents which are often very difficult to find, are included here so that one can see some of the evolution of The Classification. In addition, they give excellent dissertations on classification per se, and classification as it pertains to mortality and morbidity from the international perspective.

During the interval between the International Conference for the Sixth Revision of the *International Lists of Diseases and Causes of Death* in 1948 and the Conference for the Ninth Revision in 1975, significant changes had occurred. The 1948 Conference was convened in Paris by the Government of France. The 1975 Conference was convened by the World Health Organization in Geneva. The senior author was a representative of the United States to the 1975 Conference. Twenty-nine nations participated in construction of *ICD-6*, forty-eight in *ICD-9*. But the most significant health event was that it was during this interval that the *International Classification* came into widespread use for clinical purposes, primarily in the United States and Canada.

Introduction to ICD-6

BULLETIN OF THE WORLD HEALTH ORGANIZATION
SUPPLEMENT 1

MANUAL

OF THE

INTERNATIONAL
STATISTICAL CLASSIFICATION
OF DISEASES, INJURIES,
AND CAUSES OF DEATH

Sixth Revision of the International Lists
of Diseases and Causes of Death

Adopted 1948

Volume 1

WORLD HEALTH ORGANIZATION

Geneva, Switzerland
1949

The title page from Volume I of *International Statistical Classification of Diseases, Injuries, and Causes of Death, Sixth Revision.* World Health Organization, 1949.

General Principles

Classification is fundamental to the quantitative study of any phenomenon. It is recognized as the basis of all scientific generalization and is therefore an essential clement in statistical methodology. Uniform definitions and uniform systems of classification are prerequisites in the advancement of scientific knowledge. In the study of illness and death, therefore, a standard classification of disease and injury for statistical purposes is essential.

There are many approaches to the classification of disease. The anatomist, for example, may desire a classification based on the part of the body affected. The pathologist, on the other hand, is primarily interested in the nature of the disease process. The clinician must consider disease from these two angles, but needs further knowledge of etiology. In other words, there are many ares of classification and the particular axis selected will be determined by the interests of the investigator. A statistical classification of disease and injury will depend, therefore, upon the use to be made of the statistics to be compiled.

The purpose of a statistical classification is often confused with that of a nomenclature. Basically a medical nomenclature is a list or catalogue of approved terms for describing terms recording clinical and pathological observations. To serve its full function, it should be extensive, so that any pathological condition can be accurately recorded. As medical science advances, a nomenclature must expand to include new terms necessary to record new observations. Any morbid condition that can be specifically described will need a specific designation in a nomenclature.

This complete specificity of a nomenclature prevents it from serving satisfactorily as a statistical classification. When one speaks of statistics, it is at once inferred that the interest is in a group of cases and not in individual occurrences. The purpose of a statistical compilation of disease data is primarily to furnish quantitative data that will answer questions about groups of cases.

This distinction between a statistical classification and a nomenclature has always been clear to medical statisticians[*] The aims of statistical classification of disease cannot be better summarized than in the following paragraphs written by William Farr[1] nearly a century ago: [*See Introduction, U.S. Mortality Statistics, 1907, Government Printing Office, Washington, 1909, 21.]

> "The causes of death were tabulated in the early Bills of Mortality (Tables mortuaires) alphabetically; and this course has the advantage of not raising any of those nice questions in which it is vain to expect physicians and statists to agree unanimously. But statistics is eminently a science of classification and it is evident, on glancing at the subject cursorily, that any classification that brings together in groups diseases that have considerable affinity, or that are liable to be confounded with each other, is likely to facilitate the deduction of general principles.

> "Classification is a method of generalization. Several classifications may, therefore, be used with advantage; and the physician, the pathologist, or the jurist, each from his own point of view, may legitimately classify the diseases and the causes of death in the way that he thinks best adapted to facilitate his inquiries, and to yield general results.

> "The medical practitioner may found his main divisions of diseases on their treatment as medical or surgical; the pathologist, on the nature of the morbid action or product; the

anatomist or the physiologist on the tissues and organs involved; the medical jurist, on the suddenness or the slowness of the death ; and all these points well deserve attention in a statistical classification.

"In the eyes of national statistics the most important elements are, however, brought into account in the ancient subdivision of disease. into plagues, or epidemics and endemics, into diseases of common occurrence (sporadic diseases), which may be conveniently divided into three classes, and into injuries the immediate results of violence or of external causes."

A statistical classification of disease must be confined to a limited number of categories which will encompass the entire range of morbid conditions. The categories should be chosen so that they will facilitate the statistical study of disease phenomena. A specific disease entity should have a separate title in the classification only when its separation is warranted because the frequency of its occurrence, or its importance as a morbid condition, justifies its isolation as a separate category. On the other hand, many titles in the classification will refer to groups of separate but usually related morbid conditions. Every disease or morbid condition, however, must have a definite and appropriate place as an inclusion in one of the categories of the statistical classification. A few items of the statistical list will be residual titles for other and miscellaneous conditions which cannot be classified under the more specific titles. These miscellaneous categories should be kept to a minimum.

Before a statistical classification can be put into actual use, it is necessary that a decision be reached as to the inclusions for each category. These terms should be arranged as a tabular list under each title, and an alphabetical index should be prepared. If medical nomenclature were uniform and standard, such a task would be simple and quite direct. Actually the doctors who practice and who will be making entries in medical records or writing medical certificates of death were, educated at hundreds of medical schools and over a period of more than fifty years. As a result, the medical entries on sickness records, hospital records, and death certificates are certain to be of mixed terminology which cannot be modernized or standardized by the wave of any magician's wand. All these terms, good and bad, must be provided for as inclusions in a statistical classification.

The construction of a practical schema of classification of disease and injury for general statistical use involves various compromises. Efforts to provide a statistical classification upon a strictly logical arrangement of morbid conditions have failed in the past. The various titles will represent a series of necessary compromises between classifications based on etiology, anatomical site, age, and circumstance of onset, as well as the quality of information available on medical reports. Adjustments must also be made to meet the varied requirements of vital statistics offices, hospitals of different types, medical services of the armed forces, social insurance organizations, sickness surveys, and numerous other agencies. While no single classification will fit the specialized needs for all these purposes, it should provide a common basis of classification for general statistical use.

Historical Review

Early history.

Sir George H. Knibbs,[2] the eminent Australian statistician, credited Francois Bossier de Lacroix (1706-1777), better known as Sauvages, with the first attempt to classify diseases systematically. Sauvages' comprehensive treatise was published under the title *Nosologia*

Methodica. A contemporary of Sauvages was the great methodologist Linnaeus (1707-1778), one of whose treatises was entitled *Genera Morborum*. At the beginning of the 19th century, the Classification of disease in most general use was one by William Cullen (1710-1790), of Edinburgh, which was published in 1785 under the title Synopsis Nosologiae Methodicae.

The statistical study of disease, however, began for all practical purposes with the work of John Graunt on the London Bills of Mortality a century earlier. The kind of classification which this pioneer had at his disposal is exemplified by his attempt to estimate the proportion of liveborn children who died before reaching the age of six years, no records of age at death being then available. He took all deaths classed as thrush, convulsions, rickets, teeth and worms, abortives, chrysomes, infants, livergrown, and overlaid and added to them half the deaths classed as smallpox, swine pox, measles, and worms without convulsions. Despite the crudity of this classification his estimate of a 36 per cent mortality before the age of six years appears from later evidence to have been a good one. While three centuries have contributed something to the scientific accuracy of disease classification, there are many who doubt the usefulness of attempts to compile statistics of disease, or even causes of death, because of the difficulties of classification. To these, one can quote Professor Major Greenwood:[3]

"The scientific purist, who will wait for medical statistics until they are nosologically exact, is no wiser than Horace's rustic waiting for the river to flow away."

Fortunately for the progress of preventive medicine, the General-Register Office of England and Wales, at its inception in 1837, found in William Farr (1807-1883) — its first medical statistician — a man who not only made the best possible use of the imperfect classifications of disease available at the time, but laboured to secure better classification and international uniformity in their use.

Farr found the classification of Cullen in use in the public services of his day. It had not been revised so as to embody the advances of medical science, nor was it deemed by him to be satisfactory for statistical purposes. In the first Annual Report of the Registrar-General, therefore, he discussed the principles that should govern a statistical classification of disease and urged the adoption of a uniform classification in the following paragraph that has been quoted so regularly in both the British and American Manuals of the International List of Causes of Death :

"The advantages of a uniform statistical nomenclature, however imperfect, are so obvious, that it is surprising no attention had been paid to its enforcement in Bills of Mortality. Each disease has, in many instances, been denoted by three or four terms, and each term has been applied to as many different diseases: vague, inconvenient names have been employed, or complications have been registered instead of primary diseases. The nomenclature is of as much importance in this department of inquiry as weights and measures in the physical sciences, and should be settled without delay."[4]

Both nomenclature and statistical classification received constant study and consideration by Farr in his annual "Letters" to the Registrar-General published in the Annual Reports of the Registrar-General. The utility of a uniform classification of causes of death was so strongly recognized at the first International Statistical Congress, held at Brussels in 1853, that it requested Dr. William Farr and Dr. Marc d'Espine, of Geneva, to prepare "une nomenclature uniforme des causes de deces applicable a tous les pays."[5] At the next Congress, at Paris in

1855, Farr and d'Espine submitted two separate lists which were based on very different principles. Farr's classification was arranged under five groups: Epidemic diseases, Constitutional (general) diseases, Local diseases arranged according to anatomical site, Developmental diseases, and diseases that are the direct result of violence. D'Espine classified diseases according to their nature (gouty, herpatic, haematic, etc.). The Congress adopted a compromise list of 139 rubrics. In 1864, this classification was revised at Paris "sur le modele de cello de W. Farr," and was subsequently revised in 1874, 1880, and 1886. Although there was never any universal acceptance of this classification, the general arrangement, including the principle of classifying diseases by anatomical site, proposed by Farr has survived as the basis of the International List of Causes of Death.

Adoption of International List of Causes of Death.

The International Statistical Institute, the successor to the International Statistical Congress, at its meeting in Vienna in 1891, charged a committee, of which Dr. Jacques Bertillon (1851-1922), Chef des Travaux statistiques de la vile de Paris, was chairman, with the preparation of a classification of causes of death. It is of interest to note that Bertillon was the grandson of Dr. Achille Guillard, a noted botanist and statistician, who had introduced the resolution requesting Farr and d'Espine to prepare a uniform classification at the First Statistical Congress in 1853. The report of this committee was presented by Bertillon at the meeting of the International Statistical Institute at Chicago in 1893 and adopted by it.

The classification prepared by Bertillon was based on the classification of causes of death used by the City of Paris, which, since its revision in 1885, represented a synthesis of English, German, and Swiss classifications. The classification was based on the principle, adopted by Farr, of distinguishing between general diseases and those localized to a particular organ or anatomical site. In accordance with the instructions of the Vienna Congress made at the suggestion of Dr. L. Guillaume, the Director of the Federal Bureau of Statistics of Switzerland, Bertillon included three classifications: the first, an abridged classification of 44 titles; the second, a classification of 99 titles; and the third, a classification of 161 titles.

The Bertillon Classification of Causes of Death, as it was at first called, received general approval and was adopted by several countries, as well as by many cities. The classification was first used in North America by Dr. Jesus E. Monjaras for the statistics of San Luis de Potosi, Mexico.[6] In 1898, the American Public Health Association, at its meeting in Ottawa, Canada, recommended the adoption of the Bertillon Classification by registrars of Canada, Mexico, and the United States. The Association further suggested that the classification be revised every ten years.

At the meeting of the International Statistical Institute at Christiania in 1899, Dr. Bertillon presented a report on the progress of the classification, including the recommendations of the American Public Health Association for decennial revisions. The International Statistical Institute then adopted the following resolution:

"The International Statistical Institute, convinced of the necessity of using in the different countries comparable nomenclatures :

"Learns with pleasure of the adoption by all the statistical offices of North America, by some of those of South America, and by some in Europe, of the system of cause of death nomenclature presented in 1893;

"Insists vigorously that this system of nomenclature be adopted in principle and without revision, by all the statistical institutions of Europe;

"Approves, at least in its general lines, the system of decennial revision proposed by the American Public Health Association at it's Ottawa session (1898)

"Urges the statistical offices who have not yet adhered, to do so without delay , and to contribute to the comparability of the cause of death nomenclature."[7]

The French Government therefore convoked at Paris, in August 1900, the first International Conference for the revision of the Bertillon or International Classification of Causes of Death. Delegates from 20 countries attended this Conference. A detailed classification of causes of death consisting of 179 groups and an abridged classification of 35 groups were adopted on 21 August 1900. The desirability of decennial revisions was recognized, and the French Government was requested to call the next meeting in 1910. Actually the next conference was held in 1909, and the Government of France called succeeding conferences in 1920, 1929, and 1938.

Dr. Bertillon continued as the guiding force in the promotion of the International List of Causes of Death, and the revisions of 1900, 1910, and 1920 were carried out under his leadership. As Secretary-General of the International Conference, he sent out the provisional revision for 1920 to more than 500 persons, asking for comments. His death in 1922 left the International Conference without a guiding hand.

At the 1923 session of the International Statistical Institute, M. Michel Huber, Bertillon's successor in France, recognized this lack of leadership and introduced a resolution for the International Statistical Institute to renew its stand of 1893 in regard to the International Classification of Causes of Death and to co-operate with other International organizations in preparation for subsequent revisions. The Health Organization of the League of Nations had also taken an active interest in vital statistics and appointed a Commission of Statistical Experts to study the classification of diseases and causes of death, as well as other problems in the field of medical statistics. Dr. E. Roesle, Chief of the Medical Statistical Service of the German Health Bureau and a member of the Commission of Expert Statisticians, prepared a monograph that listed the expansion in the rubrics of the 1920 International List of Causes of Death that would be required if the classification was to be used in the tabulation of statistics of morbidity. This careful study was published by the Health Organization of the League of Nations in 1928.[8] In order to co-ordinate the work of both agencies, an international commission, known as the "Mixed Commission ", was created with an equal number of representatives from the International Statistical Institute and the Health Organization of the League of Nations. This Commission drafted the proposals for the Fourth (1929) and the Fifth (1938) revisions of the International List of Causes of Death.

The Fifth Decennial Revision Conference.

The Fifth International Conference for the Revision of the International List of Causes of Death, like the preceding conferences, was convened by the Government of France and was held at Paris in October 1938. The Conference approved three lists: a detailed list of 200 titles, an intermediate list of 87 titles and an abridged list of 44 titles. Apart from bringing the lists up to date in accordance with the progress of science, particularly in the chapter on infective and parasitic diseases, and changes in the chapters on puerperal conditions and on accidents, the Conference made as few changes as possible in the contents, number, and even in the numbering of the items. A list of causes of stillbirth was also drawn up and approved by the Conference.

As regards classification of diseases for morbidity statistics the Conference recognized the growing necessity for a corresponding list of diseases to meet the statistical needs of widely differing organizations, such as health insurance organizations, hospitals, military medical services, health administrations, and similar agencies. The following resolution, therefore, was adopted

"2. International Lists of Diseases.

"In view of the importance of the compilation of international lists of diseases corresponding to the international lists of causes of death:

"The Conference recommends that the Joint Committee appointed by the International Institute of Statistics and the Health Organization of the League of Nations undertake, as in 1029, the preparation of international lists of diseases, in conjunction with experts and representatives of the organizations specially concerned.

"Pending the compilation of international lists of diseases, the Conference recommends that the various national lists in use should, as far as possible, be brought into line with the detailed International List of Causes of Death (the numbers of the chapters, headings and subheadings in the said List being given in brackets)."[9]

The Conference further recommended that the United States Government continue its studies of the statistical treatment of joint causes of death in the following resolution:

"3. Death Certificate and Selection, of Cause of Death where more than One Cause is given (Joint Causes).

"The Conference,

"Whereas, in 1929, the United States Government was good enough to undertake the study of the means of unifying the methods of selection of the main cause of death to be tabulated in those cases where two or more causes are mentioned on the death certificate,

"And whereas, the numerous surveys completed or in the course of preparation in several countries reveal the importance of this problem, which has not yet been solved,

"And whereas, according to these surveys, the international comparability of death rates from the various diseases requires, not only the solution of the problem of the selection of the main tabulated cause of death, hut also the solution of a number of other questions;

"(1) Warmly thanks the United States Government for the work it has accomplished or promoted in this connection

"(2) Requests the United States Government to continue its investigations (luring the next ten years, in co-operation with other countries and organizations, en a slightly wider basis, and

"(3) Suggests that, for these future investigations, the United States Government should set(up a subcommittee comprising representatives of countries and organizations participating in the investigations undertaken in this connection."[10]

Previous Classifications of Diseases for Morbidity Statistics.

In the discussion so far, classification of disease has been presented almost wholly in relation to cause-of-death statistics. Farr,[11] however, recognized that it was desirable "to extend the same system of nomenclature to diseases which, ..though not fatal, cause disability in the population, and now figure in the tables of the diseases of armies, navies, hospitals, prisons, lunatic asylums, public institutions of every kind, and sickness societies, as well as in the census of countries like Ireland, where diseases of all the people are enumerated." In his "Report on Nomenclature and Statistical Classification of Diseases " presented to the Second International Statistical Congress, he therefore included in the general list of diseases the greater part of those diseases that affect health as well as diseases that are fatal. At the Fourth International Statistical Congress, held at London in 1860, Florence Nightingale[12] urged the adoption of Farr's classification of diseases for the tabulation of hospital morbidity in a paper entitled "Proposals for a Uniform Plan of Hospital Statistics."

At the First International Conference at Paris in 1900 to revise the Bertillon Classification of Causes of Death, a parallel classification of diseases for use in statistics of sickness was adopted. Such a parallel list was also adopted at the second conference in 1909. The extra categories for nonfatal diseases were formed by subdivision of certain rubrics of the cause-of-death classification into two or three disease groups, each of these being designated by a letter. The translation in English of the Second Decennial Revision, published by the U.S. Department of Commerce and Labor in 1910, was entitled International Classification of Causes of Sickness and Death. Later revisions incorporated some of the groups into the detailed International List of Causes of Death. The Fourth International Conference adopted a classification of illness which differed from the detailed International List of Causes of Death only by the addition of further subdivisions of 12 titles. These international classifications of illnesses, however, have failed to receive general acceptance, as they provided only a limited expansion of the basic cause-of-death list.

In the absence of a uniform classification of diseases that could be used satisfactorily for statistics of illness, many countries have found it necessary to prepare such lists. These should not be confused with disease nomenclatures such as the Nomenclature of Diseases of the Royal College of Physicians of London or the Standard Nomenclature of Disease now published by the American Medical Association. The former traces its lineage back to a resolution of the Royal College of Physicians of London on 9 July 1857, but the first edition of this nomenclature did not appear until 1869. Its purpose, as pointed out in the preface of this edition, was to provide authoritative medical terminology "for perfecting the statistical registration of diseases, with a view to the discovery of statistical truths concerning their history, nature, and phenomena, the want of a generally recognized Nomenclature of Diseases has long been felt as an indispensable condition ". The Nomenclature has been revised periodically (1885, 1886, 1906, 1918, 1931, and 1947) and has afforded a continual basis of authority for British physicians in the use of medical terms.

Until recently, there had been no similar authoritative nomenclature in the United States. Numerous hospital nomenclatures, such as that of the Bellevue and Allied Hospitals and that of the Massachusetts General Hospital, have had extensive use. In 1919, the U.S. Bureau of the Census published a Standard Nomenclature of Diseases and Pathological Conditions, Injuries, and Poisonings for the United States which was an attempted consolidation of eight nomenclatures then largely in use. Early in the history of the American Medical Association efforts were made in the direction of a nomenclature. An American Nomenclature of Diseases was actually prepared in 1872, but the work was discontinued until the Association took over the Standard Nomenclature of Disease in 1937. The work on this latter Nomenclature was initiated on 22 March 1928, when the National Conference on Nomenclature of Disease was formed under the sponsorship of the New York Academy of Medicine. The basic plan of this Nomenclature was adopted at the Second National Conference on Nomenclature, on 24 November 1930. The first printing appeared in 1932, the first edition in 1933, and a second edition in 1935. In 1937, the American Medical Association took over the responsibility of periodic revisions, and as a result of the Fourth National Conference on Nomenclature, held in 1940, the third edition, which included a Standard Nomenclature of Operations as well, appeared in 1942. Such standard nomenclatures, as pointed out in the preface to the first edition of the British Nomenclature, are a great aid in the "statistical registration of diseases," but cannot, because of their very nature, serve as statistical classifications.

On the other hand, many countries found it necessary to prepare lists of diseases for the statistical tabulation of causes of illness. A Standard Morbidity Code was prepared by the Dominion Council of Health of Canada and published in 1936. The main subdivisions of this code represented the eighteen chapters of the 1929 Revision of the International List of Causes of Death, and these were subdivided into some 380 specific disease categories. At the 1938 International Conference, the Canadian delegate introduced a modification of this list for consideration as the basis for an international list of causes of illness. Although no action was taken on this proposal, the Fifth International Conference adopted the resolution previously quoted.

In 1944, provisional classifications of diseases and injuries were published in Britain and the United States for use in the tabulation of morbidity statistics. Both classifications were more extensive than the Canadian list, but, like it, followed the general order of diseases as given in the International List of Causes of Death. The British classification was prepared by the Committee on Hospital Morbidity Statistics of the Medical Research Council which was created in January 1942. It is entitled A Provisional Classification of Diseases and Injuries for Use in Compiling Morbidity Statistics.[13] It was prepared for the purpose of providing a scheme for collecting and recording statistics of patients admitted to hospitals of Great Britain, using a standard classification of diseases and injuries. It has been in use by the Ministry of Health in the classification of all Emergency Medical Service records, the Ministry of Pensions, hospitals, and other agencies in England.

Somewhat earlier, the Surgeon-General of the U.S. Public Health Service and the Director of the U.S. Bureau of the Census published, in the Public Health Reports for 30 August 1940, a list of diseases and injuries for tabulation of morbidity statistics.[14] The code was prepared by the Division of Public Health Methods of the Public Health Service in co-operation with a committee of consultants appointed by the Surgeon-General. A Manual for Coding Causes of Illness according to a Diagnosis Code for Tabulating Morbidity Statistics, consisting of the diagnosis code, a tabular list of inclusions, and an alphabetical index, was published in 1944. The code is in use in several hospitals, in a large number of voluntary hospital insurance plans and medical care plans, and in special studies by other agencies in the United States.

United States Committee on Joint Causes of Death

In compliance with a resolution of the Fifth International Conference, the Secretary of State of the United States in 1945 appointed the U.S. Committee on Joint Causes of Death under the chairmanship of Dr. Lowell J. Reed, Vice-President and Professor of Biostatistics of the Johns Hopkins University. Members and consultants of this committee included representatives of the Canadian and British Governments and the Health Section of the League of Nations. Recognizing the general trend of thought with regard to morbidity and mortality statistical lists, this committee decided that before taking up the matter of joint causes, it would be advantageous to consider classifications from the point of view of morbidity and mortality, since the joint-cause problem pertains to both types of statistics.

The committee also took cognizance of that part of the resolution of the last International Conference on International List of Diseases that recommended that the "various National Lists in use should, as far as possible, be brought in line with the detailed International List of Causes of Death." It recognized that the classification of sickness and injury is closely linked with the classification of causes of death. The view that such lists are fundamentally different arises from the erroneous belief that the International List is a classification of terminal causes, whereas it is in fact based upon the morbid condition which initiated the train of events ultimately resulting in death. The committee believed that, in order to utilize fully both morbidity and mortality statistics, not only should the classification of diseases for both purposes be comparable, but if possible there should be a single list.

Furthermore, an increasing number of statistical organizations are utilizing medical records involving both sickness and death. Even in organizations which compile only morbidity statistics, fatal as ``well as nonfatal cases must be coded. A single list, therefore, greatly facilitates the coding operations in such offices. It also provides a common base for comparison of morbidity and mortality statistics, which does not now exist. A subcommittee was therefore appointed, which, during the period 10 December 1945 to 11 February 1946, prepared a preliminary draft of a "Proposed Statistical Classification of Diseases, Injuries and Causes of Death." This work received the approval of the full' committee on 11 February 1946. The classification was then subjected to trials and review by various agencies and individuals in Canada, England and the United States. After making further modifications based on these studies, the U.S. Committee met in Ottawa, Canada, on 10 March 1947, and approved a final draft of the proposed classification.

Preparation of the Sixth Decennial Revision of the International List

The International Health Conference held in New York City in June and July 1946 entrusted the Interim Commission of the World Health Organization with the responsibility of "reviewing the existing machinery and of undertaking such preparatory work as may be necessary in connection with:

"(i) the next decennial revision of 'The International Lists of Causes of Death' (including the lists adopted under the International Agreement of 1934, relating to Statistics of Causes of Death); and

"(ii) the establishment of International Lists of Causes of Morbidity."

To meet this responsibility, the Interim Commission decided at its second session, in November 1946, to set up for these purposes a committee of experts, which was appointed in

January 1947, as the "Expert Committee for the Preparation of the Sixth Decennial Revision of the International Lists of Diseases and Causes of Death." The members of the Expert Committee, together with the officers elected at its first session, held in Ottawa, Canada, in March 1947, were:

P. Stocks, M.D., F.R.C.P., D.F.H. (Chairman), Chief Statistician (Medical). General Register Office of England and Wales;

W. T. Fales, Sc.D. (Vice-Chairman), Director, Statistical Section, Baltimore City Health Department; Research Associate, School of Hygiene, Johns Hopkins University, Baltimore, Md., U.S.A.;

Julia E. Backer, Sc.D., Chief, Demographic Section, Central Statistical Office, Oslo, Norway;

S. T. Bok, M.D., Professor in Medicine, University of Leiden; Chief, Section for Statistics, Institute for Preventive Medicine, Leiden, Netherlands;

D. Curiel, Dr.P.H., Medical Chief, Division of Epidemiology and Vital Statistics, Ministry of Health and Social Welfare, Caracas, Venezuela;

P. F. Denoix, M.D., Chief, Technical Services and Section for Cancer, Institut national d'Hygiene, Paris, France;

M. Kacprzak, M.D., D.P.H., Professor of Hygiene, Director, State School of Hygiene; President, National Health Council, Warsaw, Poland;

J. Wyllie, M.D., D.P.H., Professor of Preventive Medicine, Queen's University, Kingston, Ont., Canada;

N——,* Medical Statistician, Union of Soviet Socialist Republics. [*Absent from first, second and third sessions.]

Adviser to Expert Committee.

H. L. Dunn, M.D., Ph.D., Chief, National Office of Vital Statistics; Secretary for Mortality Code, U.S. Committee on Joint Causes of Death, Washington, D.C., U.S.A.

Secretariat.

Marie Cakrtova, M.D., Dr.P.H.. Medical Officer. World Health Organization, Interim Commission , Geneva, Switzerland;

J. T. Marshall, Assistant Dominion Statistician, Acting Director, Social Welfare Statistics Division, Dominion Bureau of Statistics, Ottawa, Canada.

This committee, in carrying out its task and taking full notice of the prevailing opinion concerning morbidity and mortality classification, reviewed and revised, at its first session, the above-mentioned classification which had been prepared by the United States Committee on Joint Causes of Death and made available to the Expert Committee for its consideration.

The work of the first session was embodied in (a) International Statistical Classification of Diseases, Injuries, and Causes of Death: Introduction and List of Categories (document WHO.IC/MS/1) and (b) International Statistical Classification of Diseases, Injuries, and Causes of Death: Tabular List of Inclusions (document WHO.IC/ MS/7). The first was circulated to seventy-two governments for review and comments. The second document was distributed primarily to members of the Expert Committee and to Governments which had participated in the work of the U.S. Committee on Joint Causes of Death.

At its second session, held in Geneva, Switzerland, 21-29 October 1947, the Expert Committee considered the replies of the various governments and their national administrations and prepared a revised version of both documents incorporating such changes in the classification as appeared to improve its utility and acceptability. At this session, the committee was assisted by the following subcommittee, which had been appointed to compile a comprehensive alphabetical index in co-operation with the governmental agencies of Canada, the United Kingdom and the United States of America.

Subcommittee on Index.

S. D. Collins, Ph.D. (Chairman), Head Statistician, Division of Public Health Methods, United States Public Health Service, Washington, D.C., U.S.A.;

I. M. Moriyama, Ph.D., Chief, Mortality Analysis Section, National Office of Vital Statistics, United States Public Health Service, Washington, D.C., U.S.A.;

Winifred O'Brien, R.N., Supervisor, Nosology Section, Dominion Bureau of Statistics, Ottawa, Canada;

A. H. T. Robb-Smith, M.D., Nuffield Reader in Pathology, University of Oxford, England

J. T. Marshall (Secretary), Assistant Dominion Statistician; Acting Director, Social Welfare Statistics Division, Dominion Bureau of Statistics, Ottawa, Canada.

At this session, the committee also considered the structure and uses of special lists of causes for tabulation and publication of morbidity and mortality statistics and studied other problems related to the international comparability of mortality statistics such as form of medical certificate and rules for classification. It recommended that these subjects be placed on the agenda of the Sixth Decennial Revision Conference.

Sixth Decennial Revision Conference

The International Conference for the Sixth Revision of the International Lists of Diseases and Causes of Death was convened in Paris by the Government of France, for 20-30 April 1948, under the terms of the Agreement of 7 October 1938 signed at the close of the Fifth Revision Conference. The Conference, opened by His Excellency, M. Georges Bidault, French Minister for Foreign Affairs, was composed of delegates from the following twenty-nine countries

Belgium	Greece	Norway
Bulgaria	Guatemala	Poland
Canada	Hungary	Portugal
Chile	Iceland	Siam
Cuba	India	Sweden
Czechoslovakia	Ireland	Switzerland
Denmark	Italy	United Kingdom
Ecuador	Luxemburg	United States of
Ethiopia	Mexico	America
France	Netherlands	Venezuela

Its secretariat was entrusted jointly to the competent French administrations and to the World Health Organization, which had carried out the preparatory work under the terms of the Arrangement concluded by the governments represented at the International Health Conference in 1946. The proposals of the Expert Committee and its viewpoints were presented to the Conference by the Chairman and Vice-Chairman of the Committee and by its Rapporteur, Dr. A. H. T. Robb-Smith.

The Conference approved the Classification, prepared by the Expert Committee of the World Health Organization, as the Sixth Revision of the International Lists of Diseases and Causes of Death. It considered the application of the Classification in the compilation, tabulation and publication of statistics of Morbidity and mortality. In this connexion, the Conference recommended that the List of Three-digit Categories (Detailed List) be used in coding medical records of sickness and death, and that a uniform Medical Certificate of Cause of Death and Rules for the Selection of the Underlying Cause of Death be adopted. It also approved the following special lists for the tabulation and publication of statistics:

    (1) an "intermediate" list of 150 causes for tabulation of morbidity and mortality by age groups and other demographic characteristics;

    (2) an "abbreviated" list of 50 causes for tabulation of mortality in administrative subdivisions;

    (3) a "special " list of 50 causes for tabulation of morbidity for social insurance purposes.

It was further recommended that the World Health Assembly adopt suitable regulations under Article 21 (b) of its Constitution which would embody the recommendations of the Expert Committee and of the Conference and ensure international application of the classification. The first World Health Assembly, in Geneva, Switzerland, adopted such Regulations in July 1948, a copy of which is to be found at the end of this book.

The Sixth Decennial Revision Conference marked the beginning of a new era in international vital and health statistics. In addition to the adoption of a single comprehensive list of diseases, injuries and causes of death, it recommended the adoption of a far-reaching programme of international co-operation in the field of vital and health statistics.

The following methods of international co-operation were suggested:

    (a) establishment by the World Health Assembly of an Expert Committee on Health Statistics entrusted with the study of problems in the field of health statistics, including recording of births, diseases and deaths;

    (b) establishment by the different governments of national committees for the purpose of coordinating statistical activities within the country, and to serve as links between the national medical. statistical institutions and the Expert Committee on Health Statistics of the World Health Organization

    (c) decentralization of studies of certain statistical problems of public health importance to interested national committees on health statistics and other national agencies with a view to transmission of the results of such studies to the Expert Committee of the World Health Organization for international discussion and utilization

    (d) development of the statistical service of the World Health Organization to such technical competence as to enable it not only to carry out the statistical functions within the Organization and to implement the recommendations of the Expert Committee on Health Statistics, but also to furnish consulting services to national health administrations and statistical agencies;

    (e) convening by the World Health Organization, when occasion arises, of international technical conferences on problems of vital and health statistics

    (f) co-operation, in the execution of the work mentioned above, with the interested organs of the United Nations and its specialized agencies.

Finally, the Sixth Revision Conference entrusted to the Expert Committee which had undertaken the preparatory work for the Conference the establishment of the final forms of the:

(a) International Statistical Classification of Diseases, Injuries, and Causes of Death, and of the Intermediate, Abbreviated and Special Lists, incorporating in them as far as possible, but without changing their basic structure, amendments proposed in the discussion of the Conference;

(b) Medical Certificate of Cause of Death;

(c) Rules for selecting the underlying cause of death, when multiple causes are mentioned on the certificate;

(d) Tabulations for presenting multiple causes of death.

The Expert Committee at its third session, held in Geneva, Switzerland, 4-7 May 1948, and also attended by the Index Subcommittee, considered the suggestions of the Sixth Revision Conference and decided to recommend to the World Health Assembly the publication of the International Statistical Classification of Diseases, Injuries, and Causes of Death in the form of the present manual.

During all stages of the work connected with the Sixth Revision of the International Lists of Diseases and Causes of Death, effective co-operation had been maintained with the United Nations Statistical Office and the International Labour Organization. The second session of the Expert Committee was attended by an observer from each of these organizations. The International Labour Organization was also represented at the Revision Conference and at the third session of the Expert Committee. The Special List of 50 Causes for Tabulation of Morbidity for Social Security Purposes is based on a proposal of the Inter-American Committee on Social Security which was submitted by the International Labour Office to the Expert Committee for review and study.

International Statistical Classification of Diseases, Injuries, and Causes of Death

A list of diseases and injuries to be used for the classification of causes of both illness and death must necessarily differ in content from that of previous International Lists designed primarily for coding causes of death. The work of research groups in Great Britain and the United States, as well as in other countries, has shown clearly that the general structure of previous International Lists was a useful frame around which a morbidity classification for statistical purposes could be developed. Furthermore, the basic structure of these lists has withstood the test of well over half a century of use in numerous countries throughout the world. The very fact that the general arrangement has not been changed substantially in that time suggests that it is difficult to improve upon it as a working basis for disease statistics.

The present classification represents an expansion of the disease rubrics of the previous International Lists to provide specific categories for nonfatal diseases and injuries. In this process of expansion, provision has been made so as to permit comparability of certain categories with important titles of the Fifth Revision of the International List. It is not essential, however, that there should be strict comparability fur each individual subdivision. It must be remembered that when one compares the frequency of a disease or cause of death new and twenty years ago, one is not really comparing the actual frequency of that particular disease, but the frequency with which a particular term is used to describe a disease status by observers differing in their education and medical outlook by a period of twenty years.

In order to preserve, as much as possible, continuity of mortality rates by cause and age, the Sixth Decennial Conference repeated the recommendation which had been made at the previous Conference in 1938. The Conference recommended that deaths for the country as a whole in the year 1949 or 1950 should be coded according to the Detailed List of 1948 and also according to the Fifth Revision of the International List of 1938, and that dual tabulations of these data should be published in such a way as to indicate the changes resulting from the application of the new List. In giving an outline of the general principles underlying the present classification, it is well to consider again the purpose of a statistical classification which is to provide a list of disabilities for compiling statistics and not a nomenclature of diseases and Injuries. In other words, not every condition receives a particular rubric or number, but there is a category to which every condition can be referred, and this has been achieved by the method of selective grouping. For instance, a broad group of conditions such as the psychoses is given a two-figure number and is then divided into nine categories corresponding to fairly well defined types of psychoses, and lastly there is a tenth or residual category to which the psychoses which are not already characterized or are ill defined can be allocated. The principles of determining what conditions should be specified as definite categories are based on frequency, importance, and clarity of characterization of the condition. The question as to how satisfactory these categories are will be tested under the principle that the number of conditions allocated to the miscellaneous or residual category must not be unduly large.

List of Three-digit Categories (Detailed List)

The taxonomic philosophy of the present classification is somewhat eclectic, as no strictly systematic classification is really practicable ; but in general, the broad groups have followed the principles of the previous International Lists of Causes of Death. The classification deals first with diseases caused by well-defined infective agents; these are followed by categories for neoplasms, allergic, endocrine, metabolic and nutritional diseases. Most of the remaining diseases are arranged according to their principal anatomical site, with special sections for mental diseases, complications of pregnancy and childbirth, certain diseases of early infancy, and senility and ill-defined conditions including symptoms. The last section provides a dual classification of injuries. Although the general order of the classification follows that of the previous International Lists of Causes of Death, departures have been made from it whenever it seemed expedient, in order to secure a better arrangement of related categories, or to provide expansion required in meeting the needs -of morbidity statistics.

The Detailed List presented on pages 1-42 consists of a list of 612 categories of diseases and morbid conditions, plus 153 categories for classification of the external cause of injury and 189 categories for characterization of injuries according to the nature of the lesion. A decimal system of numbering has been adopted in which the detailed categories of the classification are designated by three-digit numbers. In many instances, the first two digits of the three-digit number designate important or summary groups that are significant. The third digit divides each group into categories which represent specific disease entities or a classification of the disease or condition according to some significant axis such as anatomical site. Further, the detailed or three-digit categories have not been numbered consecutively, but numbers have been omitted in order that the summary character of the first two digits could be preserved wherever they are meaningful. No additional three- digit categories should be introduced in the classification except when the list is revised by international agreement. The numbering system has been designed purposely as a closed system; that is, the third digit under each broad group begins with "0" and continues consecutively for the number of categories in that group.

The decimal system represents a departure from the combined number and letter subdivisions that characterized the numbering system used in previous revisions of the International Lists of Causes of Death. The numbering system adopted in the classification results in greater flexibility and utility since (1) it provides a large number of broad groups which represent significant disease entities or disease groups, (2) it permits the introduction of new categories at later revisions without upsetting the basic numbering of other categories, and (3) it provides economy of operation, both clerical and mechanical. The latter is of particular importance in statistical organizations using modern tabulating equipment and handling large volumes of records.

In the present scheme there are seventeen main sections, as compared with eighteen sections of the Fifth Revision of the International List of Causes of Death. Senility and ill-defined conditions have been combined into a single section instead of representing two main groups as in the 1938 List. Section "V. Chronic Poisoning and Intoxication" of the Fifth Revision has been eliminated, and the conditions included in that section are assigned elsewhere in the present classification. In its place, a new major group, "V. Mental, Psychoneurotic, and Personality Disorders," has been established.

The section on "Accidents, Poisonings, and Violence" has always been one of the more troublesome in the previous International Lists. The difficulties arise because there are to be considered several axes of classification of statistical interest — namely, circumstances of accident or means of injury, and nature of injury. Each of these represents important aspects of injuries, although In a particular analysis one axis may be more important than another. As a consequence of the simultaneous interest in more than one aspect of injury, this section has always represented compromises that were unsatisfactory, usually because the categories were not mutually exclusive.

In building a single code for use in morbidity and mortality statistics, this problem has therefore been attacked boldly and a dual classification adopted. As an integral part of the classification, morbid conditions resulting from injuries, poisonings and other external causes have been classified according to both the external circumstances giving rise to the injury, expressed in the classification as the "External cause," and to the kind of injury (for example: fracture, open wound, or burns) designated in the classification as the "Nature of injury." The code numbers 800-999 have been assigned to the categories in both instances, but the capital letter is prefixed to the number in case of the classification by external cause and the capital letter "N" is prefixed to the number if the classification is based on the nature of the injury. Both classifications should be considered as integral parts of the International Statistical Classification of Diseases, Injuries, and Causes of Death, and morbid conditions arising from injuries and violence should be coded according to both classifications.

Too much importance should not be attached to the broad section headings of the code. Their significance has been minimized by not including the seventeen sections as integral parts of the numbering scheme. This procedure seemed desirable because the broad sections of the earlier International Lists of Causes of Death have never represented a consistent enough collection of disease conditions to form statistically stable and usable categories. Every revision in the past has shifted diseases from one section to another in such a fashion that the groups have seldom remained comparable over long periods of years.

Tabular List of Inclusions and Four-digit Subcategories

The list of categories in the *International Statistical Classification of Diseases, Injuries, and Causes of Death* gives the framework of the classification, but it is necessary to know in detail the diagnostic terms which are included within each category before the classification can be put to practical use. Although many of the category titles are sufficiently precise to indicate the group of conditions contained therein, other titles leave room for considerable differences in individual interpretation, and satisfactory international comparison of statistics based on the classification cannot he attained without uniformity in the content of each category.

The third part of the present manual, therefore, consists of a tabular list of the inclusions contained in each category of the Detailed List. Many of the three-digit categories are herein subdivided into four-digit categories. Although these subcategories do not appear in the Detailed List, and may be considered optional, they arc none the less important and will be most useful to countries and organizations wishing to make comprehensive studies of the causes of illness and disability. If more detail is desired than that provided for, additional rubrics can be established by utilizing the fourth digit. For example, no four-digit subcategories are indicated in the section dealing with neoplasms. The fourth digit may be used in this case to designate the type of new growth. If such subdivisions are created, it is recommended that letters instead of numbers be employed, especially in publication, to indicate that the item is not a part of the International Classification. Such four-digit subcategories, of course, must include only those conditions that are included in the three-digit category of which it forms a subdivision.

It is neither possible nor desirable to include in the Tabular List of Inclusions all the terms which may appear on medical and death records. An attempt has been made, however, to show most of the diagnostic terms given in the standard or official nomenclatures, as well as terms commonly used in different countries. Furthermore, it was found necessary to include many obsolete and unsatisfactory terms still stated on medical records and death certificates. The more objectionable of these terms, as well as infrequent diagnoses, have been excluded from the Tabular List of Inclusions and appear only in the Alphabetical Index which constitutes volume 2 of the Manual.

Since many countries, such as the Scandinavian countries and some of those of continental Europe, use a larger number of Latin and Latinized names of diseases than is the custom in French- or English-speaking countries, it was thought advisable to include a number of Latin synonyms of such terms as cannot be easily recognized from the English or French text. Furthermore, it is expected that a supplementary alphabetical index of Latin synonyms will be published for the benefit of countries using Latin medical terminology.

Application of Statistical Classification to Morbidity and Mortality Statistics

The *International Statistical Classification of Diseases, Injuries, and Causes of Death* represents only a first step in the actual compilation of statistics of causes of illness and death. Before applying the classification to actual data, it is necessary to decide what purpose is to be served by the statistics. The problem is complex, because frequently in both sickness and death more than one morbid process is involved. As a consequence, in many countries more than one-half of medical certificates of death and an even larger proportion of hospital and other records of illness and disability contain mention of more than one cause. The first problem which arises, therefore, is whether the statistics are to deal with the count of persons who are sick or have died, or of conditions that produced the illness or death. Both kinds of statistics are important attributes of morbidity and mortality, and warrant study.

Application to causes of death.

Since the early records of death usually contained only a single cause, a few simple rules sufficed to secure uniform selection of the cause of death. The usual mortality table, therefore, is based on individuals who have died, assigning a single cause to each death. As a larger and larger proportion of the certificates of death contained multiple causes, the problem of selection became more important in securing comparable statistics.

Bertillon, in presenting the first revision of the International List of Causes of Death in 1900, laid down certain principles for the selection of the primary cause of death. The decisions of the United States Bureau of the Census in the application of these principles were compiled and incorporated into the United States Manual of Joint Causes of Death, published originally in 1914, and revised in 1925, 1933, and 1940 to conform to successive revisions of the International List. In addition to the United States, several other countries have used this manual during recent years as a guide to the selection of the cause of death to be tabulated.

From 1902 until 1939, the General Register Office of England and Wales used specific rules for the selection of the underlying cause of death, but they were more flexible than the ones implied in the United States Manual of Joint Causes of Death. In 1940, England began to employ the procedure of taking as the cause to be tabulated the underlying cause of death as stated by the certifying physician, except in instances where the order of entries on the medical certificate was obviously erroneous. This change in procedure had come about through the adoption in England in 1928 of a new form of medical certificate which permitted the certifying physician or surgeon to signify more clearly the order of events leading up to death.

The Fifth Decennial Revision Conference, as has been pointed out earlier, requested the United States Government to continue its previous investigations on the joint-cause problem in co-operation with other countries and organizations. As a result of this request, the United States Committee on Joint Causes of Death submitted to the Expert Committee for the Preparation of the Sixth Decennial Revision and to the Revision Conference a report on the problem of joint causes of death. [14]

The studies of the United States Committee and of the Expert Committee led to the approval by the Sixth Revision Conference of the International Medical Certificate of Cause of Death and Rules for the Selection of the Underlying Cause of Death which are presented in a later section of this manual. Both committees recognized further the importance of multiple-cause tabulations and recommended that one multiple-cause tabulation, similar to that suggested by the Expert Committee, be prepared by each country around the census year (see page 368).

Application to causes of illness and disability.

Morbidity is far less definite than mortality, and represents a dynamic rather than a static phenomenon. The occurrence of death is a definite event, and the number of such events can be counted. An illness, on the other hand, varies from a minor deviation from normal health, which does not interfere with the performance of regular duties or activities, to the chronic case which calls for bedside or custodial care for an indefinite period. Furthermore, an individual afflicted with a disease may experience only one period of illness during the interval of observation, or may have repeated illnesses from the same disease. In addition, during the same period of illness, an individual may suffer from two or more distinct diseases. Thus, the basic problem as to what is to be counted becomes very complex, and it can be easily seen that the application of the present classification to morbidity statistics cannot be laid down as precisely and relatively simply as in mortality. The application will vary, depending on the kind of morbidity experience to be studied and on the purposes to be served by the statistics.

The rapid expansion of health insurance and medical care plans, together with scientific studies of the incidence of sickness In the population, led many students of morbidity to develop certain rules which would permit bringing out one or another morbidity aspect of particular interest.

In the previously mentioned provisional classification of diseases and injuries issued by the Medical Research Council of Great Britain,'2 coding rules are given according to which the condition to be classified is " the final diagnosis of the principal disease or injury on account of which the patient sought treatment." The main interest here is centered on the condition which brought the individual under medical care. Some consideration is also given to the classification of "principal complication," "principal accessory acute disease," and "principal accessory chronic disease."

More general rules for the selection of the principal cause of illness are given in the *Manual for Coding Causes of Illness 13* issued by the U.S. Public Health Service. This manual further points out that the interest in morbidity statistics often centres on the frequency of specific diseases, whether they are the major factor in the illness or are complications, sequelae or concurrent conditions. Thus, for many studies, tabulation of all these diagnoses is important; for example, in pneumonia the cases that follow influenza and the acute communicable diseases will be counted, as well as primary pneumonia.

It would appear obvious, therefore, that before rules for classification of morbidity data can be prepared for international use, more consideration must be given by all countries to the various aspects of morbidity and to the methods of studying any particular aspect depending on the specific purpose to be served by the statistics.

The World Health Organization will be available to assist national administrations and agencies in this work and to co-ordinate the work of the countries which are interested.

Special Lists of Causes for Tabulation

The Sixth Revision Conference emphasized the importance of always coding morbidity and mortality records according to the Detailed List of three-digit categories (with or without the four-digit subcategories). Only by following this procedure will the benefits of the classification become effective.

In the presentation or publication of either mortality or morbidity statistics, the number of rubrics that can be used is limited. The selection of what categories or groups of categories will be used is dependent upon the purpose of the statistical table, and undoubtedly a great variety of special lists can be developed which utilize the three- and four-digit categories of the classification in different ways.

In a later section of the manual, there are given three lists for tabulation of morbidity and mortality data by cause to meet general needs of this kind. These lists are:

List A.   Intermediate List of 150 Causes for Tabulation of Morbidity and Mortality.

List B.   Abbreviated List of 50 Causes for Tabulation of Mortality.

List C.   Special List of 50 Causes for Tabulation of Morbidity for Social Security Purposes.

It is essential for comparability of statistics that these lists should be used in publications in the form indicated, without any further condensation or regrouping which would distort their baste structure. This limitation, however, does not prevent presentation of statistics in greater detail, provided that any extensions of these lists allow reconstitution of the original groups by simple addition of the new titles. It is important In publishing statistics according to these lists, or any other more extensive list which may serve better the specific purpose at hand, that the table clearly indicate what categories of the detailed list make up each group of causes.

References

1   Registrar-General of England and Wales. *Sixteenth Annual Report, 1856*, Appendix, 75-76

2   Knibbs, Sir G. H. The International Classification of Disease and Causes of Death and its revision. *Med. J. Aust.* 1929, **1**, 2-12

3   Greenwood, M. Medical statistics from Graunt to Farr. *Biometrika*, 1942, **32**, 204

4   Registrar-General of England and Wales. *First Annual Report, 1839*, 99

5   Registrar-General of England and Wales. *Sixteenth Annual Report, 1856*, Appendix, 73

6   Bertillon, J. Classification of the causes of death. (Abstract). *Trans. 15th Int. Cong. Hyg. Demog.*, Washington, 1912, 52-55

7   *Bull. Inst. int. Statist.* 1900, **12**, 280

8   Roesle, E. *Essai d'une statistique comparative de la morbidité devant servir à établir les listes spéciales des causes de morbidité.* Geneva, 1928. (League of Nations Health Organization, document C.H. 730)

9   Institut international de Statistique. *Nomenclatures internationales des Causes de Décès, 1938.* La Haye, 1940

10 Registrar-General of England and Wales. *Sixteenth Annual Report, 1856*, Appendix, 75

11 Fourth International Statistical Congress, London, 1860. Programme

12 Medical Research Council. *Special Report Series No. 248*, London, 1944

13 U.S. Public Health Service. *Miscellaneous Publication No. 32*, Washington, 1944

14 Report of the United States Committee on Joint Causes of Death. World Health Organization, document WHO.IC/MS/11.Rev.2, Geneva, 1948 (mimeographed ; not on sale)

Introduction to ICD-9

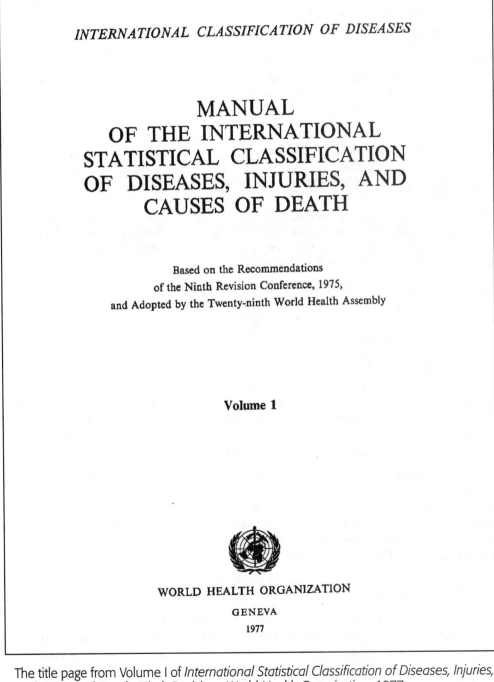

INTERNATIONAL CLASSIFICATION OF DISEASES

MANUAL
OF THE INTERNATIONAL
STATISTICAL CLASSIFICATION
OF DISEASES, INJURIES, AND
CAUSES OF DEATH

Based on the Recommendations
of the Ninth Revision Conference, 1975,
and Adopted by the Twenty-ninth World Health Assembly

Volume 1

WORLD HEALTH ORGANIZATION
GENEVA
1977

The title page from Volume I of *International Statistical Classification of Diseases, Injuries, and Causes of Death, Ninth Revision*. World Health Organization, 1977.

General principles

A classification of diseases may be defined as a system of categories to which morbid entities are assigned according to some established criteria. There are many possible choices for these criteria. The anatomist, for example, may desire a classification based on the part of the body affected whereas the pathologist is primarily interested in the nature of the disease process, the public health practitioner in aetiology and the clinician in the particular manifestation requiring his care. In other words there are many axes of classification and the particular axis selected will be determined by the interest of the investigator. A statistical classification of disease and injury will depend, therefore, upon the use to be made of the statistics to be compiled.

Because of this conflict of interests, efforts to base a statistical classification on a strictly logical adherence to any one axis have failed in the past. The various titles will represent a series of necessary compromises between classifications based on aetiology, anatomical site, circumstances of onset, etc., as well as the quality of information available on medical reports. Adjustments must also be made to meet the varied requirements of vital statistics offices, hospitals of different types, medical services of the armed forces, social insurance organizations, sickness surveys, and numerous other agencies. While no single classification will fit all the specialized needs, it should provide a common basis of classification for general statistical use; that is storage, retrieval and tabulation of data.

A statistical classification of disease must be confined to a limited number of categories which will encompass the entire range of morbid conditions. The categories should be chosen so that they will facilitate the statistical study of disease phenomena. A specific disease entity should have a separate title in the classification only when its separation is warranted because the frequency of its occurrence, or its importance as a morbid condition, justifies its isolation as a separate category. On the other hand, many titles in the classification will refer to groups of separate but usually related morbid conditions. Every disease or morbid condition, however, must have a definite and appropriate place as an inclusion in one of the categories of the statistical classification. A few items of the statistical list will be residual titles for other and miscellaneous conditions which cannot be classified under the more specific titles. These miscellaneous categories should be kept to a minimum.

It is this element of grouping in a statistical classification that distinguishes it from a nomenclature, a list or catalogue of approved names for morbid conditions, which must be extensive in order to accommodate all pathological conditions. The concepts of classification and nomenclature are, nevertheless, closely related in the sense that some classifications (e.g. in zoology) are so detailed that they become nomenclatures. Such classifications, however, are generally unsuitable for statistical analysis.

The aims of a statistical classification of disease cannot be better summarized than in the following paragraphs written by William Farr[1] a century ago:

"The causes of death were tabulated in the early Bills of Mortality *(Tables mortuaires)* alphabetically; and this course has the advantage of not raising any of those nice questions in which it is vain to expect physicians and statisticians to agree unanimously. But statistics is eminently a science of classification; and it is evident, on glancing at the subject cursorily, that any classification that brings together in groups diseases that have considerable affinity, or that are liable to be confounded with each other, is likely to facilitate the deduction of general principles.

"Classification is a method of generalization. Several classifications may, therefore, be used with advantage; and the physician, the pathologist, or the jurist, each from his own point of view, may legitimately classify the diseases and the causes of death in the way that he thinks best adapted to facilitate his inquiries, and to yield general results.

"The medical practitioner may found his main divisions of diseases on their treatment as medical or surgical; the pathologist, on the nature of the morbid action or product; the anatomist or the physiologist on the tissues and organs involved; the medical jurist on the suddenness or the slowness of the death; and all these points well deserve attention in a statistical classification.

"In the eyes of national statists the most important elements are, however, brought into account in the ancient subdivision of diseases into plagues, or epidemics and endemics, into diseases of common occurrence (sporadic diseases), which may be conveniently divided into three classes, and into injuries, the immediate results of violence or of external causes."

Historical Review

Early history

Francois Bossier de Lacroix (1706-1777), better known as Sauvages, first attempted to classify diseases systematically. Sauvages' comprehensive treatise was published under the title *Nosologia Methodica*. A contemporary of Sauvages was the great methodologist Linnaeus (1707-1778), one of whose treatises was entitled *Genera Morborum*. At the beginning of the 19th century, the classification of disease in most general use was one by William Cullen (1710-1790), of Edinburgh, which was published in 1785 under the title *Synopsis Nosologiae Methodicae*.

The statistical study of disease, however, began for all practical purposes with the work of John Graunt on the London Bills of Mortality a century earlier. In an attempt to estimate the proportion of liveborn children who died before reaching the age of six years, no records of age at death being available, he took all deaths classed as thrush, convulsions, rickets, teeth and worms, abortives, chrysomes, infants, livergrown, and overlaid and added to them half the deaths classed as smallpox, swine pox, measles, and worms without convulsions. Despite the crudity of this classification his estimate of a 36 per cent mortality before the age of six years appears from later evidence to have been a good one. While three centuries have contributed something to the scientific accuracy of disease classification, there are many who doubt the usefulness of attempts to compile statistics of disease, or even causes of death, because of the difficulties of classification. To these, one can quote Major Greenwood[2]: "The scientific purist, who will wait for medical statistics until they are nosologically exact, is no wiser than Horace's rustic waiting for the river to flow away ".

Fortunately for the progress of preventive medicine, the General Register Office of England and Wales, at its inception in 1837, found in William Farr (1807-1883) — its first medical statistician — a man who not only made the best possible use of the imperfect classifications of disease available at the time, but laboured to secure better classification and international uniformity in their use.

Farr found the classification of Cullen in use in the public services of his day. It had not been revised so as to embody the advances of medical science, nor was it deemed by him to be satisfactory for statistical purposes. In the first Annual Report of the Registrar General, therefore, he discussed the principles that should govern a statistical classification of disease and urged the adoption of a uniform classification.

Both nomenclature and statistical classification received constant study and consideration by Farr in his annual "Letters" to the Registrar General published in the Annual Reports of the Registrar General. The utility of a uniform classification of causes of death was so strongly recognized at the first International Statistical Congress, held at Brussels, in 1853, that it requested William Farr and Marc d'Espine, of Geneva, to prepare "une nomenclature uniforme des causes de deces applicable a tous les pays."[3] At the next Congress, at Paris in 1855, Farr and d'Espine submitted two separate lists which were based on very different principles. Farr's classification was arranged under five groups: Epidemic diseases, Constitutional (general) diseases, Local diseases arranged according to anatomical site, Developmental diseases, and diseases that are the direct result of violence. D'Espine classified diseases according to their nature (gouty, herpetic, haematic, etc.). The Congress adopted a compromise list of 138 rubrics. In 1864, this classification was revised at Paris "sur le modele de celle de W. Farr," and was subsequently revised in 1874, 1880, and 1886. Although there was never any universal acceptance of this classification, the general arrangement, including the principle of classifying diseases by anatomical site, proposed by Farr, has survived as the basis of the International List of Causes of Death.

Adoption of International List of Causes of Death

The International Statistical Institute, the successor to the International Statistical Congress, at its meeting in Vienna in 1891, charged a committee, of which Jacques Bertillon (1851-1922), Chef des Travaux statistiques de Ia ville de Paris, was chairman, with the preparation of a classification of causes of death. It is of interest to note that Bertillon was the grandson of Achille Guillard, a noted botanist and statistician, who had introduced the resolution requesting Farr and d'Espine to prepare a uniform classification at the First Statistical Congress in 1853. The report of this committee was presented by Bertillon at the meeting of the International Statistical Institute at Chicago in 1893 and adopted by it. The classification prepared by Bertillon was based on the classification of causes of death used by the City of Paris, which, since its revision in 1885, represented a synthesis of English, German, and Swiss classifications. The classification was based on the principle, adopted by Farr, of distinguishing between general diseases and those localized to a particular organ or anatomical site. In accordance with the instructions of the Vienna Congress made at the suggestion of L. Guillaume, the Director of the Federal Bureau of Statistics of Switzerland, Bertillon included three classifications: the first, an abridged classification of 44 titles; the second, a classification of 99 titles; and the third, a classification of 161 titles.

The Bertillon Classification of Causes of Death, as it was at first called, received general approval and was adopted by several countries, as well as by many cities. The classification was first used in North America by Jesus E. Monjaras for the statistics of San Luis de Potosi, Mexico.[4] In 1898, the American Public Health Association, at its meeting in Ottawa, Canada, recommended the adoption of the Bertillon Classification by registrars of Canada, Mexico, and the United States. The Association further suggested that the classification be revised every ten years.

At the meeting of the International Statistical Institute at Christiania in 1899, Bertillon presented a report on the progress of the classification, including the recommendations of the American Public Health Association for decennial revisions. The International Statistical Institute then adopted the following resolution:

> "The International Statistical Institute, convinced of the necessity of using in the different countries comparable nomenclatures:

> "Learns with pleasure of the adoption by all the statistical offices of North America, by some of those of South America, and by some in Europe, of the system of cause of death nomenclature presented in 1893:

> "Insists vigorously that this system of nomenclature be adopted in principle and without revision, by all the statistical institutions of Europe;

> "Approves, at least in its general lines, the system of decennial revision proposed by the American Public Health Association at its Ottawa session (1898);

> "Urges the statistical offices who have not yet adhered, to do so without delay, and to contribute to the comparability of the cause of death nomenclature."[5]

The French Government therefore convoked at Paris, in August 1900, the first International Conference for the revision of the Bertillon or International Classification of Causes of Death. Delegates from 26 countries attended this Conference. A detailed classification of causes of death consisting of 179 groups and an abridged classification of 35 groups were adopted on 21 August 1900. The desirability of decennial revisions was recognized, and the French Government was requested to call the next meeting in 1910. Actually the next conference was held in 1909, and the Government of France called succeeding conferences in 1920, 1929, and 1938.

Bertillon continued as the guiding force in the promotion of the International List of Causes of Death, and the revisions of 1900, 1910, and 1920 were carried out under his leadership. As Secretary-General of the International Conference, he sent out the provisional revision for 1920 to more than 500 persons, asking for comments. His death in 1922 left the International Conference without a guiding hand.

At the 1923 session of the International Statistical Institute, Michel Huber, Bertillon's successor in France, recognized this lack of leadership and introduced a resolution for the International Statistical Institute to renew its stand of 1893 in regard to the International Classification of Causes of Death and to co-operate with other international organizations in preparation for subsequent revisions. The Health Organization of the League of Nations had also taken an active interest in vital statistics and appointed a Commission of Statistical Experts to study the classification of diseases and causes of death, as well as other problems in the field of medical statistics. E. Roesle, Chief of the Medical Statistical Service of the German Health Bureau and a member of the Commission of Expert Statisticians, prepared a monograph that listed the expansion in the rubrics of the 1920 International List of Causes of Death that would be required if the classification was to be used in the tabulation of statistics of morbidity. This careful study was published by the Health Organization of the League of

Nations in 1928.[6] In order to co-ordinate the work of both agencies, an international commission, known as the "Mixed Commission," was created with an equal number of representatives from the International Statistical Institute and the Health Organization of the League of Nations. This Commission drafted the proposals for the Fourth (1929) and the Fifth (1938) revisions of the International List of Causes of Death.

The Sixth, Seventh and Eighth Revisions

The International Health Conference held in New York City in 1946 entrusted the Interim Commission of the World Health Organization with the responsibility of undertaking preparatory work for the next decennial revision of the International Lists of Causes of Death and for the establishment of International Lists of Causes of Morbidity[7]. The International Conference for the Sixth Revision of the International Lists of Diseases and Causes of Death was convened in Paris in April 1948 by the Government of France and its secretariat was entrusted jointly to the competent French administrations and to the World Health Organization which had carried out the preparatory work under the Arrangement concluded by the governments represented at the International Health Conference in 1946 [7].

The Sixth Decennial Revision Conference marked the beginning of a new era in international vital and health statistics. Apart from approving a comprehensive list for both mortality and morbidity and agreeing on international rules for selecting the underlying cause of death it recommended the adoption of a comprehensive programme of international co-operation in the field of vital and health statistics, including the establishment of national committees on vital and health statistics for the purpose of coordinating statistical activities in the country and to serve as a link between the national statistical institutions and the World Health Organization[8].

The International Conference for the Seventh Revision of the International Classification of Diseases was held in Paris under WHO auspices in February 1955[9]. In accordance with a recommendation of the WHO Expert Committee on Health Statistics[10] this revision was limited to essential changes and amendments of errors and inconsistencies.

The Eighth Revision Conference convened by WHO met in the Palais des Nations, Geneva, from 6 to 12 July 1965[11]. This revision was of a more radical nature than the Seventh but left unchanged the basic structure of the Classification and the general philosophy of classifying diseases according to their aetiology rather than a particular manifestation.

Report of the International Conference for the Ninth Revision

The International Conference for the Ninth Revision of the Inter- national Classification of Diseases convened by the World Health Organization met at WHO headquarters in Geneva from 30 September to 6 October 1975. The Conference was attended by delegations from 46 Member States:

Algeria	Nigeria
Australia	Norway
Austria	Poland
Belgium	Portugal
Brazil	Saudi Arabia
Canada	Singapore

Chad
Denmark
Egypt
Finland
France
German Democratic Republic
Germany, Federal Republic of
Guatemala
Hungary
India
Indonesia
Ireland
Israel
Italy
Japan
Libyan Arab Republic
Luxembourg
Netherlands, Kingdom of the

Spain
Sudan
Sweden
Switzerland
Thailand
Togo
Trinidad and Tobago
Tunisia
Union of Soviet Socialist Republics
United Arab Emirates
United Kingdom of Great Britain
    and Northern Ireland
United Republic of Cameroon
United States of America
Venezuela
Yugoslavia
Zaire

The United Nations, the Organization for Economic Cooperation and Development, the International Labour Organisation, and the International Agency for Research on Cancer sent representatives to participate in the Conference, as did the Council for International Organizations of Medical Sciences and ten other international non-governmental organizations concerned with dental health, dermatology, gynaecology and obstetrics, mental health, neurosurgery, ophthalmology, paediatrics, pathology, radiology, and rehabilitation of the disabled.

The Conference was opened by Dr. A. S. Pavlov, Assistant Director-General, on behalf of the Director-General. Dr Pavlov reviewed the history of the LCD, reminding delegates that it had developed from an International List of Causes of Death, first agreed in 1893. WHO took over responsibility with the Sixth Revision and its concern with the ICD is written into its Constitution. Since WHO took over, there had been a great extension of use of the ICD for the indexing and retrieval of records and for statistics concerning the planning, monitoring and evaluation of health services, besides its traditional use in epidemiology.

The Conference elected the following officers:

Chairman:	Dr. R. H. C. Wells (Australia)
Vice-Chairmen:	Dr. J. M. Avilan-Rovira (Venezuela)
	Dr. G. Cerkovnij (USSR)
	Dr. I. M. Moriyama (United States of America)
	Mr. G. Paine (United Kingdom)
Rapporteurs:	Dr. M. A. Heasman (United Kingdom)
	Dr. (Mlle) M. Guidevaux (France)
Secretariat:	Dr. A. S. Pavlov (Assistant Director-General, WHO)
	Mr. K. Uemura (Director, Division of Health Statistics, WHO)

Dr. K. Kupka (Chief Medical Officer, International Classification of Diseases, WHO) (Secretary)

Mr. H. G. Corbett (Statistician, International Classification of Diseases, WHO)

Professor G. G. Avtandilov (USSR) (Temporary Adviser)

The Conference adopted an agenda dealing with the Ninth Revision of the International Classification of Diseases, with several provisional supplementary classifications intended for use in conjunction with it, and with allied topics.

1. Ninth Revision of the International Classification of Diseases

1.1 Review of activities in the preparation of the proposals for the Ninth Revision

The procedures leading up to the Ninth Revision commenced in 1969 with the calling of a Study Group. The work had been planned and carried out so that the proposals before the Conference were in a much more advanced state of preparation than had been the case at earlier revisions. The intention was to have the completed manual, with its alphabetical index, in the hands of users in good time to allow for adequate training and familiarization in countries before its introduction. The progress of preparations for revision had been guided by further meetings of the Study Group and by meetings of Heads of Centres for Classification of Diseases. The first meeting of the Study Group considered that the revision ought to be a limited one.

It soon became clear, however, that a much more radical revision was being demanded by specialists in many fields of medicine. Views were sought from individual consultants, international specialists bodies, the WHO Centres for Classification of Diseases and headquarters units. Regional offices arranged meetings so that representatives of Member States could give their views. The third meeting of the Study Group considered proposals incorporating views from all these sources, and on the basis of their recommendations draft proposals were circulated to Member States in mid-1973. Comments on the proposals were considered by the WHO Expert Committee on Health Statistics in June 1974[12], and the final proposals before the Conference were the results of its recommendations. Delegates from several countries spoke in support of the revision as proposed.

In particular it was reiterated that clinical pressures had demanded an extensive revision at this stage on the grounds that the structure of several of the ICD chapters was out of touch with modern clinical concepts. The delegation from Sweden, on behalf of the five Nordic countries (Denmark, Finland, Iceland, Norway and Sweden), put forward the view that the problems and cost associated with so extensive a change would be substantial since these countries had established a 5-digit version based on the ICD-8 which was widely used in computerized health information systems. They considered that this 5-digit version met to a large extent the clinical demands for greater specificity which the Ninth Revision was aiming at.

The Conference noted the concern of the Nordic countries but, recognizing the need pointed out by several countries to satisfy clinical requirements by structural changes as well as by providing increased specificity, in general supported the scope of the proposed revision as presented to the Conference.

1.2 History and development of uses of the ICD

The Conference was reminded of the impressive history of the classification. Its origins lay in a list of causes of death, which was used for many years. At the Sixth Revision, the classification was extended to cover non-fatal conditions. Later the classification had been shown to be useful for the purposes of hospital indexing, particularly if adapted by means of some extra subdivision. More recently adaptations had been made for use in medical audit systems. The Ninth Revision proposals include a device designed to improve its suitability for use in statistics for the evaluation of medical care. For the future, it would have to be decided what kind of adaptation of the ICD would render it usable for Health Insurance Statistics, and whether it was possible to adapt it as a basis for central payment for medical services. All these uses tended to push the classification in the direction of more detail. At the other end of the scale it had to be remembered that there were demands from countries and areas were such sophistication was irrelevant but which nevertheless would like a classification based on the ICD so as to assess their progress in healthcare and in the control of sickness.

1.3 General characteristics of the proposed Ninth Revision

The general arrangement of the proposals for the Ninth Revision considered by the Conference was much the same as in the Eighth Revision, though with much additional detail. Care had been taken to ensure that the categories were meaningful at the 3-digit level. There were certain innovations:

(i)   Optional fifth digits were provided in certain places: for example, for the mode of diagnosis in tuberculosis, for method of delivery in Chapter XI, for anatomical site in musculoskeletal disorders and for place of accident in the E code.

(ii)   An independent 4-digit coding system was provided to classify histological varieties of neoplasm, prefixed by the letter M (for morphology) and followed by a fifth digit indicating behaviour. This code was for optional use in addition to the normal code indicating topography.

(iii)   The role of the E code for external causes had changed. In the Sixth, Seventh and Eighth Revisions, Chapter XVII consisted of two alternative classifications, one according to the nature of the injury (the N code) and one according to external cause (the E code). In the Ninth Revision it was proposed to drop the N prefix and consider only the nature of injury as part of the main classification. The E code becomes a supplementary classification to be used, where relevant, in conjunction with codes from any part of the classification. For mortality statistics, however, the E code should still be used in preference to Chapter XVII in presenting underlying causes of death, when only one is used.

(iv)   The Ninth Revision proposals included dual classification of certain diagnostic statements. The Conference heard that the system had been introduced into the 1973 proposals after it had become obvious that there was a demand to classify diseases according to important manifestations, e.g. to classify numps encephalitis to a category for encephalitis. It would have been unwise to change the whole axis of the ICD to this basis, so the first proposal was to make the positioning according to manifestation alternative to the traditional placing according to aetiology. As a result of criticism, it is now proposed that the "traditional" aetiology codes, those marked with a ///+/// should be considered primary, and the new codes, positioned in the classification according to manifestation and marked with an *, should be secondary, for use in applications concerned with the planning and evaluation of medical care. This system applies only to diagnostic statements that contain information about both etiology and manifestation and when the latter is important in its own right.

(v)   Categories in the Mental Disorders Chapter include descriptions of their content with a view to overcoming the particular difficulties in this field, where international terminology is not standard.

The V code (formerly the Y code) continues to appear in Volume 1.

These characteristics of the proposed revision were accepted by the Conference.

1.4 Adoption of Ninth Revision of the International Classification of Diseases

The Conference,

Having considered the proposals prepared by the Organization on the recommendations of the Expert Committee on Health Statistics[13],

Recognizing the need for a few further minor modifications to meet the comments on points of detail submitted by Member States during the Conference,

Recommends that the revised Detailed List of Categories and Sub-Categories in Annex I to this report constitute the Ninth Revision of the International Classification of Diseases. [The Annexes to the Report are not reproduced here. They are represented by the contents of this Volume.]

2. Classification of Procedures in Medicine

In response to requests from a number of Member States, the Organization had drafted a classification of therapeutic, diagnostic and prophylactic procedures in medicine, covering surgery, radiology, laboratory and other procedures. Various national classifications of this kind had been studied and advice sought from hospital associations in a number of countries. The intention was to provide a tool for use in the analysis of health services provided to patients in hospitals, clinics, outpatient departments, etc.

The Conference congratulates the Secretariat on this important development and

Recommends that the provisional procedures classifications should be published as supplements to, and not as integral parts of, the Ninth Revision of the International Classification of Diseases. They should be published in some inexpensive form and, after two or three years' experience, revised in the light of users' comments.

3. Classification of Impairments and Handicaps

The ICD provided the means of classifying current illness or injury; the classification of procedures provided a means of coding the treatment or other services consumed by the patient. There remained a need to classify impairments and the consequent handicaps or disadvantages.

This was an area in which much development was occurring and a draft classification had been prepared by the Organization although this was to a large extent experimental and exploratory. It had been drafted after much consultation with agencies responsible for social services and rehabilitation.

The Conference having considered the classification of Impairments and Handicaps believes that these have potential value and accordingly

Recommends that the Impairments and Handicaps classifications be published for trial purposes as a supplement to, and not as an integral part of, the Ninth Revision of the International Classification of Diseases.

4. *Adaptations of ICD for the Use of Specialists*

The Conference noted three adaptations of the ICD which had been designed for the use of specialists.

The first was an adaptation for oncology — ICD-O. Coding was on three axes indicating the topography, morphology and behaviour of tumours. The 4-digit topography code was based on the list of sites of the malignant neoplasm section of Chapter II of the Ninth Revision of the ICD, but was to be used for any type of neoplasm. To this would be added a 4-digit code indicating histological variety of neoplasm, and a single-digit code indicating behaviour. It was intended that the code should be used by centres requiring to record extra detail about tumours, as an alternative to the Ninth Revision of ICD, with which it was entirely compatible. (A conversion guide would be available, enabling translation of codes by computer if desired.)

Other adaptations had been produced for dentistry and stomatology and for ophthalmology. Each of these contains, in a small volume, all conditions of interest to the specialist, selected from all chapters of the ICD, and provides additional detail by means of a fifth digit.

5. *Lay Reporting*

The Conference discussed the problem of securing badly needed morbidity and mortality statistics in countries still suffering from a lack of sufficiently qualified personnel. There was a divergence of opinion concerning the system of classification to be used where information about sickness or causes of death is necessarily furnished by persons other than physicians. Some delegates considered that the International Classification of Diseases in some simplified form (e.g. one of the tabulation lists) would serve this purpose while others believed that a system independent of the ICD needed to be established.

A small working party, consisting of delegates from Member States with experience of the problem, was convened to consider the question in more detail and in the light of its report

The Conference,

Realizing the present problem involved in the full utilization of ICD by the developing countries in most of the regions;

Recognizing the need for introducing a system which could provide useful and objective morbidity and mortality data for efficient health planning;

Appreciating the field trials conducted in some countries for collection of morbidity and mortality information through non-medical health or other personnel and the experience thus obtained;

Noting the concern of the World Health Organization for development and promotion of health services, particularly in the developing countries, as contained in resolutions EB55.R16[14], WHA28.75[15], WHA28.77[16] and WHA28.88[17],

Recommends that the World Health Organization should

(1)   become increasingly involved in the attempts made by the various developing countries for collection of morbidity and mortality statistics through lay or paramedical personnel;

(2)   organize meetings at regional level for facilitating exchange of experiences between the countries currently facing this problem so as to design suitable classification lists with due consideration to national differences in terminology;

(3)   assist countries in their endeavour to establish or expand the system of collection of morbidity and mortality data through lay or paramedical personnel.

6. *Statistics of Death in the Perinatal Period and Related Matters*

The Conference considered with interest the reports of the Scientific Group on Health Statistics Methodology relating to Perinatal Events [18] and the recommendations of the Expert Committee [12] on this subject. These were the culmination of a series of special WHO meetings attended by specialists from many disciplines. It had become clear that a review of the situation was needed in the light of certain developments in medical sciences, notably those leading to the improved survival of infants born at a very early gestational age.

After discussion, the Conference

Recommends that, where practicable, statistics in relation to perinatal deaths should be derived from a special certificate of perinatal death (instead of the normal death certificate) and presented in the manner set out in Annex II, which also includes relevant definitions. This annex also includes recommendations in respect of maternal mortality statistics.

7. *Mortality Coding Rules*

The Conference was made aware of the problems arising in selecting the underlying cause of death where this was the result of factors connected with surgical or other treatment. It was proposed that where an untoward effect of treatment is responsible for death then this should be coded rather than the condition for which the treatment was given. Although there were views expressed by some delegates that this interfered with the traditional underlying cause concept, the Conference preferred the former view and accordingly

Recommends that the modification rule in Annex III be added to the existing rules for selection of cause of death for primary mortality tabulation.

The Conference was also informed that additional guidelines for dealing with certificates of death from cancer had been drafted and were being tested in several countries. If the tests showed that the guidelines improved consistency in coding, they would be incorporated into the Ninth Revision.

8. *Selection of a Single Cause for Statistics of Morbidity*

No rules had hitherto been incorporated into the LCD concerning the tabulation of morbidity. Routine statistics are normally based upon a single cause and the Conference considered that the application of the ICD to routine morbidity statistics had reached a point where international recommendations for selection of a single cause for presentation of morbidity statistics was appropriate and accordingly

Recommends that the condition to be selected for single-cause analysis for healthcare records should be the main condition treated or investigated during the relevant episode of hospital or other care. If no diagnosis was made, the main symptom or problem should be selected instead. Whenever possible, the choice should be exercised by the responsible medical practitioner or other healthcare professional and the main condition or problem distinguished from other conditions or problems.

It is desirable that, in addition to the selection of a single cause for tabulation purposes, multiple condition coding and analysis should be attempted wherever possible, particularly for data relating to episodes of healthcare by hospitals (inpatient or outpatient), health clinics and family practitioners. For certain other types of data, such as from health examination surveys, multiple cause analysis may be the only satisfactory method.

9. *Short Lists for Tabulation of Mortality and Morbidity*

Difficulties had become apparent in the use of the present short lists A, B, C and D for the tabulation of mortality and morbidity. Their construction and numbering was such that confusion often arose and comparability of statistics based on different lists presented some difficulties. Proposed new lists were presented to the Conference in which totals were shown for groups of diseases and for certain selected individual conditions. Minimum lists of 55 items were recommended for the tabulation of mortality and morbidity and countries could add to these further items from a basic list of 275 categories.

The Conference

Recommends that the Special Tabulation Lists set out in Annex IV to this report should replace the lists for tabulation of morbidity and mortality and should be published as part of the International Classification of Diseases together with appropriate explanation and instruction as to their use.

10. *Multiple Condition Coding and Analysis*

The Conference noted with interest the extended use of multiple condition coding and analysis in a number of countries with a variety of ends in view. One example was the study of the interrelationship of various conditions recorded on a death certificate; another was to permit computer selection of the underlying cause of death. The Conference also noted the value of a store of multiple-coded national data on mortality and morbidity. The Conference expressed encouragement of such work but did not recommend that the ICD should contain any particular rules or methods of analysis to be followed.

11. *Different Disease-Coding Systems*

The Conference was reminded of the existence of other disease classifications and reviewed their attributes as a preliminary to discussion of the possible form of the Tenth Revision. Some of these classifications are developments from the International Classification of Diseases; others are multi-axial, enabling retrieval from different viewpoints but not primarily designed with the presentation of routine statistics in mind. In others, a unique code is given to each disease or term, enabling retrieval of specific conditions and assembly into alternative classifications according to need. These developments seemed to indicate some desire for greater flexibility and to raise doubts as to whether a single multi-purpose classification was any longer practicable. It was felt that multi-axial classification often destroyed the ability to retrieve disease terms. Allocating a unique code to a disease or term might be one way of over-coming problems caused by changes in classification.

12. *The Tenth Revision of the International Classification of Diseases*

The Conference recognized the need to make an early start in planning the next revision of the classification and discussed a number of questions that needed to be settled before detailed work could begin. The most fundamental point was that the Organization's programme was no longer confined to disease classification alone. Many other reasons, social and economic, for contact with health services were now included in the main classification and supplementary classifications of procedures in medicine and of impairments and handicaps had been added. These needed to be further developed and incorporated into a comprehensive and coordinated system of classifications of health information. The name of the Organization's programme should reflect the wider scope of its activities

Standardization of nomenclature on a multilingual basis was essential for conformity in diagnosis, and glossaries similar to the one developed for psychiatry might be provided for other specialities where diagnostic concepts were unclear. A lack of balance in the Eight Revision, which contained 140 categories for infectious diseases but only 20 for the whole of perinatal morbidity, had been retained in the Ninth Revision because ot its essentially conservative nature, but such a restriction should not necessarily hold for the next revision.

It was acknowledged that conflicts existed between the need for a fairly broad classification for the purposes of international comparisons and the desire for a very high degree of specificity for diagnostic indexing and for epidemiological research, and between the requirements of a classification usable at the community level in developing countries and one suitable for a national morbidity programme with access to a computer. The structure of the Tenth Revision was another question for urgent decision; should the present uni-axial system be retained or should there be a move to a multi-dimensional approach; should the coding and classification elements be separated so that the former could remain constant while the latter could be revised at shorter intervals than at present?

The view of the Conference was that these questions should be decided within the next two or three years by the construction and trial of model classifications of various types. It was recognized that this would be an additional task to the normal work of the Organization in this area and would require the provision of extra resources.

The Conference recognized the great value of the work already done and still being done on ICD; it also recognized the rapidly increasing demands for more flexibility than is available in the present structure of this classification.

The Conference,

Noting that the ICD, despite the present constraints upon resources, which it completely absorbs, is one of the most influential activities of WHO,

Recommends that:

(1)　WHO should continue its work in developing revisions of the ICD and related classifications and that the Organization's activity in connexion with the revision of the ICD should be expanded;

(2)　the ICD programme should be given sufficient resources to enable it simultaneously to explore the needs for new departures in the realm of health classifications and how these can be met without detracting from the present revision process; the programme should also be enabled to carry out extensive field trials of the various alternative approaches that exist or which may emerge.

The Conference expressed the hope that efforts would be made to retain the continuity of expertise that had been developed in the Organization, in the centres for classification of diseases and among numerous organizations and individuals throughout the world.

13. Publication of the Ninth Revision

The Conference was informed that, although the Tabular List of the ICD (Volume 1) in English and French could be made available in published form by the end of 1976, it was unlikely that the Alphabetical Index (Volume 2) could be published before the middle of 1977. The Russian and Spanish versions should follow the English and French fairly closely.

Member States intending to publish national language versions would receive pre-publication copies of the various parts of the classification as and when they were completed by the Secretariat to enable them to adhere as nearly as possible to this timetable.

Several delegates pointed out that the late appearance of the alphabetical indexes at the Eight Revision had resulted in a high rate of coding errors during the first year of use.

Because of the large amount of work still to be done before the Ninth Revision can be published and because the training of coders requires that both volumes, including the alphabetical index, should be in the hands of users some 12 months before it is due to come into use,

The Conference

Recommends that the Ninth Revision of the International Classification of Diseases should come into effect on 1 January 1979.

14. Familiarization and Training in the Use of the Ninth Revision

There were many aspects of the proposed revision, besides the change in the categories themselves, which would require very careful explanation to coders and to users of statistics based on the ICD. It was planned that familiarization courses would be organized by the WHO regional offices, to help Member countries in planning their own courses. The Conference noted with interest that WHO hoped to prepare a set of training material covering an instructional course for coders of approximately two weeks, to make sure that the instruction was as consistent as possible. WHO would also make available explanatory material for users of statistics.

Adoption of the Ninth Revision

The Twenty-ninth World Health Assembly, meeting in Geneva in May 1976, adopted the following resolution with regard to the Manual of the International Classification of Diseases (Resolution WHA29.34)[19].

The Twenty-ninth World Health Assembly,

Having considered the report of the International Conference for the Ninth Revision of the International Classification of Diseases,

1.   *Adopts* the detailed list of three-digit categories and optional four- digit sub-categories recommended by the Conference as the Ninth Revision of the International Classification of Diseases, to come into effect as from 1 January 1979;

2.   *Adopts* the rules recommended by the Conference for the selection of a single cause in morbidity statistics;

3.   *Adopts* the recommendations of the Conference regarding statistics of perinatal and maternal mortality, including a special certificate of cause of perinatal death for use where practicable;

4.   *Requests* the Director-General to issue a new edition of the *Manual of the International Statistical Classification of Diseases, injuries and Causes of Death.*

The Assembly adopted a further resolution concerning activities related to the International Classification of Diseases (Resolution WHA29.35)[20].

The Twenty-ninth World Health Assembly,

Noting the recommendations of the International Conference for the Ninth Revision of the International Classification of Diseases in respect of activities related to the Classification,

1.   *Approves* the publication, for trial purposes, of supplementary classifications of Impairments and Handicaps and of Procedures in Medicine as supplements to, but not as integral parts of, the International Classification of Diseases;

2.   *Endorses* the recommendation of the Conference concerning assistance to developing countries in their endeavour to establish or expand the system of collection of morbidity and mortality statistics through lay or paramedical personnel;

3.   *Endorses* the request made by the Executive Board in resolution EB57.R34[21] to the Director-General that he investigate the possibility of preparing an International Nomenclature of Diseases as an improvement to the Tenth Revision of the International Classification of Diseases.

Manual of the Ninth Revision

Conventions used in the Tabular List

The Tabular List makes special use of parentheses and colons which needs to be clearly understood. When parentheses are used for their normal function of enclosing synonyms, alternative wordings or explanatory phrases, square brackets [...] are employed. Round brackets (...) are used to enclose supplementary words which may be either present or absent in the statement of a diagnosis without affecting the code number to which it is assigned. Words followed by a colon [:] are not complete terms, but must have one or other of the understated modifiers to make them assignable to the given category. "NOS" is an abbreviation for "not otherwise specified" and is virtually the equivalent of "unspecified" and "unqualified".

As an example of the use of the above conventions, category 464.0, Acute laryngitis, includes the following terms:

Laryngitis (acute):
      NOS
      Haemophilus influenzae [H. influenzae]
      oedematous
      pneumococcal
      septic
      suppurative
      ulcerative

This signifies that to this category should be assigned laryngitis, with or without the adjective "acute" , if standing alone or if accompanied by one or other of the modifiers: Haemophilus influenzae [of which H. influenzae is an alternative wording], oedematous, pneumococcal, septic, suppurative, or ulcerative. Influenzal, streptococcal, diphtheritic, tuberculous, and chronic laryngitis will be found in other categories.

Dual classification of certain diagnostic statements

The Ninth Revision of the ICD contains an innovation in that there are two codes for certain diagnostic descriptions which contain elements of information both about a localised manifestation or complication and about a more generalised underlying disease process. One of the codes — marked with a dagger (/+/) — is positioned in the part of the classification in which the diagnostic description is located according to normal ICD principles, that relating to the underlying disease, and the other — marked with an asterisk (*) — is positioned in the chapter of the classification relating to the organ system to which the manifestation or complication relates. Thus tuberculous meningitis has its dagger code in the chapter for infectious and parasitic diseases, and its asterisk code in the nervous system chapter.

The necessity for this arose from the desire of specialists and those concerned with statistics of medical care to have certain manifestations which are medical-care problems in their own right classified in the chapters relating to the relevant organ system. The ICD has traditionally classified generalised diseases and infectious disease entities which may affect several parts of the body to special chapters of the classification, and their manifestations are normally assigned to the same place, so that until now tuberculous meningitis has been classifiable only to the infectious and parasitic diseases chapter.

The dagger and asterisk categories are in fact alternative positionings in the classification for the relevant conditions, enabling retrieval or statistical analysis from either viewpoint. It is, however, a principle of LCD classification that the dagger category is the primary code and that the asterisk code is secondary, so it is important where it is desired to work with the asterisk code, and both are used, to use some special mark or a predetermined positioning in the coded record, to identify which is the dagger, and which the asterisk, code for the same entity.

The criteria adopted in the Ninth Revision are that asterisk categories are provided:

(i)   if the manifestation or complication represents a medical-care problem in its own right and is normally treated by a specialty different from the one which would handle the underlying condition, and

(ii)   if the information about both the manifestation and the underlying condition is customarily contained in one diagnostic phrase (such as "diabetic retinitis"), or

(iii)   if the category relating to the manifestation is subdivided according to the cause — an example is arthropathy in which the subdivisions relate to broad groups of causes.

Other underlying condition/manifestation combinations exist which do not cause coding and retrieval problems and have therefore not been incorporated in the "dagger and asterisk" system. Examples are:

(i)   situations where the two elements are customarily recorded as discrete diagnostic phrases and can be dealt with simply by coding the two terms separately, e.g. certain types of anaemia which may be the consequence of other diseases; the classification of the anaemia is usually according to its morphological type and does not depend on the cause;

(ii)   where the manifestation is an intrinsic part of the basic disease and is not regarded as a separate medical-care problem; for example, cholera, dysentery, etc. in the infectious and parasitic diseases chapter do not have asterisk categories in the digestive system chapter; lower genito-urinary tract manifestations of venereal diseases, in the infectious and parasitic diseases chapter, do not have asterisk categories in the genito-urinary diseases chapter, although gonococcal salpingitis and orchitis do;

(iii)   where the LCD has traditionally classified the condition according to the manifestation, e.g. anaemia due to enzyme defect.

The areas of the Classification where the dagger and asterisk system operates are limited; there are about 150 rubrics of each in which asterisk- or dagger-marked terms occur. They may take one of three different forms:—

(i)   if the symbol († or *) and the alternative code both appear in the title of the rubric, all terms classifiable to that rubric are subject to dual classification and all have the same alternative code, e.g.

049.0† Lymphocytic choriomeningitis (321.6*)

Lymphocytic:
          meningitis (serous)
          meningoencephalitis (serous)

321.2* Meningitis due to ECHO virus (047.1 †)

Meningo-eruptive syndrome

(ii)   if the symbol appears in the title but the alternative code does not, all terms classifiable to that rubric are subject to dual classification but they have different alternative codes (which are listed for each term), e.g.

074.2† Coxsackie carditis

Aseptic myocarditis ofCoxsackie:

newborn (422.0*)endocarditis (421.1*)

myocarditis (422.0*)
pericarditis (420.0*)

420.0* Pericarditis in diseases classified elsewhere

Pericarditis (acute):
    Coxsackie (074.2†)
    meningococcal (036.4†)
    syphilitic (093.8†)

Pericarditis (acute):
    tuberculous (017.8†)
    uraemic (585†)

(iii)   if neither the symbol nor the alternative code appear in the title, the rubric as a whole is not subject to dual classification but individual inclusion terms may be; if so, these terms will be marked with the symbol and their alternative codes, e.g.

078.5Cytomegalic inclusion disease

Cytomegalic inclusion virus hepatitis† (573.1*)
Salivary gland virus disease

424.3Pulmonary valve disorders

Pulmonic regurgitation:
    NOS
    syphilitic* (093.2†)

The use of asterisk coding is entirely optional. It should never be employed in coding the underlying cause of death (only dagger coding should be used for this purpose) but may be used in morbidity coding and in multiple-condition coding whether in morbidity or mortality. Any published tabulations, whether according to the detailed list or one of the short lists, of frequencies based on asterisk coding should be clearly annotated "Based on LCD asterisk coding".

Role of the E Code

As explained in the Report of the International Revision Conference (see paragraph 1.3 (iii), page XVI), the E Code is now a supplementary classification that may be used, if desired, to code external factors associated with morbid conditions classified to any part of the main classification. For single-cause tabulation of the underlying cause of death, however, the E Code should be used as the primary code if, and only if, the morbid condition is classifiable to Chapter XVII (Injury and Poisoning).

Gaps in the numbering system

It will be noticed that certain code numbers have not been used, leaving gaps in the numbering system. The reason for this practice was to avoid unnecessary changes in code numbers familiar to coders who have been using the Eighth Revision. For example, gangrene (category 445 in the Eighth Revision) has been moved to category 785.4; in order to avoid changing the code numbers of categories 446 (Polyarteritis nodosa and allied conditions), 447

(Other disorders of arteries and arterioles) and 448 (Diseases of capillaries), it was preferred to leave the code number 445 unused in the Ninth Revision.

Glossary of mental disorders

A glossary describing and defining the content of rubrics in Chapter V (Mental Disorders) was published separately from the Eighth Revision of the International Classification of Diseases. In the Ninth Revision, the glossary has been incorporated into the Classification itself (see pages 177-213).

The glossary descriptions are not intended as an aid for the lay coder, who should code whatever diagnostic statement appears on a medical record according to the provisions of the Tabular List and Alphabetical Index. Their purpose is to assist the person making the diagnosis, who should do so on the basis of the descriptions rather than the category titles, which may differ in meaning from place to place.

Adaptations of the ICD

Several adaptations or applications of the ICD to specific specialties have been published or are in preparation. They are briefly described below.

Dentistry and Stomatology

The "Application of the ICD to Dentistry and Stomatology" (ICD-DA), based on the Eighth Revision of the ICD, was prepared by the Oral Health Unit of WHO and first published in 1969. It brings together those LCD categories that include "diseases or conditions that occur in, have manifestations in, or have associations with the oral cavity and adjacent structures." It provides greater detail by means, of a fifth digit, but the numbering system is so organized that the relationship between an ICD-DA code and the ICD code from which it is derived is immediately obvious and frequencies for ICD-DA categories can be readily aggregated into ICD categories.

ICD-DA has been revised to concord with the Ninth Revision of the LCD and this revision was published by the World Health Organization in 1977.

Oncology

The "International Classification of Diseases for Oncology" (ICD-O) was published by the World Health Organization in 1976. Developed in collaboration with the International Agency for Research on Cancer (WHO) and the United States National Cancer Institute, with input from many other countries and extensive field trials, the ICD-O is intended for use in cancer registries, pathology departments and other agencies specializing in cancer.

ICD-O is a dual-axis classification, providing coding systems for topography and morphology. The topography code uses for all neoplasms the same three- and four-digit categories that the Ninth Revision of ICD uses for malignant neoplasms (categories 140-199), thus providing increased specificity of site for other neoplasms, where the ICD provides a more restricted topographical classification or none at all.

The morphology code is identical to the neoplasms section of the morphology field of the Systematized Nomenclature of Medicine (SNOMed) 21 and is compatible with the 1968 Edition of the Manual of Tumor Nomenclature and Coding (MOTNAC) 22 and the Systematized Nomenclature of Pathology (SNOP) [23]. It is a five-digit code, the first four digits identifying the histological type and the fifth the behaviour of the neoplasm (malignant, in situ, benign, etc.). The ICD-O morphology code also appears in this Volume (see pages 667-690) and in the Alphabetical Index.

In addition to the topography and morphology codes, ICD-O also includes a list of tumour-like lesions and conditions. A table explaining the method of converting ICD-O codes into LCD codes will be published in due course.

Ophthalmology

The International Council of Ophthalmology, supported by ophthalmological groups in many countries, has prepared a Classification of Disorders of the Eye, based on the Ninth Revision of the ICD.

In addition to the ICD section "Disorders of the eye and adnexa" (categories 360-379), it includes all other ICD categories that classify eye disorders, from infectious diseases to injuries. It is a five-digit classification, being identical with ICD at the three- and four-digit level but introducing additional detail at the fifth digit for the use of specialists.

The classification was published in the "International Nomenclature of Ophthalmology" by the American Academy of Ophthalmology and Otolaryngology 24 in 1977, which also includes definitions or short descriptions of all terms, synonyms and equivalent terms in French, German and Spanish, and reference terms to facilitate literature retrieval.

WHO Centres for Classification of Diseases

Six WHO Centres have been established to assist countries with problems encountered in the classification of diseases and, in particular, in the use of the ICD. They are located in institutions in Paris (for French language users), São Paulo (for Portuguese), Moscow (for Russian) and Caracas (for Spanish); there are two Centres for English language users, in London and, for North America, in Washington, DC., USA. Communications should be addressed as follows:—

Head, WHO Centre for Classification of Diseases
Office of Population Censuses and Surveys
St. Catherine's House
10 Kingsway
London WC2B 6JP
United Kingdom

or

Head, WHO Center for Classification of Diseases for North America
National Center for Health Statistics
US Public Health Service
Department of Health, Education and Welfare
Washington. DC.,
United States of America

REFERENCES

1. Registrar General of England and Wales, *Sixteenth Annual Report, 1856,* Appendix, 75-76

2. Greenwood, M. (1948) *Medical statistics from Graunt to Farr.* Cambridge, p. 28

3. Registrar General of England and Wales, *Sixteenth Annual Report, 1856,* Appendix, p. 73

4. Bertillon, J. (1912) Classification of the causes of death. (Abstract). *Trans. 15th Int. Cong. Hyg. Demog.,* Washington, pp. 52-55

5. *Bull. Inst. int. Statist. 1900,* **12**, 280

6. Roesle, E. (1928) *Essai d'une statistique comparative de la morbidité devant servir à établir les listes spéciales des causes de morbidité.* Geneva (League of Nations Health Organization, document C. H. 730)

7. *Off. Rec. Wld Hlth Org.,* 1948, 2, 110

8. *Off. Rec. Wld Hlth Org.,* 1948, **11**, 23

9. World Health Organization (1955) *Report of the International Conference for the Seventh Revision of the International Lists of Diseases and Causes of Death,* Geneva (unpublished document WHO/HS/7 Rev. Conf./17 Rev. 1)

10. *Wld Hlth Org. techn. Rep. Ser.,* 1952, **53**

11. World Health Organization (1965) *Report of the International Conference for the Eighth Revision of the International Classification of Diseases,* Geneva (unpublished document WHO/HS/8 Rev. Conf./11.65)

12. World Health Organization, Expert Committee on Health Statistics (1974) *Ninth Revision of the International Classification of Diseases,* Geneva (unpublished document WHO/ICD9/74.4)

13. *Off. Rec. Wld Hlth Org.,* 1975, **223**, 10

14. *Off. Rec. Wld Hlth Org.,* 1975, **226**, 42

15. *Off. Rec. Wld Hlth Org.,* 1975, **226**, 44

16. *Off. Rec. Wld Hlth Org.,* 1975, **226**, 53

17. World Health Organization, Scientific Group on Health Statistics Methodology related to Perinatal Events (1974), Geneva (unpublished document ICD/PE/74.4)

18. *Off. Rec. Wld Hlth Org.,* 1976, **233**, 18

19. *Off. Rec. Wld Hlth Org.,* 1976, **233**, 18

20 *Off. Rec. Wld Hlth Org.,* 1976, **231**, 25

21. College of American Pathologists (1976), *Systematized Nomenclature of Medicine*, Chicago, Illinois

22. American Cancer Society, Inc. (1968), *Manual of Tumor Nomenclature and Coding*, New York, NY

23. College of American Pathologists (1965), *Systematized Nomenclature of Pathology*, Chicago, Illinois

24. American Academy of Ophthalmology and Otolaryngology (1977), *International Nomenclature of Ophthalmology*, 15 Second Street, S.W., Rochester, Minnesota 55901

B

Standard Nomenclature of Diseases & Operations

PRIOR TO THE MID-1950S, hospitals usually coded their diagnoses and operations using the *Standard Nomenclature of Diseases and Operations (SNDO)*. [1] "Snowdough," as it was called by physicians and medical record professionals, presented problems in both the coding process and in the retrieval of information.

The Difficulties of Coding with SNDO

Actually, what was called "coding" was really taking the English term used by the physician and putting it into a "standardized language representation of the disease" — a process called "transformation."[2] The "standardized language" (not a "standard term" or "preferred term" as one would think of those phrases) then was coded by using its concatenation of code numbers. The code for a transformed term decodes into the transformed term, not back to the original English of the entity term.

SNDO is a "structured code," meaning that each digit or character in a given position has a fixed meaning. This is discussed further below.

---

1. *SNDO* was initiated in 1928 by the National Conference on Nomenclature of Disease, which included representatives from most of the leading medical and public health organizations in the U.S. The first edition was entitled *Standard Classified Nomenclature of Disease* (published in 1933, with a preliminary printing in 1932). A second edition came out in 1935. In 1937, the American Medical Association took on responsibility for its periodic revision, and in 1942 published the 3rd Edition, *Standard Nomenclature of Diseases and Standard Nomenclature of Operations* (Edwin P. Jordan, MD, editor). For the 4th Edition (1952), the name was simplified to *Standard Nomenclature of Diseases and Operations*, with Richard J. Plunkett, MD, and Adaline C. Hayden, RRL, editors. The 5th and final edition appeared in 1961 with the same title, Edward T. Thompson, MD, replacing Plunkett as senior editor.

2. See "Modular Languages," page 83.

Structured classification One of the attributes of a structured classification is that codes are long, because of the necessity of holding certain positions in the code open even though, in many instances, a given meanings will not use that position. And frequently, the coding is awkward.

Transformation coding *SNDO* is no exception; its codes were long and awkward, requiring that the diagnosis or operation be *transformed* into coded descriptions along two (and sometimes three or more) axes (for more about axes, see page 133). Every condition was required to be transformed (labeled) along its first axis, (1) topography (portion of the body affected) and its second axis, (2) etiology (cause of the disorder). And many needed also the recording of (3) manifestations, found in a "supplementary code."

Topography could require up to five or six or more digits, etiology likewise, and manifestations several more. Digits were not only decimal, but also "x" and "y" in places (the reason for this was that punch cards had twelve rows representing "0 through 9" and also "x" and "y"). Decimal points were also used, and their location was, at times, significant. Other suggestions (or requirements) were also found. For example, "mental deficiency" was accompanied by a note to include intelligence quotient (IQ) when available, although where in the sequence of numbers, and how to tell that the numerical IQ was not a numerical code from one of the other axes, were not specified. Additionally, there was a list of "non-diagnostic terms for the hospital record."

SNDO was organized in seven sections:

Schema of the Classification Here the topographic and the etiologic naming schemes and the accompanying codes were given.

Nomenclature of Diseases In this section (remember, the volume was entitled "nomenclature"), all the "known" diseases were named. Each was found under the code number given the disease term, rather than in an alphabetical list. This was a "tabular list." Later in the volume is an alphabetic index of disease terms.

Supplementary Terms These could modify any of the diagnoses in the Nomenclature section.

Standard Nomenclature of Operations This really was a classification rather than a nomenclature, and a broad classification at that. Each operation category consisted, like diagnoses, of a topographic component taken from the same schema, followed by a "-" and the numerals 0-8, which placed every "type" of procedure then envisioned into one of the nine categories, such as "incision," "endoscopy,"" and the like. In the field of surgery, new procedures and techniques appear daily, and virtually all hospitals seriously interested in indexing them had to expand on this classification, if they used it at all.

Index to Nomenclature of Disease It is of interest that when a diagnostic term was found, the reader was directed to the page number where it was found, rather than to its code. This led to a report that at least one hospital solved its disease index problem by coding to the page number rather than to the code for the diagnosis itself! This, of course, introduced a new and unintended axis into the classification. The medical record librarian in that hospital was said to be uncommonly efficient in finding the cases the doctor wanted. The "new classification" was only discovered when a visitor knowledgeable in *SNDO* asked the origin of the unfamiliar numbers.

Index to Nomenclature of Operations This index also referred the user to the page number. It was here that procedures known by their "inventors," e.g., a "Braun graft," could also be found.

Appendix to the Standard Nomenclature and International Statistical Classification This appendix is discussed in some length below in the section entitled "The International Classification."

As to the way the system worked, a "basic" *SNDO* code was required to have two segments: (1) first, a segment designating the anatomic location of the disease (its *topography*) by an alphanumeric code, followed by "-" which indicated the start of (2) the second segment, also a series of alphanumeric characters, which showed the cause of the disease (its *etiology*).

Topography There were eleven main topographic divisions:[3]

> 0++- Body as a whole (including the psyche and the body generally), not a particular system exclusively

1++- Integumentary System (including subcutaneous areolar tissue, mucous membranes of orifices, and the breast)

2++- Musculoskeletal system

3++- Respiratory system

4++- Cardiovascular system

5++- Hemic and lymphatic system

6++- Digestive system

7++- Urogenital system

8++- Endocrine system

9++- Nervous system

x++- Organs of special sense

Etiology Thirteen major divisions of etiology were used:

-0++ Diseases due to prenatal influence

-1++ Diseases due to a lower plant or animal parasite

-2++ Diseases due to a higher plant or animal parasite

-3++ Diseases due to intoxication

-4++ Diseases due to trauma or physical agent

-50++ Diseases secondary to circulatory disturbance

-55++ Diseases secondary to disturbance of innervation or of psychic control

-6++ Diseases due to or consisting of static mechanical abnormality (obstruction, calculus, displacement or gross change in form) due to unknown causes

-7++ Diseases due to disorder of metabolism, growth or nutrition

---

3. In these illustrations of the sections of *SNDO* on topography and etiology, two typographic conventions are used: "++" indicates the use of succeeding digits, sometimes four or five, which gave increasing detail; occasionally decimal subdivisions were used to give further information. "-" indicated the end of the topographic or beginning of the etiologic segment respectively.

-8++ New growths

-9++ Diseases due to unknown or uncertain cause with the structural reaction (degenerative, infiltrative, inflammatory, proliferative, sclerotic or reparative) manifest; hereditary and familiar diseases of this nature

-x++ Diseases due to unknown or uncertain cause with the functional reaction alone manifest; hereditary and familial diseases of this nature

-y++ Diseases of undetermined cause

Supplementary Terms The supplementary terms, which could be used to modify any portion of the term, each began with a leading character which meant that it pertained to the topographic section of the schema which began with that digit, so each supplementary code beginning with "0" referred to the body as a whole, and so on. Beyond that digit, the codes were arbitrary in meaning, i.e., they could not be synthesized by using intrinsic meanings of their component digits. The supplementary term codes were usually three digits in length, but sometimes four. The character "-" was also used to show the beginning of the "field" or segment containing supplementary terms.

"x" and "y" Usually "x" and "y" were used as "11" and "12" when the ten decimal digits "0" to "9" didn't give enough categories. Although few hospitals at this time used punch cards in handling medical record data, this took advantage of the fact that IBM cards had twelve rows of holes, designated "x", "y", and "0-9". (In the etiology classification, this expansion was not sufficient, as can be seen above, and instead of "5", the "first digit" could be either "50" or "55", each with a different meaning.) Thus:

x as the first "digit" in a code means "Organs of special sense"

x within the topography "field" can mean "11", an expansion of the ten decimal digits 0-9

x following "-" (i.e., introducing the etiological component of the code) means "Diseases due to unknown or uncertain cause with the functional reaction alone manifest; hereditary and familial diseases of this nature"

y could be used under some circumstances to expand the ten decimal digits (0-9) to "12" y   following "-" means "Diseases of undetermined cause"

-    separated the "fields": topography from etiology; etiology from supplementary terms

"y" or "Y" "y" or "Y" was also used to indicate lack of information in both the topographic and the etiologic fields. "Undiagnosed disease of the heart" would be coded as "410-y00": 410- being the topographic designation for "heart, general," and the etiologic code of -y00 signifying an undetermined cause. A lesion known merely to involve an unidentified portion of the digestive tract would receive the topographic code "6y0-+++".

A complete ignorance of the nature of a disease, both as to location and cause, would be indicated by "y00-y00". It is not surprising that it became itself a diagnosis — "YO-YO's disease" became a well known term among medical record librarians and physicians and, of course, a valid code.

Where the above methods did not suffice, at various places in the codes the user was instructed to affix a decimal point at the end of the topography or etiology, followed by a code, e.g., ".x1" meant "with psychotic reaction" when used in the "Diseases of the psychobiologic unit" codes.

A disease with several codable manifestations, shown by their supplementary codes, required the repetition of the topography-etiology section for each of the manifestations. Thus, for a disease with three such manifestations, three lengthy codes, differing only in the last three or four digits, would be needed.

Several results of this coding scheme should be pointed out:

- A complete code could be very long, perhaps 20 characters.

- Codes would vary in length, depending on how many characters were needed for each of its components.

- The "-" was critically important in telling whether a given series of characters meant a site, an etiology, or a manifestation. (Holding the maximum possible number of spaces open for each of these three attributes, and labeling the three "fields" appropriately, would have eliminated the ambiguity and the need for "-", but it was not a feasible option at the time.)

Code "Synthesis" The final paragraph of the Preface reads:

> General—For diagnoses which are not found listed or for which specific provision for coding has not been made, e.g., as in the "Regional Classification," it is requested that the user communicate with the editors. Please do not try to improvise new code numbers or titles.

It is unlikely that these inquiries were numerous, or the admonition often heeded, because the very nature of such a "modular classification" invited the physician or medical record librarian simply to synthesize the code and not bother with a protracted dialog with strangers in Chicago. Such creation of a code number seemed reasonable enough when the coder knew how the classification worked, the topography of the condition, its etiology, and any supplementary information that should be included.

But few saw the problem this would produce. The fact of the matter was that equally competent classifiers could (and did) end up with different codes for the same diagnosis — and virtually all codes were "legal."[4]

Retrieval Problems

The coding problems — especially having varying codes for a single diagnosis — resulted in serious difficulties when groups of medical records were sought for studying treatments and operations. Since the medical records were indexed using the *SNDO* codes to represent (in transformed language, of course) the diagnoses and operations, these codes were the only place the medical record professional could look to find the desired cases. This brings us to the *International Classification*.

SNDO-4 and ICD

An innovation in the Fourth Edition of *SNDO* (1952) was that the authors included, for each diagnostic term in its "Nomenclature of Diseases" section, the code for the category of the *International Statistical Classification of Diseases, Injuries and Causes of Death, Sixth Revision (ISC-6, later ICD)* into which that diagnosis would fall. Thus the user of the book could look up the term and find preceding it its

---

4.   For more about "legal" codes, see "Validity," page 131.

SNDO code and, in parentheses at the right margin of the page, its *ICD-6* code.

In the Appendix to *SNDO-4*, all of the published *SNDO* nomenclature codes were collected in a "tabular list" under the category of *ICD-6* where they fell. The Appendix was entitled:

"List of 3-Digit and 4-Digit Categories
of the
International Statistical Classification
With Standard Numbers Included in Each International Category"

Occasionally, there was only one *SNDO* code below the *ICD* number. But more frequently there were many. Some lists occupied an entire page. There were, for example, 101 *SNDO* codes which might have been given to varieties of "strabismus" (crossed eyes), which was a single category, Code 384, in *ICD-6*.

On the following pages are illustrations from *SNDO-4* showing its treatment of diabetes mellitus — first, the *SNDO* coding (with *ICD* codes in parentheses), and second, the *ICD* cross-reference in the Appendix, with the *SNDO* codes listed under the *ICD* code.

Figure B.1 *SNDO-4* (illustrative page)

378   ENDOCRINE SYSTEM

DISEASES OF THE INSULAR TISSUE

See also Diseases of the Pancreas, *page 274*

871–   Insular tissue

—7 DISEASES DUE TO DISORDER OF METABOLISM, GROWTH OR NUTRITION
Record primary diagnosis when possible

871–771	Diabetes mellitus with hyperthyroidism	*(260) (252.0)*
871–772	Diabetes mellitus with hypothyroidism	*(260) (253)*
871–776	Diabetes mellitus with hyperpituitarism	*(260) (272)*
871–777	Diabetes mellitus with hypopituitarism	*(260) (272)*
871–781	Diabetes mellitus with hyperadrenalcorticalism	*(260) (274)*
871–782	Diabetes mellitus with hypoadrenalcorticalism	*(260) (274)*
871–770	Diabetes mellitus with hyperfunction of chromaffin tissue	*(260) (274)*
871–785	Diabetes mellitus	*(260)*
871–784	Hyperinsulinism, without tumor	*(270)*

—8 NEW GROWTHS

871–8091	Adenocarcinoma of insular tissue. *Specify behavior (page 78)*	*(157)*
871–8091A	Adenoma of insular tissue	*(270)*
871–8044F	Functioning islet cell adenocarcinoma of insular tissue	*(157)*
871–8044A	Functioning islet cell adenoma of insular tissue	*(270)*
871–8074F	Non-functioning islet cell adenocarcinoma of insular tissue	*(157)*
870–8074A	Non-functioning islet cell adenoma of insular tissue	*(270)*
871–8...	Unlisted tumor of insular tissue. *Specify neoplasm and behavior (page 78)* (malignant, *157*; benign, *270*; unspecified, *270*)	

—9 DISEASES DUE TO UNKNOWN OR UNCERTAIN CAUSE WITH THE STRUCTURAL REACTION MANIFEST

871–953	Sclerosis of insular tissue due to unknown cause	*(270)*
871–953.6	With diabetes mellitus	*(260)*

—X DISEASES DUE TO UNKNOWN OR UNCERTAIN CAUSE WITH THE FUNCTIONAL REACTION ALONE MANIFEST

871–x10	Diabetes mellitus without known cause or structural change	*(260)*

Page 378 from "Nomenclature of Diseases," *Standard Nomenclature of Diseases and Operations, Fourth Edition.* American Medical Association, 1952.

Figure B.2 *SNDO-4 Appendix* (illustrative page)

892   APPENDIX

DISEASES OF THYROID GLAND *(250–254)*

250   Simple goitre
810–739
810–943

251   Nontoxic nodular goitre

810–8024B	810–8091A	810–8...*
810–8065A	810–8094A	810–952
810–8078A	810–8095B	

† Excludes benign neoplasm of cartilage of thyroid *(212)*.

252   Thyrotoxicosis with or without goitre
252.0   Toxic diffuse goitre

132–771	810–300*	871–771*
410–771	810–771	x11–771
785–771	810–776*	
803	810–943.6	

252.1   Toxic nodular goitre

810–8047A
810–952.6

253   Myxœdema and cretinism

13.–772	810–016	810–7722
22x–771*	810–3001*	810–777*
410–772	810–415.6	810–911
501–772	810–471.6	871–772*
785–772	810–7721	x20–772*

254   Other diseases of thyroid gland

810–093	810–190	810–942
810–100.2	810–600.8	810–y00
810–100	810–942.1	

This title excludes thyroglossal cyst *(759.3)*.

DIABETES MELLITUS *(260)*

260   Diabetes mellitus

0..–785.1	871–771	907..–785
0..–785.9	871–772	975–785
114–785	871–776	98..–785
13.–785	871–777	x12–785
360–785	871–781	x15–785
571	871–782	x201–785
712–7x9	871–785	x20–785.x
713–785.9	871–953.6	x20–785
774–785	871–x10	x23–785
871–770	906–785	x2x–785.5

Page 892 from "Nomenclature of Diseases," *Standard Nomenclature of Diseases and Operations, Fourth Edition*. American Medical Association, 1952.

This feature of the Fourth Edition of *SNDO*, along with the Appendix to the book, proved to be the bridge between coding with *SNDO* and the use of the *International Statistical Classification (ISC)* for hospital disease indexing (which became predominant in the mid-1950s), despite the note in the preface to *SNDO:*

> Note: The International List code numbers have been included in this edition solely for the purpose of allowing for their use as a cross-coding to[5] Standard Nomenclature for large scale statistical surveys. It is not our intention that they should in any way replace the "Standard" code numbers for use in the recording of hospital records or as a substitute for "Standard" for use in clinical research.

With a code structured as is *SNDO*, with each digit and its position having explicit meanings, common sense would indicate that decoding would, in each instance, come up with the term which had been coded. In the above figure, the listing for "Diabetes Mellitus" shows that is not necessarily the case, because such translations among codes are not one-way streets. Following this route, here's the decoding for two of the codes:

"114-785" decoded as

114(topography) "Skin proper (cutis)"

785(etiology) "Decreased function of the insular tissue of the pancreas"

In the "Nomenclature of Diseases" section of the book, the diagnosis for 114-785 is given as "Xanthoma diabeticorum."

"871-771" decoded as

871(topography) "Pancreas, insular tissue"

771(etiology) "Disturbance of thyroid gland, increased or perverted function."

Under "Nomenclature..." the diagnosis for 871-771 turns out to be "diabetes mellitus with hyperthyroidism."

This feature of *SNDO*, the incorporation of the International codes, was recognized by ingenious medical record librarians as the best available tool for organizing the retrieval of series of cases requested by physicians,

---

5.   This should have read "from," since such cross-coding is a one-way street; the broader class can never be "cross-coded" into the more specific.

a task which had hitherto been most formidable. When a physician asked for "all the cases of diabetes mellitus," for example, the Appendix[6] was a ready reference of *most* of the Standard codes under which the cases might have been indexed. The record librarians' previous recourse had been to somehow develop such lists themselves, a terribly laborious process. Furthermore, their lists could never be truly verified, because there was no way to prevent or detect either inventive, but logical, coding not found in the book, or outright coding errors.

Obviously, not every one of the possible combinations is medically possible, but unless someone compiles a list of what is possible in the real world of medicine, i.e., a list of valid or "legal" codes, it will be impossible to control the input to any system using such codes in order to insure that the input makes sense. Computer systems regularly provide validation rules for data elements, e.g., a numeric field is not permitted to receive alphabetic characters, a field for dollars and cents is not permitted to have more than two places to the right of the decimal point, or, more to this point, a numerical field for months cannot have a number higher than 12. A little mentioned, but highly significant, factor in the swing from *SNDO* to *ICDA* was that virtually *any* combination of numbers of the correct length was, so far as the viewer and the data processing world was concerned, a legal code in *SNDO*, yet it could easily be absolute clinical nonsense. And there was no way to devise any set of rules which could be applied to solve or avoid this problem. *ICDA*, on the other hand, had a finite, auditable, list of valid codes, and any invalid code could be blocked from use by programming of the computer. A quantum improvement in data quality was the immediate result of the switch.

The Final Edition: SNDO-5

This use of the International codes did not go unnoticed by the authors of *SNDO* who, in the Fifth Edition, dropped the International table, and countered with the American Medical Association's own *Abridged Statistical Classification for Clinical Indexing*. The introductory statement indicates that "Generally the first two digits are identical with

---

6.   This despite the fact that the Appendix was not indexed, so the only way to find anything was to browse looking for the relevant *ICD* category. But that was far easier than the previous methods of selecting the codes for the retrieval of series of cases.

the first two digits of the topographic code and the last two digits identical with the first two digits of the etiologic categories ... " This was indeed a generality; code 5800 of this statistical classification is labeled "Diseases of the ear," although the ear, in the topographic schema is code "x71" and "00" in the etiologic classification signifies "Diseases due to abnormality of bone development."

Meanwhile, medical records professionals had simply said to themselves "why not just use the *ICD* code from the right side of the *SNDO* book in the first place and not have to go through the 'double coding'." And that's what several leaders did.[7]

Whether or not the new *SNDO* "clinical indexing" classification was useful is a moot point. The switch to the International had begun in the mid-fifties with two events: The first was adoption of the 6th Revision for hospital indexing by the Professional Activity Study (PAS) after PAS had given the *International Classification* some increase in specificity by incorporation of the subdivisions and modifications developed in Columbia-Presbyterian Medical Center in New York and the United States Public Health Service Hospital in Baltimore.[8] This use in prestigious hospitals and in PAS stimulated the second event, a collaborative study made by the American Hospital Association (AHA), which showed the superiority of the *International Classification* for indexing medical records.[9] As a result of this study, the United States Public Health Service in 1960 issued "Publication 719" entitled on the spine *Diagnostic Index*, and on the title page *International Classification*

---

7. From the very first, however, they made certain modifications to increase the specificity of the *ICD: ICD* had a single pigeonhole (260) for diabetes mellitus, as illustrated; the users gave this 7 subdivisions. *ICD* lumped acute myocardial infarction into code 420.1, a mixed bag entitled "Heart disease specified as involving the coronary arteries." The medical record personnel gave two unused digits to "myocardial infarction" and "coronary insufficiency." And so on.

8. These were the work of Dorothy Kurtz, CRL, in the Columbia-Presbyterian Medical Center in New York and Loyola Voelker, CRL, in the United States Public Health Service Hospital in Baltimore.

9. "Efficiency in Hospital Indexing of the Coding Systems of the International Statistical Classification and Standard Nomenclature of Diseases and Operations," *Journal of the American Association of Medical Record Librarians*, Vol 10 No 3 June 1959.

of Diseases Adapted for Indexing of Hospital Records and Operation Classification.

No further editions of *SNDO* appeared after the Fifth Edition in 1961, which was already in press when the AHA study was published.

C

Diagnosis Related Groups

DIAGNOSIS RELATED GROUPS (DRGs) is the classification of episodes of hospital care used in the billing system in the United States. They were first employed in the Medicare Prospective Payment System (PPS) beginning in 1983 following a trial in New Jersey the preceding year. They have since been generally adopted by other payers.

The work leading to the development of DRGs was begun at Yale University in 1967 by Professor Robert B. Fetter of the Department of Administrative Sciences and Professor John D. Thompson of the Department of Epidemiology and Public Health of the School of Medicine. Physicians in the local university hospital asked for help with utilization review, thinking that perhaps industrial experience in quality and cost controls could be applied in the hospital.

The studies by Fetter, Thompson, and their group led to the conviction that the products of hospital care, i.e., the "bundles" of services provided to the individual patients, could be defined as to their resource demands and consumption, and information about them managed in such a manner that the result would be a useful tool for hospital and medical care management. Application in the reimbursement process was *not* the initial purpose of developing the classification.

The key to the system is the grouping scheme. The grouping system which emerged had four requirements:

- It must start with information routinely collected on hospital abstracts. This came from the Uniform Hospital Discharge Data Set (UHDDS) (see page 141). Included in UHDDS are the principal diagnosis, additional diagnoses, procedures, age, sex, length of stay, and discharge status.

- The patients must be grouped into a manageable number of classes.

- Each class must have within it similar patterns of resource intensity, i.e., length of stay and charges.

- Each class must be clinically coherent — must have similar types of patients from the clinical perspective.

The groupings have undergone a number of revisions over the years in order to make them more useful, for example, more sensitive to the intensity of care required by individual patients and the severity of illness. And the principles have been applied in Ambulatory Visit Groups (AVGs), Ambulatory Patient Groups (APGs), Patient Dependency Groups (PDGs) for long term care patients, Resource Intensity Measures (RIMs) for nursing care, and in other contexts. DRGs have also been placed in use in other countries.

In brief, each patient's computer abstract — in which diagnoses and procedures are expressed as *ICD-9-CM* codes — is processed through a computer program called GROUPER which allocates the case to one of about 480 Diagnosis Related Groups using the following logic:

- Each case, on the basis of its principal diagnosis, falls into one of roughly 25 mutually exclusive Major Diagnostic Categories (MDCs).

- Then, for the MDCs in which operating room surgery is a possible treatment, the case is put into a subset of those with such surgery.

Further splitting then occurs:

- For surgical patients, the type of surgery, age, and substantial comorbidities and complications (CCs), principal diagnoses, and non-operating room procedures are the factors considered.

- For medical patients, the principal diagnosis, age, additional diagnoses, certain non-operating room procedures, and discharge status are considered.

The system is periodically reviewed, and changes made in the definitions of each factor used in the distribution of cases in the DRGs. Over a dozen such reviews have occurred. The final number of classes, pigeonholes, is about 480 (a number which can change slightly as the system is periodically refined). See the illustration on page 424 for a sample of DRG codes.

The Prospective Payment System for Medicare uses DRGs to determine the payment for each patient. For each patient, the hospital receives an amount for the DRG into which that patient falls. Each DRG has a relative value which represents its "cost" as a proportion of the average cost of all DRGs. This relative value is multiplied by a national standardized operating payment amount, adjusted by factors including location of the hospital, its size, and others. The payment has been calculated on the assumption that individual patients with low and high resource consumption will average out, but special provisions have been made for "outliers."

The initial DRGs were developed in the late 1960s and early 1970s when the diagnostic and procedure information was coded in the UHDDS to one of the two versions of the *International Classification* then in use, the *Hospital Adaptation of ICDA (H-ICDA)*, published by the Commission on Professional and Hospital Activities (CPHA), or the *Eighth Revision of International Classification of Diseases Adapted for Use in the United States (ICDA)*, USPHS Publication 1693. CPHA was one source of the clinical data used during the early development of DRGs. When *ICD-9-CM* replaced the two earlier adaptations of the *International Classification of Diseases, 8th Revision (ICD-8)*, it was necessary again to obtain a large sample of hospital discharge abstracts and hospital bills and revise the algorithm for placing cases into DRGs so that the proper pricing for each DRG could be determined. This process has to be carried out every time there is a change in the category coded information in the input to the system. For an alternative, see "Entity Coding," page 277.

Figure C.1 DRG & MDC Codes (Examples)

App. 23: Diagnosis Related Groups (DRGs)
Major Diagnostic Category (MDC)

1   Diseases and disorders of the nervous system
2   Diseases and disorders of the eye
3   Diseases and disorders of the ear, nose, and throat
4   Diseases and disorders of the respiratory system
5   Diseases and disorders of the circulatory system
6   Diseases and disorders of the digestive system
7   Diseases and disorders of the hepatobiliary system and pancreas
8   Diseases and disorders of the musculoskeletal system and connective tissue
9   Diseases and disorders of the skin, subcutaneous tissue, and breast
10 Endocrine, nutritional, and metabolic diseases and disorders
11 Diseases and disorders of the kidney and urinary tract
12 Diseases and disorders of the male reproductive system
13 Diseases and disorders of the female reproductive system
14 Pregnancy, childbirth, and the puerperium
15 Newborns and other neonates with condition originating in perinatal period
16 Diseases and disorders of blood and blood-forming organs
17 Myeloproliferative disorders
18 Infectious and parasitic diseases
19 Mental diseases and disorders
20 Substance use and substance-induced organic mental disorders
21 Injuries, poisonings, and toxic effects of drugs
22 Burns
23 Factors influencing health status and other contacts with health services
24 No major diagnostic category

DRG	MDC		TITLE
1	1	S	Craniotomy, age >17 except for trauma
2	1	S	Craniotomy for trauma, age >17
3	1	S	Craniotomy, age <18
4	1	S	Spinal procedures
5	1	S	Extracranial vascular procedures
6	1	S	Carpal tunnel release
7	1	S	Peripheral and cranial nerve and other nervous system procedures, age >69 and/or C.C.
8	1	S	Peripheral and cranial nerve and other nervous system procedures, age <70 without C.C.
9	1	M	Spinal disorders and injuries
10	1	M	Nervous system neoplasms, age >69 and/or C.C.
11	1	M	Nervous system neoplasms, age <70 without C.C.
12	1	M	Degenerative nervous system disorders
13	1	M	Multiple sclerosis and cerebellar ataxia
14	1	M	Specific cerebrovascular disorders except transient ischemic attack
15	1	M	Transient ischemic attack and precerebral occlusions
16	1	M	Nonspecific cerebrovascular disorders with C.C.
17	1	M	Nonspecific cerebrovascular disorders without C.C.
18	1	M	Cranial and peripheral nerve disorders, age >69 and/or C.C.
19	1	M	Cranial and peripheral nerve disorders, age <70 without C.C.
20	1	M	Nervous system infection except viral meningitis
21	1	M	Viral meningitis
22	1	M	Hypertensive encephalopathy
23	1	M	Nontraumatic stupor and coma
24	1	M	Seizure and headache, age >69 and/or C.C.
25	1	M	Seizure and headache, age 18 to 69 without C.C.
26	1	M	Seizure and headache, age 0 to 17
27	1	M	Traumatic stupor and coma, coma >1 hour

M = medical case; S = surgical case; C.C. = comorbidity or complication; O.R. = operating room

2311

Page from *Taber's Cyclopedic Medical Dictionary.*

D

Unified Medical Language System

THE NATIONAL Library of Medicine (NLM) of the United States has as its mission

> ... to support biomedical research and to improve healthcare delivery by providing ready access to published biomedical information ...

In 1986, NLM established a long-term research and development project to build the Unified Medical Language System® (UMLS®). Although UMLS is a United States effort, it has strong international collaboration. The goal of UMLS is to "improve the ability of computer programs to 'understand' the biomedical meaning in user inquiries and, with this understanding, to retrieve and integrate the most relevant machine-readable information for users."

There are two chief barriers which UMLS seeks to overcome:

- The same concepts are expressed in different ways in different machine-readable sources and by different people.

- Useful information is distributed among many disparate databases and systems.

Another way to express the goal of UMLS is to describe it as a bridge between concepts, as expressed in various ways by various individuals (users, inquirers) and the information sources where the information is stored. To do this NLM, the UMLS project, has developed three "UMLS Knowledge Sources." They are:

Metathesaurus The first Knowledge Source, the Metathesaurus®, is an ever-growing collection of biomedical terms from machine-readable "controlled" sources which are studied and related to the biomedical concepts which they represent. The term sources include biomedical vocabularies such as *SNOMED*, classifications, such as *ICD-9-CM* and the *Read Clinical Classification System (Read Codes; now called NHS Codes)* and MeSH®,[1] databases, such as MEDLINE,[2] and also diagnostic expert systems such as DXplain, Iliad, and QMR (Quick Medical Reference), and factual databases such as drugs, toxicology, and protein and nucleic acid sequences. Both expert decisions and algorithms are used to determine to which concept each term pertains. The Metathesaurus files contain a good deal of explanatory and reference material about the terms and the concepts. Each concept is a "main term" in the thesaurus, along with which are given he terms used to express the concept in various vocabularies, such as synonyms, lexical variations, and translations for that term.

Of course, a given term may pertain to more than one concept. For example, the word "dressing" is both a bandage and a part of the verb "to dress," and thus is in two concepts, and the context in which it appears is important. The intended use of the thesaurus is that the term coming in from the sources, such as patient records, bibliographic citations, and elsewhere will link to the concept, and that the concept will be the starting point in the link from the inquiry of the user to the source of the desired information. By 1995, the Metathesaurus had grown to 222,927 concepts named by 478,562 biomedical terms from 31 source vocabularies. In 1999, the count of concepts was 626,893 and of biomedical terms was 1,358,891 from about 50 source vocabularies.

---

1.   MeSH® (Medical Subject Headings®) is the annual authority list for the subject analysis of the biomedical literature in the National Library of Medicine (NLM). The list is divided into two sections, an alphabetical list of the subjects along with their reference code numbers (MeSH numbers), and a tabular list, called a tree structure, in which the subjects are categorized and subdivided, often to several levels, according to the hierarchical arrangement of the classification. Any document in the literature will be classified under as many subjects as are logically necessary. The list is published by NLM but may only be obtained from the National Technical Information Service of the United States Department of Commerce.

2.   MEDLINE is a biomedical database containing bibliographic material from thousands of medical journals. It was developed and is maintained by the National Library of Medicine and is available to individuals and medical libraries. Searches are carried out through NLM's Medical Literature Analysis and Retrieval System (MEDLARS). A number of other biomedical databases are also offered by NLM, including CHEMLINE, a chemical dictionary, CATLINE, a book catalog, and DIRLINE, an organization database. The name, MEDLINE, is derived from "MEDLARS-on-line."

Details can be found in a Fact Sheet, periodically brought up to date, which is available from NLM or on the Internet. (Fact Sheets are provided for each component and for UMLS itself.)

Semantic Network The second Knowledge Source of UMLS is the Semantic Network. Its purpose is to provide a system for categorizing objects, i.e., the concepts in the Metathesaurus, and of identifying the relationships which link various concepts with each other. In early 2000 there are 153 semantic types and 53 relationships between them. The primary relationship is called an "isa" relationship, from the two words "is" and "a." Thus a dog "isa" mammal "isa" animal and the relationships defined by isa are hierarchical. Each level in a hierarchy inherits the characteristics of the level above. Dogs have all of the characteristics of the higher level, mammal. Mammals have all the characteristics of animals.

Specialist Lexicon The third Knowledge Source of UMLS is the Specialist Lexicon, which contains 108,000 lexical records with over 186,000 strings in the English language. Each lexical item may be a single word or a multi-word term. For each item, the lexicon gives the parts of speech, the various forms of the word, spelling variations, and other information about how the term in its various forms and usages fits into the construction of sentences in English. The sources of the items have been the UMLS Test Collection of MEDLINE citation records, items which occur in the Metathesaurus and Dorland's Illustrated Medical Dictionary, and frequently used words from the general English vocabulary. Like the other components of UMLS, the Specialist lexicon is available in machine-readable form for use by developers of information systems.

UMLS is designed to support user applications which are under development by a variety of institutions and organizations.

Thus UMLS does not provide a source of language for the biomedical community. Its Metathesaurus is, rather, a collector of the language used in the biomedical community, and an organization of the language according to the biomedical concepts expressed. Its identification of biomedical concepts may well become the standard reference.

Further information can be obtained about UMLS from NLM. Fact Sheets about the project and each of its components are periodically updated, and an increasing amount of information, including the Fact Sheets, is being placed on the Internet. See at http://www.nlm.nih.gov.

Inquiries are welcomed by

Betsy L. Humphreys
UMLS Project Officer
National Library of Medicine
8600 Rockville Pike
Bethesda MD 20894

FAX 301-496-4450

http://www.nlm.nih.gov/research/umls

E

SNOMED International

THE INTRODUCTION to the third edition of *SNOMED International: Systematized Nomenclature of Human and Veterinary Medicine (SNOMED III)* [1] states that it is a "structured nomenclature and classification of the terminology used in human and veterinary medicine." It is a system based on transformation coding — each concept, or portion of a concept, is transformed into a structured term within a coded component of *SNOMED*.[2] The components, such as topography and morphology, in *SNOMED* are called modules. Terms from several modules are linked together to form a complete concept, a diagnosis, for example. Decoding then retrieves the terms into which the original term was transformed rather than the original language.

SNOMED III, the third edition of *SNOMED*, had its origin in the *Systematized Nomenclature of Pathology (SNOP)*, originated by Arthur Wells, MD, published in 1965. This was expanded to the *Systematized Nomenclature of Medicine*. The second edition of that volume, *SNOMED II*, appeared in 1979. A parallel volume, the *Systematized Nomenclature of Veterinary Medicine, SNOVET*, was published in 1984, following which the two were merged, and *SNOMED III* was published in 1993 (revised in 1999). The growth in content has been impressive. The seven modules in *SNOMED II* have been increased to eleven modules, and its 44,500 records to over 156,000 (of course, some of the added terms came from *SNOVET*). *SNOMED* is the result of many

---

1. *SNOMED International: Systematized Nomenclature of Human and Veterinary Medicine*, published by the College of American Pathologists (1992). David Rothwell, MD, coauthor, and Gordon Briggs, of the College of American Pathologists, graciously provided a copy of *SNOMED III* and the browser for use in studying *SNOMED III*, which by 1999 had progressed to Version 3.5 with the addition of more terms in a number of the modules.

2. See "Transformation Coding," page 127.

years of hard work by many dedicated individuals and the investment of many resources — a herculean task.

Authors are Roger A. Côté, MD, FCAP, David J. Rothwell, MD, FCAP, James L. Palotay, DVM, Ronald S. Beckett, MD, FCAP, and Louise Brochu. The work is being carried out under an International Committee, which includes, in addition to the original authors from Canada and the United States, members from Brazil, China, Czechoslovakia, Denmark, Germany, Hungary, Italy, Japan, Mexico, and Switzerland. Translation is occurring into about a dozen languages. Publication is by the College of American Pathologists as a four-volume set of books (plus a loose-leaf volume for updates and errata). Volumes I and II are numeric, giving for each module the contents in numeric sequence. Volumes III and IV are alphabetic indexes to the numeric volumes, a separate index for each module. The four volumes total about 3,700 pages, 8.5 x 11 in size. An electronic form is also available. The electronic form also carries the codes from *SNOMED II*, where appropriate, permitting machine translation for those who previously used *SNOMED II*, as well as other information not in the printed version.

Structure

SNOMED International (3.5) is organized as a set of eleven modules, each of which is divided into Chapters or Sections. (The electronic version has 12 modules, the last being "Pharmaceutical and Manufacturing.") The Introduction to *SNOMED* lists the modules in the printed version, the number of terms in each, and the lengths of their "termcodes" as shown in the table below.

Note that an additional character is sometimes required for the suffix "V" to indicate that the term is a veterinary one. For example, the code D4-10740V is "splayleg in piglets." This is used, incidentally, in modules in addition to D (the diagnosis/disease module). The number of V codes in the D module alone is 3,409, which reduces the number of human disease codes available by that number.

Figure E.1 Structure of SNOMED III

Designator	Module	Description	Number of characters in Term Code[a]	Number of Records in 1993	Number of Records in 1999
T	Topography	A functional anatomy for human and veterinary medicine	5	12,385	13,165
M	Morphology	Terms used to name and describe structural changes in disease and abnormal development	5	4,991	5,898
F	Function	Terms used to describe the physiology and pathophysiology of disease processes	5	16,352	19,355
L	Living Organisms	Living organisms of etiological significance in human and animal disease	5	24,265	24,821
C	Chemicals, Drugs, and Biological Products	Including a separate module of Pharmaceutical Manufacturers	5	14,075	14,859
A	Physical Agents, Activities, and Forces	A compilation of physical agents and activities, physical hazards, and the forces of nature	5	1,355	1,601
J	Occupations	Developed by, and used in permission from, the International Labour Office in Geneva, Switzerland	5	1,886	1,949
S	Social Context	Social conditions and relationships of importance to medicine	5	433	1,070

Figure E.1 Structure of SNOMED III *(continued)*

Designator	Module	Description	Number of characters in Term Code[a]	Number of Records in 1993	Number of Records in 1999
D	Diseases/ Diagnoses	A classification of the recognized clinical conditions encountered in human and veterinary medicine	6	28,622	41,494
P	Procedures	A classification of healthcare procedures	6	25,000 (est)	30,796
G	General Linkage/ Modifiers	Linkages, descriptors, and qualifiers to link or modify terms from each module	4	1,176	1,594
			Totals	130,540	156,602

a. An additional character

SNOMED III shows its heritage from pathology in the maturity of its modules on Topography, Morphology, Etiology (now divided into "Living Organisms," "Chemicals, Drugs, and Biological Products," and "Physical Agents, Forces, Activities"), and Function.[3]

The Introduction ends with a final paragraph:

> *SNOMED III* is a detailed, finely grained, semantically typed, comprehensive, and computer-processible terminology used in both human and veterinary medicine. Terms are placed in a data structure in such a way that both simple and complex diagnostic entities and their manifestations can be represented. It will permit the composition of new terms from existing ones giving precise characterization to the new term.

---

3.   As the authors recognize, some of the modules, those with the oldest history, such as Topography, Morphology, Function, and Procedures are far more mature and complete than the newer modules, such as Occupation and Social Context, which must be considered rudimentary.

SNOMED III is a standardized vocabulary/data dictionary and data structure suitable for use in the computer-based patient record.

Modules

Each module is briefly described here, and some comments specific to the module are included.

Topography (T)

This module is one of the oldest in the system, having been used since the publication of the *Systematized Nomenclature of Pathology (SNOP)*. It has been somewhat reorganized from previous versions, and includes veterinary terms (with the suffix "v").

The first thirteen sections deal with body systems, integumentary, musculoskeletal, and so on. The fourteenth section covers topographic regions, such as head and neck. The fifteenth section is devoted to cellular and subcellular structures, and the last section covers products of conception and embryonic structures.

A possible cause of confusion, recognized by the authors, is that the Topography module

> ... retains specific termcodes for paired anatomic structures (e.g., both), for laterality (e.g., left and right) and combined codes (e.g., gastroduodenal). The terms "both," "left," and "right" also appear in the G - General Linkage/Modifier module of *SNOMED*, thus creating ambiguity, e.g., two possible representations for the same concept. We recognize this as a problem though not a major one. When this occurs, conventions can and should be established on how to index these terms, and for that matter all other terms, consistently.

Topography codes from the *International Classification of Diseases for Oncology (ICD-O)* are included in this module.

Morphology (M)

Morphology is also one of the original modules.[4] In its introduction, the increasing detail given with the successive characters in the termcodes, a convention used throughout *SNOMED III* is illustrated:

---

4. Morphology is the science of form and structure.

... the coded representation of terms carries within the code contextual information related to that term.

To illustrate this, consider the term fibrocystic disease and its coded representation in *SNOMED III* M-74320:

"M" tells the term is a descriptor of a morphologic entity;

"7" that the condition belongs to the family of conditions related to growth and maturation alterations;

"4" that the condition belongs to the family of terms related to dysplasia;

"3" that the condition belongs to the family of terms related to cystic diseases; and

"20" specifies the discrete term fibrocystic disease.

The Sections of the Morphology module are

1. General Morphologic Terms
2. Traumatic Abnormalities
3. Congenital Anomalies
4. Mechanical Abnormalities
5. Types of Inflammation
6. Degenerative Abnormalities
7. Cellular and Subcellular Abnormalities
8. Growth, Maturation, and Non-neoplastic Proliferations
9. International Classification of Neoplasms — This Section is, by agreement with the World Health Organization, an exact duplicate of the *International Classification of Diseases for Oncology (ICD-O)*, 1990. Cross references are given to the topographic terms in *SNOMED III*.
10. Specific Veterinary Tumors

A significant change from *SNOMED II* was the moving of terms which represented specific diseases from this module to the Diseases/Diagnoses (D) module.

In some instances, an M term carries a cross reference to topography.

This module also offers an optional fifth-digit behavior code for neoplasms, and an optional sixth-digit code for their histologic grading and differentiation.

Function (F)

This was the third of the original modules. It is a series of extensive sections with the following headings:

1. General Biological Functions, Patient States, and Nursing Diagnoses
2. Biological Functions and Units of the Musculoskeletal System
3. Respiratory System
4. Cardiovascular System
5. Integumentary System
6. Digestive System
7. Biological Functions and Units, and Phenomena of Metabolism and Nutrition
8. Functions and Disturbances of the Psyche and Sexual States
9. Biological Functions of the Nervous System
10. Hormones, Vitamins, and Receptor Sites
11. Biological Functions and Factors of the Immune System
12. Biological Functions and Functional Units of the Hematopoietic System
13. Genetic, Molecular, and Cellular Units and Functions
14. Biological Functions, Units, and Symptoms of the Special Senses

Note the inclusion in this module of nursing diagnoses.

The Function module is cross-referenced to the International Union of Biochemistry (IUB) codes for enzymes.

Living Organisms (L)

The Etiology module found in earlier versions of *SNOMED* has been split up into three modules in *SNOMED III*, this module, the "Chemicals... (C)" module, and the "Physical Agents...(P)" module. In this L module the organisms are classified "according to the Five Kingdom Classification of Living Things:

I   Monera: Bacteria, Actinomyces and Cyanobacteria (blue-green algae/bacteria), and viruses

II Fungi: Zygomycota, Dikaryomycota, and colorless algae; Prototheca

III Protists: Protozoans, brown, red, and green algae
IV Plantae: All plants
V Animalia: Coelenterates, worms, mollusks, insects, reptiles, birds, mammals

However, this classification is not apparent in the organization of the module's numeric volume which is divided into 14 sections, 0 through C, none of which bear headings which appear to relate to these five kingdoms. The alphabetic index to this module carefully includes both common names for organisms and their biological names, although they are found in separate sections with no indication that they are synonyms.

Living organisms of all kinds are found in this module, because any organism may, under certain circumstances, be either the victim or the aggressor. And in this chapter there is no distinction between human and veterinary, i.e., no "v" modifier, because of this fact.

Chemicals, Drugs, and Biological Products (C)

This is the second of the three new modules which, together, replace the former Etiology module. Its sections cover the following. (Clearly, restricting the number of groupings in this module to 16 reflects the restraint imposed by limiting the coding to the hexadecimal notation; see "Code Details," page 443.)

1.   General Convenience Codes

2.   Elements and Basic Chemical Compounds

3.   Industrial Products

4.   Plant and Animal Products

5.   Generic Drugs, Hormones, and Vitamins

6.   General Terms, Antihistamines, and Anti-infective Drugs

7.   Central Nervous System Agents

8.   Miscellaneous Drug Categories

9.   Cardiovascular, Gastrointestinal, and Respiratory System Drugs

10. Skin, Eye, Ear, Nose, and Throat Drugs

11. Hormones, Vitamin Preparations, and Blood-related Drugs

12. Diagnostic Aids, Serums, Toxoids, and Vaccines

13. Proprietary Drugs and Biologicals

14. Veterinary Proprietary Drugs and Biologicals (also have the "v" modifier)

15. Animal Disease Vaccines, Toxoids, and Diagnostic Products (also have the "v" modifier)

16. Foods and Diets

Physical Agents, Forces, and Activities (A)

This module, the third of the modules into which the former Etiology module was split, has 11 sections:

1. General Physical Agents, Robots, Prostheses, and Artificial Organs

2. Hospital Medical, and Surgical Equipment (2 sections)

3. Instruments of Aggression and Protective Devices

4. Household Appliances, Devices, and Tools

5. Transport Vehicles

6. Clothing Materials and Accessories

7. Physical Activities and Recreational Equipment

8. Physical Forces

9. Physical Hazards and Hazardous Situations

10. Physical Contacts and Exposures

The module is noted as modest in scope, that it will need to be expanded. For finer detail re medical devices, the authors suggest use of the *ECRI Universal Medical Devices Nomenclature System* (Plymouth Meeting, PA).

Occupations (J)

This module is derived, with permission, from that developed by the International Labour Office (ILO) in Geneva, Switzerland as the "International Standard Classification of Occupations." It carries, in the introduction, the statement:

> As with other *SNOMED* modules, other authority lists or job classifications can be substituted, modified, or appended to this classification as need arises.

This statement is surprising, in view of the efforts being made to have *SNOMED III* accepted as the authority for nomenclature in the computer-based patient record, where it is expected to be " ... a

standardized vocabulary/data dictionary and data structure ... "
Permission to substitute (and to truncate, or use much or little detail as
desired) would seem at cross purposes to the essential standardization if
medical and veterinary information are to be readily exchanged not only
within but among countries. The latter is clearly a goal; witness the
current efforts to translate *SNOMED III* " ... into multiple languages to
allow, for example, a coded patient summary in English to be transferred
to Japan and decoded in Japanese ... "

Social Context (S)

This module is described by the authors as "embryonic," containing, as it
does, only 433 terms. The statement is made that "Social context data is
no longer considered 'soft data.'" The terms are distributed into 6
Sections:

1. Social Context: General Conditions
2. Parental and Civil States
3. Social Problems Not Due to a Mental Disorder
4. Life Style
5. Religions and Philosophies
6. Economic Status

It is of interest that the module does not contain information about
education and literacy.

Diseases/Diagnoses (D)

This module is divided into 16 Chapters, each with a title beginning
"Diagnoses related to the ... "

1. Skin and subcutaneous tissues
2. Musculoskeletal system and connective tissues
3. Respiratory system
4. Cardiovascular system
5. Congenital diseases
6. Digestive system
7. Metabolic and nutritional disorders
8. Genitourinary systems
9. Pregnancy and the perinatal period

10. Mental disorders

11. Nervous system and special senses

12. Endocrine organs

13. Hematopoietic and immune systems

14. Injuries and poisonings

15. Infectious and parasitic diseases

16. General disorders, victim status, and death

Two significant changes from *SNOMED II* in this chapter are, first, that the diagnoses which were in the Morphology module were moved into this module.

The second major change, pointed out by the authors, was

> ... the incorporation of virtually all of the *[International Classification of Diseases, 9th Revision, Clinical Modification]* ICD-9-CM terms and codes; most[5] are found in the Diseases/Diagnoses module ...

The authors go on to assert: "It will be possible for users of *SNOMED III* to use this system as the primary tool for indexing their records and, at the same time, provide the necessary *ICD-9-CM* codes required for reporting."

Study of the D module shows that in the present generation of *SNOMED* this will not be possible. One will not be able to code to *SNOMED* and then let the computer allocate the terms to their *ICD-9-CM* rubrics. This would amount to using the D module as an alphabetic index to *ICD-9-CM*.[6] But even if one could use this module instead of *ICD-9-CM*'s own alphabetic index, the apparent attempt to attach an *ICD-9-CM* code to each term in the D module was unsuccessful. Even cursory inspection discovers instances where this did not occur. For example, "placenta previa" has code 641.1 in *ICD-9-CM*. In the D module "placentia

---

5. Some were placed in the Morphology module, others in Function. A further exception is that *SNOMED III* uses *ICD-O* for neoplasms rather than the neoplasm chapter of *ICD-9-CM*.

6. Elsewhere in this volume, coding with *ICD-9-CM* is considered in detail, and the dangers of coding directly from the Alphabetic Index is thoroughly discussed; see "How We Code Today: Category Coding," page 205.

previa" is given codes D4-F3060 through D4-F3063. The 641.1 *ICD-9-CM* code has not been attached to any of these entries.

A further problem is that the D module contains a great many terms which apparently are not found in *ICD-9-CM* . These are terms which will have to be dealt with by the coder or the computer system. But they have not been assigned to an *ICD-9-CM* rubric. For example, a count of the entries on pages 124 and 125 of *SNOMED III* show that, of a total of 81 separate (preferred) terms and their termcodes, only 9 have accompanying *ICD-9-CM* codes. The user would have to code the remaining 72 terms to *ICD-9-CM* in some other manner.

No mention is made for plans for a relationship of *SNOMED III* to *ICD-10*, which was published by the World Health Organization in 1992 as the successor to *ICD-9* for use in the international exchange of statistical information about health. *ICD-10* has significant changes over *ICD-9* in structure and in content as well. See the table on page 357.

Procedures (P)

This module " ... contains both generic and specific administrative, medical, surgical, and nursing procedures as well as those performed by paraprofessionals and other providers from the entire healthcare field." It is one of the most extensive of the modules, having approximately 27,000 terms, organized into 11 Chapters.

1. Administrative Procedures and Physician Services
2. Operations and Anesthesia Procedures
3. Medical Procedures and Services
4. Laboratory Procedures
5. Radiology, Radiotherapy, Nuclear Medicine, and Ultrasound Procedures
6. Physical Medicine and Physiotherapy Procedures and Services
7. Dental Procedures and Services
8. Psychologic and Psychiatric Procedures and Services
9. Nursing and Home Care Procedures

The largest Chapter is that covering operations, which are organized in the same manner as used in the Topography and Diseases/Diagnoses modules.

A significant change from *SNOMED II* is that the fifth digits in *SNOMED II* were used to tell the specific approach for selected procedures, e.g., transabdominal or transthoracic. In *SNOMED III* this information is to be carried by using the appropriate entry from the General Linkage/Modifiers (G) module.

Unlike other parts of *SNOMED III*, the Procedures module is not cross referenced to any other procedure coding system, such as the American Medical Association's *Current Procedural Terminology (CPT)*, which is widely used for billing.

General Linkage/Modifiers (G)

This module was introduced

> ... to support two vital functions that are necessary to access and fully utilize the information content provided by the *SNOMED III* data model.

> First it is necessary to link the detailed elements found in each of the other modules in a meaningful way that will accurately reflect the medical events they are intended to represent. Syntactic linkage terms as well as a more generalized set of linkage terms are needed to achieve this. In this edition, an embryonic set of these linkage terms is provided; with wider use and with a greater experience representing in detail the content of the medical record, this set of terms is expected to expand significantly. As the needs and pressure to codify natural language increases more attention will be directed to this task.

> The second vital function of this module is related to the need to modify or qualify the diagnostic entries found in each of the other modules ... "

There are seven groups of "modifier-qualifier" terms:

1. General adjectival modifiers; "these include virtually all of the modifiers found in the 5th digit tables of *SNOMED II* plus a small number of more general medically important adjectival modifiers;"

2. Topographic modifiers reflecting position and laterality of an organ, sign, or symptom.

3.   Types of diagnoses derived during the course of a medical work-up.

4.   Severity of diagnosis

5.   Certainty of diagnosis

6.   A formative list of the accepted clinical specialties, and

7.   Stages of disease.

The Introduction goes on to state

> With this new tool, new terms can be constructed and complex terms faithfully represented by the elements they contain. The terms present in each of the other modules contain the elements required of a medical knowledge system. The terms in the General Linkage/Modifier module will glue these informational units to one another in a coherent manner providing the basis of a knowledge representation system for medicine.

Pharmaceutical and Manufacturing

Such a module does not appear in the Table of Contents of *SNOMED III*, but there is a twelfth "module" described as part of the electronic version and given this heading. This would appear to be the last (unlisted) Section in the "Chemicals" (C) module. The final pages of the C module numeric listing contain the appropriate information prefixed by the letter "X," e.g., "X-10002, A. H. Robins, a pharmaceutical manufacturer." The final pages of the alphabetic index to the C module (unlabeled) index this information.

Code Details

Study of the volumes indicates that, while the number of characters in the termcodes is technically correct, the actual length which must be accommodated is somewhat larger, because of modifiers and other factors. In computer use, it is larger still, depending on the wishes of the user, who may want the computer record to carry added, related information. Four types of such information are "Class" (see below), *ICD-9-CM* codes, American Hospital Formulary Service (AHFS) codes, and MFG codes (manufacturers codes for proprietary drugs). The allowances for these supplementary codes are shown in the table below.[7]

---

7. This table was developed from the description of *SNOMED International, Electronic Version.*

Figure E.2　Structure of SNOMED Codes

Structure of SNOMED III

Module		Number of Characters							
Designator	Module Title	Chapters, Sections	Term-code	Modifier[a]	Class[b]	ICD-9-CM[c]	AHFS[d]	MFG[e]	Total Char.
T	Topography	16	8	5	2	15	–	–	30
M	Morphology	10	8	5	2	15	–	–	30
F	Function	16	8	5	2	15	–	–	30
L	Living Organisms	13	8	5	2	–	–	–	15
C	Chemicals, Drugs, & Biological Products	16	8	5	2	–	10	100	125
A	Physical Agents, Forces, & Activities	11	8	5	2	–	–	–	15
J	Occupations	12	8	5	2	–	–	–	15
S	Social Context	6	8	5	2	15	–	–	30
D	Diseases/Diagnoses	15	8	5	2	16	–	–	31
P	Procedures	11	8	5	2	–	–	–	15
G	General Modifiers	7	8	5	2	–	–	–	15

a　Modifiers, e.g., laterality, severity, certainty of diagnosis, states of disease.

b　Class, e.g., the "type of medical term" as used in English, e.g., "preferred term," "synonym."

c　Two ICD-9-CM codes are included, in two 8-character fields, "for the dagger asterisk format of ICD." Note that this format is not a part of ICD-9-CM.

d　American Hospital Formulary Service

e　Manufacturer's codes for proprietary drugs.

The first expansion over the number of characters given in Table 1, above, is that apparently the module designator, e.g., "T," followed by a hyphen "-," i.e., "T-," must prefix each code, thus adding a minimum of 2 characters. In some instances the module designator is two characters, e.g., in Diseases/Diagnoses and Procedures, and thus 3 characters would be required.

A suffix is also used on occasion. For example, when a term pertains solely to veterinary medicine, a modifier, the letter "v," is used as a suffix to the Termcode.

In the Topography module, an asterisk "*" follows some of the termcodes to indicate that a cross-reference to the *International Classification of Diseases for Oncology (ICD-O)* has been provided. (This may be solely for the information of the reader and not be expected to be used as a part of the Termcode.) For example, skin of the nipple is shown as "T-02431*" and the cross reference is to *ICD-O* topography code, C44.5 (skin of the trunk). There is a further cross referencing in the Topography section which also illustrates the possibility of coding a given topography in two ways within *SNOMED III* itself: skin of the nipple has a single code "T-02431" or "T-01000," skin NOS (not otherwise specified) plus "T-04100," nipple. Because of this alternate method of coding the same entity, for information retrieval the user would have to search both for cases with the code "T-02431" and for cases with "T-01000 and T-04100."

The numeric sections of the termcodes in *SNOMED II* were in duodecimal notation (0-9, X, Y), while in *SNOMED III* they are in hexadecimal notation (0-9, A-F). Duodecimal notation offers about 250,000 codes using 5-digits, while hexadecimal offers a little over 1,000,000, thus economizing in the number of characters required. As shown in Table 1, the largest number of "records" (terms) in any module at the present time is reported to be just under 29,000 in the Diseases/Diagnoses module.

"Using SNOMED"

There is apparently no agreement on what "using *SNOMED*" means.

It is clear that the goal of *SNOMED III* is that it be accepted as the authority for nomenclature in the computer-based patient record, where it is expected to be " ... a standardized vocabulary/data dictionary and data structure ... " The idea that medical and veterinary information can be readily exchanged not only within but among countries is demonstrated by the current efforts to translate *SNOMED III* " ... into multiple languages to allow, for example, a coded patient summary in English to be transferred to Japan and decoded in Japanese ... "

Standardization of Concepts

A current article about the computer-based patient record (CPR) expands on the first of twelve key attributes of the CPR as published by the Institute of Medicine (IOM), namely that it should have a Problem List and problem-orientation of the information.[8] The authors have prepared a list of the "gold standards" for the CPR,[9] and with regard to this attribute, one factor is that the CPR should "base [the] problem description on *SNOMED III*." Conversation with the authors indicated their position that standardized terminology is essential for the successful implementation of the CPR and their view that *SNOMED III* offers the most complete list of terminology available today. They are aware, however, that *SNOMED III* does not offer problem terminology, as the term "problem" is used in healthcare.[10]

Problems with SNOMED as a Standardized Language

There are several serious problems with adopting *SNOMED* as the source of the desired standardized language or vocabulary of medicine.

---

8. Andrew, William, and Richard Dick. "On the Road to the CPR: Where Are We Now?" *Healthcare Informatics* 13, no. 5 (1996): 48-62.

9. See page 62.

10. From *Slee's Health Care Terms, Third Comprehensive Edition*, "In health care, a problem is a disease, injury, or any other condition or situation which brings an individual into contact with the health care system. Certain conditions, such as alcoholism, are not admitted by all to be diseases, but they do bring individuals to health care, as do ill-defined symptoms, behavioral problems, the need for well-person examinations, and the like. This is the usage of the term "problem" in the problem-oriented medical record (POMR).

Standardization of Terms

A number of policies, instructions, and comments in *SNOMED III* actually work *against* standardization of terminology and coding. For example, here are some comments from *SNOMED III*:

- ... It will permit the composition of new terms from existing ones giving precise characterization to the new term. *SNOMED III* is a standardized vocabulary/data dictionary and data structure suitable for use in the computer-based patient record." [In this case, there seems to be an internal contradiction.]

- [The Topography module] retains specific termcodes for paired anatomic structures (e.g., both), for laterality (e.g., left and right) and combined codes (e.g., gastroduodenal). The terms "both," "left," and "right" also appear in the G - General Linkage/ Modifier module of *SNOMED*, thus creating ambiguity, e.g., two possible representations for the same concept. We recognize this as a problem though not a major one. When this occurs, conventions can and should be established on how to index these terms, and for that matter all other terms, consistently.

- As with other *SNOMED* modules, other authority lists or job classifications can be substituted, modified, or appended to this classification as need arises ...

The point is made that the structure of the termcodes permits the user to provide *as much detail as he wishes,* and the illustration is given that "T-60000 = digestive organ, T-61000 = salivary gland NOS, T-61100 = parotid gland, T-61130 = parotid duct." One might call this "pseudo truncation" of the Termcode, i.e., providing less than the detail which could be recorded, but filling out the remaining digits with "0..." The person retrieving the information could not tell whether the full detail had been available but the coder chose to record only the gross picture, or that only the information to the detail coded had, in fact, been available. Permission to substitute (and to truncate, or use much or little detail as desired) would seem at cross purposes to the essential standardization.

Complexity in Expression of Concepts

The introductory material to *SNOMED III* makes it clear that it is to be used to express medical concepts and that, to do so, the use of terms from several modules remains a principle. The following examples serve both to illustrate how the modules are linked to equate with a diagnosis, using tuberculosis as an example, and some of the changes between the two editions. The first is from taken from *SNOMED II*, where it is stated that " ... every disorder, without exception, should carry a *SNOMED* Topography code, e.g.,

> Disorder APPENDICITIS, Topographic Site APPENDIX
>
> Disorder FEVER, Topographic Site BODY AS A WHOLE.
>
> Disorder DEPRESSION, Topographic Site PSYCHE"

The expression of a concept by the use of terms from several modules is a key feature of *SNOMED*. The following examples serve both to illustrate how the modules are linked to equate with a diagnosis, using tuberculosis as an example, and some of the changes between the two editions. The first is from taken from *SNOMED II*:

> T-28000 (Lung)
>
> + M-44060 (Granuloma)
>
> + E-2001 (*M. Tuberculosis*)
>
> + F-03003 (Fever)
>
> = D-0188 (Tuberculosis)

Constructing the same illustration in *SNOMED III* the expression comes out as

> T-28000 (Lungs)
>
> + M-44060 (miliary granuloma)
>
> + L-21801 (Mycobacterium tuberculosis hominis)
>
> + F-03003 (Increased body temperature)
>
> = DE-14800 (Tuberculosis, NOS)

or, to indicate pulmonary tuberculosis, there are two options:

DE-14813 (tuberculosis of lung with cavitation) or
DE-14814 (tuberculosis of lung with involvement of bronchus).

At this point, *SNOMED III's* Introduction goes on to state

> *SNOMED III* expands on this model [that of *SNOMED II*] by providing additional modules and categories of even greater specificity. In the new "formulation"[11] a disease or diagnosis can be given specificity by linking some or all of the other modules and in turn linking these to the procedures that were used to establish that diagnosis.

> From this vantage point, any medical encounter can be viewed as:

> A PROCEDURE performed on a SITE makes known a RESULT-FINDING

> To illustrate this model consider the following activities:

> Auscultation (PROCEDURE) performed on arm (SITE) makes known a murmur (RESULT-FINDING)

> Electrophoresis (PROCEDURE) performed on serum (SITE) makes known a monoclonal protein associated with multiple myeloma (RESULT-FINDING)

> Virtually all of the information obtained from a medical encounter can be seen from this perspective. *SNOMED III* provides a comprehensive tabulation of procedures and anatomic site termcodes each in their separate modules, procedures, and topography. The result-finding terms are distributed across the remaining *SNOMED* modules, Morphology [M], Living Organisms [L], Chemicals-Drugs [C], Function [F], Disease [D], and Physical Agents [A]. Each of these can in turn be linked to one another

---

11. "Formulation" appears to be a new term which refers to a string of terms from various modules which (1) contain entries from the PROCEDURE and SITE modules, (2) plus appropriate entries from the MLCFD modules, which then (3) are followed by the appropriate term from the General Linkage/Modifiers (G) module which indicates the relationship in which the preceding string should be considered together as a single formulation. The "formulation" equation for linking terms requires that the module designators MLCFD must always be used, as well as a final entry from the "G" module. Since not every "formulation" would require contributions from every module, the total formulation could not be deciphered unless the termcodes used were always labeled with the module designators. A number of questions could be raised about the general applicability of this model.

using the General Linkage/Modifier module [G]. The *SNOMED III* model [formulation] becomes:

{ (P) performed at (T) makes known (MLCFD) } G[12]

This "expansion" should rather be called an alternative method of expressing a concept. The formulas for the "T+M+E+F=D" (or, as now stated, "T+M+[L,C, or A]+F=D") expression and the "P+T+(MLCFD)+G are obviously quite different.

Continuity of Meanings

The meanings of terms and their termcodes are not kept constant over time. It is essential that the meanings of codes can always be determined (see "Making Meaning Precise," page 318). This could be called the issue of "generations" or versions of the systems of terms and of their codes. Some illustrations above show how both terminology and coding have changed in *SNOMED* with succeeding generations.

In healthcare coding, the generation problem is a serious one. For example, in *ICD-8*,[13] code 386 is "otosclerosis," while in *ICD-9*, code 386 is "vertiginous syndromes and other disorders of the vestibular mechanism" (otosclerosis had migrated to code 387). Several of the commonly used systems delete codes from time to time. They also move the terms they represent from one place to another. *SNOMED II* had the appendix as code T-66000, while in *SNOMED III* it is T-59200 (there is no code T-66000 in *SNOMED III* and unless one had *SNOMED II* at hand, the code T-66000 would be a complete mystery). Unless one knows which generation of the classification is being used, and has access to the coding references, one cannot know the meaning of the code.

Another problem. The assumption is often made that a given generation of a code was used during the period it was supposed to be used, i.e.,

---

12. There would appear to be strings of modules which would not require the "P" entry. Should the physician be required to tell, for example, that he learned about the patient's dizzy spells by entering "P2-01000" (History taking, NOS) or something more specific, such as "P2-01020" (History taking, limited), or give more detail by using terms and termcodes which indicated that the information was elicited by a computer-administered questionnaire?

13. *ICD-8* is the Eighth Revision of the *International Classification* (WHO) and *ICD-9* is the Ninth Revision (the base volume from which *ICD-9-CM* was developed).

adopted on a specific date and abandoned on another specific date. This assumption is hazardous. As noted elsewhere, a major developed nation was using the 7th Revision of the *International Statistical Classification* when the rest of the world had, for a number of years, been using the 8th Revision. Inspection of the coded data had not yielded this information. In another instance, users of the coded data were unaware that a large insurance company had never expanded the data fields in its computer system (an expensive process) when the coding system for diagnoses was expanded from a 4-digit code to a 5-digit code. It had simply truncated the codes — it had discarded the information carried in the 5th digit.

The only ways to deal with this problem are either to adopt a policy that, once assigned, a code is unique and will never be reused, or to add to every code a "key," designating its generation or version, i.e., whether it came from *SNOMED I* or *SNOMED II* or *SNOMED III* (in the instance of *SNOMED* this would mean to every code in every module). The first alternative, "no code can ever be reused," is by far the preferred solution.

Data Validity

It is not possible to tell whether a given *SNOMED* code is a valid code or not. On the face of it, *SNOMED* presents 150,000 terms from an authoritative source. Actually, this number is the sum of the terms which are distributed over some eleven "modules," the most extensive of which, Diseases/Diagnoses, has roughly 41,000 terms (*ICD-9-CM* has over 100,000 "diagnostic entries" in its alphabetic index). Users of the nomenclature are expected to take terms from each appropriate module and link them together to express a medical concept. The formula, as given above, is given that, for each concept, the minimum requirement is to use one code from each of four kinds of modules, and the notation given is that these are additive, and in a sense they are: give the part of the body, the structural condition, the cause of that condition, and how it affects function, and one has a diagnosis, thus:

> 1 entry from Topography (T) (12,000 terms)
> + 1 entry from Morphology (M) (5,000 terms)
> + 1 entry "causes," i.e., from Living Organism (L) (24,000 terms) or Chemicals, Drugs, and Biological Products (CC) (14,000 terms) or one from Physical Agents (P) (1,400 terms)
> + 1 entry from Function (F) (16,000 terms).
> = 1 diagnosis (concept)

But in terms of number of possible concepts, the mathematics required is multiplication, not addition, so, using any topography, any morphology, any cause, and the smallest cause list, P, the number of possible diagnoses or concepts is almost infinite:

$$12,000 \times 5,000 \times 1,400 \times 16,000 = 1,344,000,000,000,000$$

Obviously, not every one of these combinations is medically possible, but unless someone compiles a list of what is possible in the real world of medicine, i.e., a list of valid or "legal" codes, it will be impossible to control the input to any system using these codes in order to insure that the input makes sense. Computer systems regularly provide validation rules for data elements, e.g., a numeric field is not permitted to receive alphabetic characters, a field for dollars and cents is not permitted to have more than two places to the right of the decimal point, or, more to this point, a numerical field for months cannot have a number higher than 12.

A little known factor in the swing from *SNDO* to *ICDA* in the 1950s was that virtually *any* combination of numbers of the correct length was, so far as the data processing world was concerned, a legal code in *SNDO*, yet it could easily be absolute clinical nonsense. And there was no way to devise any set of rules which could be applied to solve or avoid this problem. *ICDA*, on the other hand, had a finite, auditable, list of valid codes, and any invalid code could be blocked from use by programming of the computer. A quantum improvement in data quality was the immediate result of the switch.

Other Comments

Alternative Medicine

A search for alternative medicine ("unconventional therapies" or "complementary medicine") was fruitless, although such content might be expected. The National Institutes of Health in 1992 received a commissioned report of nearly 400 pages covering the modalities and the systems of practice. The American Medical Association in 1993 published its *Reader's Guide to Alternative Health Methods*. In 1993 the World Health Organization Regional Office for the Western Pacific published the second edition of *Standard Acupuncture Nomenclature*. A search was made in *SNOMED III* "acupuncture" and it could not be found under any obvious heading. Neither was "acupuncturist" a recognized occupation.

Caregiver

The previous illustration brings up the interesting absence from *SNOMED III* of a way to code the kind of caregiver (or source of the information). Occupation of the patient and social factors are taken into account. One would think that the credence given to a diagnosis, as well as the interpretation of the diagnosis, would differ depending on whether the information were furnished by a physician, a nurse, a non-medical coroner, the patient, or a shaman. Yet the only place that such information can be indicated is by use of the Occupations (J) module. This module contains

> The International Labour Office's list of occupations. Within the *SNOMED* structure, and in accordance with the *SNOMED* philosophy, this module is essential because so many diseases and accidents are directly and indirectly related to the working environment. The increasingly important role of preventative medicine, especially within the workplace, makes it mandatory to capture and link workplace exposures to disease processes.

A search there under "osteopath" gives only 3 entries: "osteopath," "osteopathic physician," and "osteopathy teacher." "Physician" yields only "physician (general practice)," "physician, public health," and "physician, specialised." "Nurse" fares better, with 18 terms developed by modifying the word "nurse," ranging from "nurse, anaesthetist" to "nurse, specialised." But there is neither an entry for "nurse practitioner" or "physician's assistant." "Veterinarian, general" and "veterinarian, public health" are given codes. There are six codes for "veterinary:" "veterinary bacteriologist" through "veterinary surgeon (general)." "Shaman" does not appear nor does "homeopathic physician."

Even in view of the stated purpose of having an occupation classification in the system, namely, the importance of the workplace in causing problems and as a venue for preventive efforts, one would expect caregivers, with their peculiar exposure to the ill and contagious, and to potentially hazardous diagnostic and treatment modalities, to be described and given categories in far greater detail.

Synonyms

In many portions of the system, preferred terms are given, accompanied by some of their alternates or synonyms. It should be recognized that retrieval, decoding, will bring back the preferred term only. As noted below under Indexing, synonyms should be included freely for the convenience of the coder.

Classes

It will be noted that Table 2 has a column entitled "Class." The instructions state that this indicates the "type of medical term" and that it *can be used* with terms in all the modules. The meanings are given:

01 = a primary or preferred term

02 = a synonym of the primary term

03 = a term with a more specific characteristic of the primary term

05 = the adjectival form of the term, e.g., hepatic for liver. This allows for the use of automated language analysis.

New Terms

The system is designed so that the user can create new terms and complex terms, and the General Linkage/Modifier module is stated as the tool for this purpose. Presumably, this means that "unforeseen" combinations of modules are encouraged, but not the invention of new (primary) terms and termcodes themselves. It is stated in the General Instructions to the electronic version that,

> New entries to *SNOMED III* (classifications of "01") must be submitted to the *SNOMED III* Editorial Office for review and Termcode allocation. The new terms may be added temporarily to your *SNOMED* data files by including a Termcode with a "Y" as the leading character of the term number. For example to add a new Topography term to your Topography module, add a new entry coded as "T-Y0001." Include the term and any applicable references, ICD codes, etc.

A "User Response and Request for Modification" form is provided for this purpose.

No information is given as to the speed with which the Editorial Office will respond to requests that terms be added and given termcodes so that future coding and retrieving will not have to consult the "wastebasket" "Y" to insure completeness. Nor is it clear how such new terms and termcodes will be communicated to other users of the system.

New terms and alternative terms must be dealt with and given codes (though not necessarily placed in categories) as quickly as a new telephone subscriber can be given a telephone number. Classification, i.e., placing an entity within a category of one or more classifications, is an entirely different matter, one which often takes study, and which rarely is a matter requiring instant solution.

Cross Reference

This term is used frequently throughout *SNOMED III.* but its meaning is not clear. In some instances, as in the Diseases/Diagnoses module, a code of a specific appearance (nnn.n or nnn.nn) to the right of the term means the corresponding code from *ICD-9-CM.* Elsewhere the meaning is not as clear. It may mean that an alternative expression for the diagnosis is the use together of termcodes from two or more modules in a concatenated string. It would be useful for the authors to provide a definition of "cross reference," and then to make the use of the term consistent throughout the various modules.

Alphabetic Indexes

The alphabetic indexes found in Volumes III and IV are organized like the "yellow pages," like the classified section of a telephone book. Corresponding to the headings in the yellow pages, each module's index has alphabetic headings *in the order and with labels determined by the author.*

The alphabetic index (called the alphabetic concordance) to the Procedures (P) module illustrates this factor. It is organized under 11 major headings. The introduction to the module's index lists these headings alphabetically:

> Administrative Procedures (P0)
>
> Anesthesia Procedures (P1)
>
> Dental Procedures (P8)
>
> Laboratory Procedures (P3)
>
> Medical Procedures (P2)
>
> Nursing Procedures (PA)
>
> ... and so on

and the alphabetic indexes for each of these follow in the same sequence in the body of the index.

Within Medical Procedures (P2), for example, the list of major headings reads

> Acetowhitening
>
> Actinotherapy
>
> Activation
>
> Acuity
>
> Adaptation
>
> Administration [of various agents]
>
> Aerosol
>
> Aerosol-Induced
>
> Affinity
>
> Agent
>
> Aid
>
> ... and so on

Within "Activation" there are five entries (with their codes, e.g., "P2-91190"):

> Electroencephalogram with pharmacological activation, only
>
> Electroencephalogram with physical activation, only
>
> Pharmacological activation during prolonged monitoring
>   for localization of cerebral seizure focus
>
> Wada activation test for hemispheric function including
>   electroencephalographic EEG monitoring
>
> Wada activation test with EEG monitoring

The only way that a user can find these entries is to know that they will be thought of as medical procedures (heading in the yellow pages), and that the key word (subheading in the yellow pages) is "activation."

It seemed likely that chiropractic procedures would be found in this section, Medical Procedures P2. The search was fruitless. They appeared under P7- Physical Medicine Procedures, under at least two subheadings:

"Adjustment," where a number of "chiropractic adjustments of [site]" are given separate codes, and under "Chiropractic," where other adjustments by site are given codes, as are modalities, such as [chiropractic use of] diathermy and [chiropractic use of] ultrasound. Osteopathy could be found in the same section, P7, under the major heading "Osteopathic," where the terms relate to manipulations of various types. It may, of course, appear elsewhere.

A consolidated fully alphabetical index would appear to be absolutely essential for the successful use of *SNOMED III*. The single index should contain synonyms to the extent that they can be identified.

Searches

The excerpt from the Introduction, above, states that the "result-findings" which are produced by a formulation are distributed across the other six modules as appropriate. This means that the user of the alphabetic index would have to search all six of the module indexes; there is no composite alphabetic index.

The problem of locating the appropriate term and term code with the multiple, module, alphabetic indexes can be illustrated by a search for how to code "positive Babinski reflex." In *Stedman's Medical Dictionary*, this is synonymous with "positive Babinski sign." "Babinski" is not found under reflexes (or "tests," where one might also look) but it is found under "sign" with the Termcode "F-A1890." To indicate the result, a "G" code must be added: "G-A200" for positive, "G-A201" for negative.

Multiple Diagnoses

As discussed elsewhere, the actual unit of information carried in the healthcare data systems is the patient (or the patient's illness or encounter with the system). Patients have more than one diagnosis; in fact, it is the rare patient who has only one diagnosis. In the absence of a document explaining optimal use of the *SNOMED III* system in the computer-based medical record, for example, several questions arise:

- How many diagnoses would one allow (could one afford to allow) for in a given clinical record?

- How many characters should be allowed for a fully-coded "formulation?" Or for another type of string (as yet unlabeled) which is not a formulation because it does not include the Procedure module.

- How can one eliminate the redundancy which would occur when a patient had, for example, two or more diagnoses involving the same information from several modules? If the entire string of modules is needed for stating each diagnosis, the time consumed in coding the same information repeated in every string, the space required for carrying the redundant information, and the problems of framing inquiries of the data, are serious considerations.

User's Manual

It is surprising that no users' manual is available, as are such manuals for *ICD-9-CM*. An inquiry to the Education office of the College of American Pathologists resulted in the reply to the request for such a manual that the inquirer could be put in touch with users of the system.

Development of a manual for users (both coders and users of the coded material) is an urgent matter.

The College of American Pathologists maintains a World Wide Web site for *SNOMED* at http://www.snomed.org.

F

NHS Codes (Read Codes)

IN 1982, a physician named James Read, then a full time General Practitioner, "developed a simple set of mnemonic codes for his first practice computer to record those conditions which presented commonly in his practice. Over the next few years, the number of codes and the sophistication of the file structure increased to produce one of the leading coding systems for the recording of clinical care." This was the Read Clinical Classification System, most often called simply the "Read Codes."[1]

In 1987, the Joint Computing Group of the Royal College of General Practitioners and the General Medical Services Committee of the British Medical Association established a Technical Working Party to consider clinical classification systems for use in General Practice and to make recommendations to their parent bodies. The 1988 report from that group, entitled "The Classification of General Practice Data," recommended that the Read Codes be adopted for the recording of medical data in general practice, and that the United Kingdom (UK) National Health Service (NHS) should consider the application of the Read Codes in other sectors of the NHS.

In response to this recommendation, the UK Secretary of State for Health acquired the system in 1990, and the Read Codes became Crown Copyright. They are now the recommended standard in UK General Practice, and the name has been changed to the "NHS Codes."[2]

In the same year, the government established the NHS Centre for Coding and Classification (NHS CCC) in Loughborough, Leicestershire, as a

---

1. NHS Centre for Coding and Classification, *General Information,* Loughborough, England, 1994.

2. We'll continue to use "Read Codes" throughout this section, however, because it is about the development of the system, and most references are to Read Codes rather than the more recent NHS Codes.

part of the Information Management Group of the NHS Executive. Doctor Read became its Director. NHS CCC is charged with maintaining and further developing the Read Codes as "the standard coded thesaurus of clinical terms for the NHS." Funding is from the Department of Health.

In support of the CCC are representatives of the main bodies of the medical profession in the UK, the Office of Population Censuses and Surveys, the NHS Executive, the British National Formulary, and others.

Over 50 medical and paramedical groups and specialty bodies are working with NHS CCC on projects to make sure that clinicians, the primary users of the Read Codes (now NHS Codes), have their needs met. Ambitious "Clinical Terms Projects" have worked with clinical (medical) terms, and those of nursing, midwifery, visiting health, and other professions allied to medicine. A drug dictionary is also part of the system. Further detail on the scope of the system is found below. The Read Codes are to be distributed solely by Computer Aided Medical Systems Limited (CAMS). CAMS role is to support users and potential users of the NHS Codes within the NHS and also software developers who wish to use the NHS Codes. CAMS supplies demonstration software on request both within the UK and outside, conducts training programs, and consults with users and vendors.

The initial description of the Read Codes, taken from the CAMS literature, is:

> The Read Codes are a comprehensive, hierarchically arranged, thesaurus of terms used in healthcare. This has been coded, organised in file structures suitable for use in computers, cross-referenced to important national and international classifications, and is dynamic.

Effective with Version 3 of the codes, which is now in place, the codes themselves no longer carry hierarchical meanings, because the developers found it prudent to adopt a strategy which did not confine a term, such as a given diagnosis, to a single hierarchy. Although the clinical concepts and their terms are kept hierarchically, the codes are now described as purely labels for the concepts. Each code, now a 5-byte code,[3] is simply a

---

3.   The code uses both upper and lower case letters and also numerals, and thus describing it as 5-byte code is more appropriate than simply calling it a 5-character alphanumeric code. Earlier versions used a 4-byte code.

label for the preferred term for the concept expressed, and it is constructed in such a manner that its meaning cannot be decoded from the code itself; it must be looked up in a table. With this change in strategy, "pulmonary tuberculosis," for example, can now be both a "pulmonary disorder" and an "infective disorder." The codes never change (when a term goes into disuse it is labeled "obsolete," but it will always remain retrievable with no change in its meaning).

Contents of the Read Codes

A more recent description helps in understanding the scope of the Read Codes coverage of healthcare terms:

> The Read Codes cover all aspects of healthcare — all concepts that may be written in the record of any healthcare provider. Thus the Read Codes may be looked on as a dictionary of healthcare terms. Each concept identified has a preferred term, and may have any number of synonymous or eponymous terms and abbreviations.

In 1993, the main chapters of the Read Codes were listed as:

Diagnosis
Clinical, social, and family history
Symptomatology
Examination and signs
Bedside diagnostic procedures
Laboratory procedures
Radiological procedures
Prospective care
Operative and non-operative procedures
Drugs and appliances
Administration

In Version 3, the list is longer, some of the contents have been placed in different chapters, and new chapters have been added, so that the list of chapters now appears as:

Occupations
History and observations
Disorders
Investigations

Operations and procedures
Regimes and therapies
Prevention
Causes of injury and poisoning
Tumour morphology
Staging and scales
Administration
Drug
Appliance and equipment
Unit
Organisms
Anatomical site
Additional values
Attribute
Context dependent categories
Read thesaurus concept type

A further change in Version 3 is that certain terms which were classification terms, i.e., simply pigeonholes from classifications, were made obsolete. These were terms like "other specified" and "not elsewhere classified." Such pigeonholes are mandatory in a classification, which must have a place to fit everything in the universe being classified.

Version 3 responded to the need for extra detail by offering "qualifiers," i.e., Read Codes which can be linked by the computer to the main terms. Qualifiers have both attributes and values. An example given in the descriptive material is that "fixation of fracture" can be qualified by addition of a code giving the *attribute* (here the "site") and its *value*, e.g., "femur." This can be made more specific by a secondary value, i.e., a value may modify another value, e.g., "right" could modify "femur."

The coverage of terms in all aspects of healthcare is very broad, and broadening daily, in compliance with the stated objective, above, namely that the codes will encompass "all concepts that may be written in the record of any healthcare provider." Some examples:

- "Occupations" contains a growing list of job titles.

- "History and observations" includes terms recorded from taking the patient's history, examinations, assessments, and special investigations and tests. Not only are symptoms included, but such observations as "lives alone, with help available," and physical findings such as "fast heart rate" (tachycardia). Diagnoses that are made or suspected are found in the chapter on "Disorders."

- "Disorders," includes diseases, abnormalities, injuries, and other terms which have been labeled after study. There are terms, however, which might equally well have been placed in the History chapter and, in fact, some such terms are found both places in this generation of the Codes.

- "Investigations" provides for laboratory and special investigations that are performed; the results of these tests are the property of the "History and observations" chapter. An example is electrocardiography.

- "Operations and procedures" are physical acts performed on the patient for therapeutic or diagnostic purposes. Examples are "venipuncture" and "appendectomy."

- "Regimes and therapies" are non-surgical treatments and managements. Examples given are "alkaline diuresis" and "psychotherapy."

- "Prevention" deals with contraception, obstetric care, infectious disease control, and childhood examinations. Included are, for example, vaccinations and "home delivery booked."

- "Causes of injury and poisoning" reflects the corresponding chapter in *ICD-10*. The *ICD-9* "E codes" are also present, but marked as obsolete. The codes in this chapter are, of course, in the Read Code 5-byte format, but they are prefixed by an [X] to indicate that they are cross-mappable to *ICD-10*.

- "Tumour morphology" is designed to be "fully compatible with *ICD-O, ICD-9, ICD-10, SNOMED II* and *SNOMED III (SNOMED International.)*"

- "Staging and scales" is described as pertaining to a variety of tumor staging systems, and the terms are to be used as qualifiers for other tumor diagnostic terms.

- "Administration" at present has terms primarily used in general practice, such as "patient temporarily left," "offered child surveillance," and "[Form No.] signed."

- "Context of care" terms are those such as "complaining of," "offered," "action status," "ordered," and "done." Such contextual terms were formerly "embedded" with or in other terms, such as "blood test done." The earlier "combined" terms are being marked "obsolete" but are not being deleted.

- "Attributes" are terms which describe certain relationships, such as "causative agent," "direction," and "onset."

- "Values" are terms that are used in conjunction with "attributes." They are distributed into the several chapters listed below.

- "Drug" terms are all the drugs that the NHS permits to be prescribed within Primary Care, as well as other groups such as special foods and special cosmetics. There are modifiers for drugs which describe the form of the drug, dosage, and so on. In addition, the user can find both generic and brand name suppliers of the product, the packaging, and the pricing.

- "Appliances and equipment" originally contained all the "prescribable products in the Drug Tariff for England and Wales." It has been expanded to include other products used in hospitals, such as specific bandages.

- "Units" includes SI (Systeme Internationale) units and others.

- "Organisms" lists plants, animals, insects, and microorganisms "considered to be of significance to humans."

- "Anatomical sites" covers both regional and systemic anatomy.

- "Additional values" is a chapter which contains those values not fitting into the categories above.

"Read thesaurus concept type" is a label attached to every Read Code. Examples are "procedure type" and "prevention type." The list of types is being expanded.

Codes, Terming, and Encoding

The organizations responsible for implementing the Read Codes, the NHS Centre for Coding and Classification and Computer Aided Medical Systems Limited (CAMS), are dedicated to the development of a system which can and will be used routinely in the daily encounters with patients. Therefore,

> New codes and synonyms are added to each release [of the Read Codes] as a result of new work done in collaboration with the relevant national bodies or as a result of direct feed-back from users through a well established mechanism. In addition users can allocate codes that are required immediately to holding areas within the structure of the Read Codes pending incorporation into the main body with the next release.[4]

> This dynamic quality is essential if healthcare providers are to use computerised patient record systems as medicine is continually changing. New concepts and procedures evolve as do new drugs and therapeutic agents. If clinicians cannot find the terms they require represented in the language they use, they will not take advantage of these systems and all the potential benefits they bring to healthcare.

> ... Clinicians can use their own terminology to record health information, encouraging the use of clinical systems and the realisation of the benefits that these would bring.

Reflecting this philosophy, the Read Codes have adopted a new description of the process used for getting information from natural language into computer codes. The professional caregiver is expected to "record the details of clinical care" in a process called "terming." Someone else or a computer does the "encoding."

Technical Notes

The Codes

As noted above, the Read Codes are in hierarchies, first with 4 bytes, and later with 5 bytes. An example of the five levels of detail is shown in the table below.

---

4. Releases are on a quarterly schedule, except for the drug codes, which are released monthly.

Figure F.1 The Read Code Hierarchy

Level	Read Code Terms	Read Code
1	Circulatory system diseases	G . . . .
2	Ischaemic heart disease	G3 . . .
3	Acute myocardial infarction	G30 . .
4	Acute anterior myocardial infarction	G301 .
5	Acute anteroseptal myocardial infarction	G3011

The alphanumeric characters used are 0-9, A-Z, and a-z. The letters "l" and "o" and "I" and "O" are excluded to avoid misinterpretation. There are 58 options at each junction in each level of the hierarchy, which makes 656,356,768 possible codes (58 to the power of 5) in the existing framework.

Synonymous terms — including eponyms and abbreviations — have their own two character alphanumeric code. Thus each synonym is represented unambiguously by the five byte code of its preferred term and by its own two character code.

Each 5-byte code has its term "with a 30 character description with additional 60 and 198 character descriptions if required to avoid abbreviations. Additional fields are linked to each Read Code to hold mappings to other classifications and flags for a number of specialty groups to use to identify sets of codes especially useful to them and agreed by them. There are also fields to hold information about the status of each preferred term, e.g., if it is current or withdrawn or deprecated."[5]

The Database

CAMS supplies only a relational database which contains the terms, the concepts, descriptions, hierarchies, keys, specialty files, and cross-reference files. System developers incorporate this database into their applications with advice and consultation from CAMS as desired. These applications developed by suppliers will provide indexing of the files, for

---

5.   Discouraged from further use.

example, in accordance with their system designs. The database is updated quarterly (drugs monthly).

The database structure of Version 3 is described as a fully normalized relational database.[6] The change from the hierarchical structure can be illustrated by the example of a condition such as Paget's disease of the fibula. In Version 2, it was "Paget's disease — fibula." In Version 3, it is "Paget's disease of bone," with qualifiers added to give the site, "fibula." Laterality, e.g., "right," can easily be added with a second qualifier.

The relational database design makes it necessary to carry, in this illustration, only one anatomical table with all the bones listed. The site (specific bone) can be applied to any disease code where it would be relevant. Similarly the laterality codes (right, left, both) would be in only one table; they can be applied to any code to which laterality could pertain; they would be available to specify which kidney, for example. In the hierarchical database, every site to which laterality pertains would have to have three complete entries, one for right, one for left, and one for both. Thus for, say, 100 bones, under a hierarchical scheme there would have to be 300 "combined site-laterality" codes, while with the relational approach there would be 103 codes, 100 for site, 3 for laterality. The economy in data storage and the flexibility provided are very significant.

Implementation

Implementation, that is, using the Read Codes in electronic medical records (EMR) and computerized information systems, is in the hands of software developers, primarily commercial enterprises. The NHS CCC and CAMS provide a "secretariat" for the maintenance and enhancement of the code system itself and an organization for distributing the codes and consulting and training in their use in information systems and the training of developers and users.

CAMS advises that:

> Users should be able to access Read Code terms from natural language using the keys provided and also from the Read Code directly if it is known. Once a term has been selected different levels of the hierarchy

---

6.   See "Database 101," page 172.

either above or below the selected term should be able to be accessed directly by one key depression.

The Read Codes are a "quasi-closed" system. At any given time they are fixed by and are periodically and formally updated by a publicly known system. The whole Read Codes are released quarterly but the drug chapters are released monthly. Each release is date stamped to maintain an historic reference and audit trail.

Mapping

For many purposes, raw data need to be placed in the pigeonholes of a classification. And the same raw data must, for different purposes, be placed in the pigeonholes of different classifications. In the Read Clinical Classification this is called "mapping" the codes to different classifications. "Mapping tables" are supplied in Version 3 for placing the codes into the pigeonholes of the three classifications which are required in the UK for reporting:

- *International Classification of Diseases, 9th Revision, Clinical Modification (ICD-9-CM)*

- *International Statistical Classification of Diseases and Health Related Problems, Tenth Revision, (ICD-10)*

- *Office of Population Censuses and Surveys Classification of Surgical Operations and Procedures, Fourth Revision (OPCS-4)*

Local changes in these three mapping tables provided by the system are forbidden in order to insure standardized data.

The designers have also made sure that "the Read Codes are at least as detailed as, mapped to, and compatible with most widely used standard statistical national and international classifications ... " In addition to the three classifications for which mapping tables have been created, this compatibility extends also to *RCGP 1986 (The Classification and Analysis of General Practice Data)*,[7] *ICPC (International Classification of Primary Care)*,[8] *BNF (British National Formulary)*,[9] and the *ATC*

---

7.   2nd Edition, Royal College of General Practitioners, 1986.

8.   ICPC Working Party, World Organization of National Colleges, Academies, and Academic Associations of General Practitioners/Family Physicians, 1987.

9.   British Medical Association and The Pharmaceutical Society of Great Britain.

(*Anatomic Therapeutic Chemical (ATC) Classification Index*) [10] drug classification.

There is no limit to the number of such classification maps that could be developed for special purposes. Those classifications provided by the system are there because of the requirement that the cases be reported in one or more of them. Specialty bodies have begun developing classifications for their own use and the mapping from Read Codes to them is under way.

In the case of diagnosis coding, whether a given code is to be mapped into a pigeonhole of *ICD-9-CM* or *ICD-10* is determined by the coder, who makes a single selection directing the computer which mapping table to use. The maps have been already created; the process of coding directly from terms to categories (category coding, as used in the United States) has been replaced by the two-step process. The computer helps code the term; the computer then is invoked to find the correct pigeonhole into which to place the term code.

Comments

The Read Codes are transformation codes of the "preferred term"[11] variety. Synonyms go in and the preferred terms for the concepts, as they are defined in the Read Clinical Classification System, come out. There is a recognized benefit in having each concept stated in only one way.

✓ The Read Codes do not provide entity coding. Entity coding could readily be introduced as an earlier step in the coding process and the entity codes could be retained. This would preserve the original language in machine-accessible form. Then the entity codes could be mapped to the concept codes exactly as the concept codes are mapped to the various classifications.

The system handles the allocation of data to a variety of "required" classifications by providing mapping tables which place the Read Codes in the categories where they belong for each of the classifications. At

---

10. WHO Collaborating Centre for Drug Statistics Methodology, January 1992.

11. See "Preferred Terms," page 88.

present these classifications are *ICD-9-CM*, *ICD-10*, and *OPCS-4*. Classifications for other purposes can be developed at any time. This approach is more advanced than the category coding system used in the United States; it provides the flexibility to cope with classification changes and with other classifications without having to make coding changes.

It should be noted, however, that classifying a case to *ICD-9-CM*, for example, is not simply a matter of putting a diagnosis code into a category. For most of the categories, more must be known than just the diagnosis itself. The category may call for the patient's age, concomitant diagnoses, and may include special instructions to take into account other attributes of the case. Hence a simple mapping table, diagnosis to category, often will not achieve a correct assignment.

The Read Clinical Classification System is broader than other systems in that it covers a much greater portion of the information in clinical records than other systems. It translates such information as occupations, details of history, clinical observations, details of investigation, therapeutic regimes, administrative data, appliances, and equipment information into Read Codes.

As stated, the Read Codes are codes of concepts. It is not clear what provision has been made to accommodate changes in the definitions of concepts insofar as synonyms do often have subtle differences in meaning. Such changes in concept definitions are bound to occur, and it would be useful to be able to map synonyms and "arrays" of entities to various definitions of concepts, a facility which entity coding would provide.

CAMS

Computer Aided Medical Systems Limited (CAMS) has two primary roles in the Read Codes project:

1. to distribute the codes, and

2. to provide support to users and developers

It reports its activities as falling under the following headings: Basic Awareness, Pre-Implementation Advice, Training and Support, Quality Assurance and Monitoring, Development of Operational Requirements, Advanced Training — Clinical Management Audit, Functionality Compliance Reports, Development of Information Technology Strategy, and Maintenance of Skills. It provides consultance services and training, both on-site and off-site.

CAMS will supply demonstration materials and information in response to overseas as well as national inquiries. The current demonstrator of Version 3 is available on CD-ROM as a Windows application. For further information, contact:

Computer Aided Medical Systems Limited
Tannery Buildings
58-60 Woodgate
Loughborough
Leicestershire
LE11 2TQ
ENGLAND

Telephone: 01509 611006 FAX -1509 235560

e-mail: support@cams.co.uk

URL: http://www.cams.co.uk

G

International Classification of Primary Care

THE *International Classification of Primary Care (ICPC)* is the product of a working group of WONCA, the World Organization of National Colleges, Academies, and Academic Associations of General Practitioners/Family Physicians. In 1978, the World Health Organization (WHO) appointed a special group, the WHO Working Party for Development of an International Classification of Primary Care which collaborated with the WONCA working group. *ICPC* is the latest in a series of volumes:

- The first appeared in 1975 with the publication of ICHPPC: *International Classification of Health Problems in Primary Care.* Two refinements of this publication, *ICHPPC-2* and *ICHPPC-2-Defined* followed in 1979 and 1983.

- *IC-Process-PC: International Classification of Process in Primary Care,* 1986.

- *ICPC: International Classification of Primary Care,* 1987.

- A second edition of *ICPC, ICPC-2,* under the authorship of the WONCA International Classification Committee, was published in 1998. The prime motivations for the new edition were to relate it to *ICD-10,* which had been published since *ICPC* appeared in 1987, and to add inclusion and exclusion notes and additional cross-referencing.

The International Classification of Primary Care in the European Community, with a Multi-Language Layer, was published in 1993. The languages covered are English, Danish, Dutch, French, German, Italian, Portuguese, and Spanish, and mapping to *ICD-10* was also provided. A "companion" classification called the *ICPC Classification of Drugs* has been developed for European use by De Maeseneer to learn how current drugs are prescribed as related to the problems presented in general practice and the diagnoses established.

The goal of the working group was to develop a classification of an encounter with a caregiver, using, to the extent possible, the framework of the problem-oriented concept, SOAP:[1]

S	Subjective	The condition as experienced by the patient; the patient's reason for the encounter (RFE)
O	Objective	The findings of the caregiver (these are not covered in *ICPC*)
A	Assessment	The interpretation of the caregiver; the provider's assessment/diagnosis of the patient's health problems.
P	Plan	The plan for going forward; the diagnostic and therapeutic interventions undertaken in the process of care.

The WONCA group approached the classification issue from the point of view of the medical educator and the desire to have a realistic picture of the clinical, social, and other problems for which the primary care physician should be prepared. It was clear that

- The primary caregiver sees the widest spectrum of problems of any class of caregivers.

- The frequency distribution of the problems presented in primary care is quite different from that seen by specialist caregivers, or that found in the usual morbidity and mortality statistics.

- There was no source of information on these matters, and the desire to find out about them is strongly reflected in the *ICPC*" Series" of publications.

In some of the research in which *ICPC* has been used, the data system has carried information linking the encounters in series for each episode, and also informing the user of other episodes (often chronic conditions) occurring simultaneously. Chapter 7 of *ICPC* is entitled "Standardized data set for use with ICPC." It suggests (and provides codes for) data about the patient (age and sex), the provider type, and the encounter.

---

1.   Weed, L. L. *Medical Records, Medical Education, and Patient Care*, Year Book Medical Publishers, Chicago, 1969.

Such data management is essential if the potential of medical records for epidemiological study adding to the resources for evidence-based medicine is to be exploited.

The authors of *ICPC* point out that its use "allows four important issues of health services research to be addressed":

- The analysis of complete episodes

- A comprehensive epidemiological approach

- An optimal health statistical orientation

- The characterization of the different forms of professional behavior and clinical judgment by physicians.

The authors have also been careful to achieve optimal coordination with the International Classifications, *ICD-9* and *ICD-10*, and with other classifications, and a table showing the relationships is provided.

The authors point out that complete use of *ICPC* would use it in three modes:

- The RFE mode (reason for encounter), mentioned above, in which the reason for encounter is classified. There is no mention of a need to expand this list to accommodate more detail, although, as with other modes, extensions after a decimal point could be used locally.

- The Diagnostic mode, in which the caregiver classifies the assessment made. The basic ICPC classification for diagnoses is coded to a three-character rubric. It is suggested that additional detail may be desired, and that one or two digits may be added after a decimal point for local use.

- The Process mode, in which the care given is classified. Note that this mode does not record the results of treatments or care. Use of *IC-Process-PC* in conjunction with *ICPC* for recording process provides more detail in a standard form by the addition of one or two digits, taken from *IC-Process-PC* following a decimal point.

ICPC contains both a Tabular List and an Alphabetic Index, as well as instructional material on its use, advice on how to train users, and a glossary.

The Classification

ICPC is biaxial in construction, with one axis of Chapters which primarily represent bodily systems. Each Chapter has an alphabetic code. The other axis is of Components relating to the Chapter content, each Component with a 2-digit numeric code.

The seventeen Chapters are:

A	General
B	Blood, blood forming
C	Digestive
F	Eye
H	Ear
K	Circulatory
L	Musculoskeletal
N	Neurological
P	Psychological
R	Respiratory
S	Skin
T	Metabolic, endocrine, nutritional
U	Urinary
W	Pregnancy, childbearing, family planning
X	Female genital
Y	Male genital
Z	Social

The Components are:

1. Symptoms and complaints, unique to each Chapter, e.g., "pain attributed to heart" (Circulatory Chapter); "insect bite" (Skin Chapter); "problems: food and water" (Social Problems Chapter).

2. Diagnostic, screening prevention, e.g., medical examination, blood test, preventive immunizations.

3. Treatment procedures, medication, e.g., prescription, excision, local injection, listening.

4. Test results, e.g., results of procedure, letter from other provider.

5. Administrative procedure, e.g., provision of certificate.

6. Referrals and other reasons for encounter, e.g., follow-up encounter, referral

7. Diagnoses, diseases, unique to each Chapter, e.g., "urinary calculus all types/sites" (Urology Chapter); "dislocations" (Musculoskeletal Chapter); "toxic effect of other substances" (General and unspecified Chapter).

As any classification should, provision is always made for "other," i.e., items of information which do not fit into any existing category of a Chapter or Component.

Thus, the matrix of Chapters and Components has 119 cells. Components 2 through 6 are the "Standard Process Components." These are:

2   Diagnostic, screening, prevention

3   Treatment procedures, medication

4   Test results

5   Administrative procedure

6   Referrals and other reasons for encounter

The numbers of standard components for each section are shown in the table below.

Figure G.1 ICPC Structure

Count of Categories in Each ICPC Chapter, by Component

No.	Prefix	Title	Standard Process Components, Categories in Each							Total in Chapter
			1 Symptoms	2 Diagnostic	3 Treatment	4 Test Results	5 Administrative	6 Referrals	7 Diagnoses	
1	A	General	22	20	10	2	1	7	28	90
2	B	Blood, blood forming	8	20	10	2	1	7	20	68
3	D	Digestive	27	20	10	2	1	7	32	99
4	F	Eye	14	20	10	2	1	7	22	76
5	H	Ear	10	20	10	2	2	7	20	70
6	K	Circulatory	12	20	10	2	1	7	30	82
7	L	Musculoskeletal	24	20	10	2	1	7	30	94
8	N	Neurological	15	20	10	2	1	7	21	76
9	P	Psychological	27	20	10	2	1	7	14	81
10	R	Respiratory	18	20	10	2	1	7	27	85
11	S	Skin	28	20	10	2	1	7	29	97
12	T	Metab, endoc, nutritional	15	20	10	2	1	7	18	73
13	U	Urinary	12	20	10	2	1	7	15	67
14	W	Maternity, family planning	17	20	10	2	1	7	22	79
15	X	Female genital	28	20	10	2	1	7	23	91
16	Y	Male genital	18	20	10	2	1	7	18	76
17	Z	Social	27	20	10	2	1	7	-	67
		TOTALS	322	340	170	34	17	119	369	1371

Although only 1,371 categories are offered, and a total of 84 of these are "other" categories, the Alphabetical Index is stated as offering about 5,000 terms, which are "directed to" the appropriate categories. For greater detail, additional digits must be supplied following a decimal point. *IC_Process_PC* is a reference for detail for some of the process Components, e.g., endoscopy can be specified as to site; referral can be specified as to type of specialist. There is no "standard" list for adding detail to symptoms, complaints, or diagnoses.

Comments

ICPC and its companion volumes have been used extensively in research into the activities of the primary care physician in the United States, but more generally in Europe and Australia. There is little evidence that it has been adopted for routine use by family physicians or general practitioners in their daily record-keeping.

The development and research uses of *ICPC* have made a number of important contributions. Among them:

- The practice of primary care has been described in a number of countries.

- Valuable information as to the educational needs for primary care has been provided.

- Several significant contributions have been made to clinical thinking. Among them:

  - The "reason for encounter (RFE)" concept came into the literature. The RFE is not the same as Weed's "problem," because the encounters may be the results of symptoms, be stated as existing diagnoses, or as requests for specific services.

  - The episode is the logical unit of clinical information. An episode is defined as "a problem or illness in a patient over the entire period of time from its onset to its resolution." The episode formed the basic unit of investigation in several research studies mounted by the WONCA group and its members. An episode can be described, recorded, and displayed as one or more encounters in a series.

- An important use has been made of *ICPC* in the "encounter mode" by being careful to reach agreement with the patient as to the presenting symptoms and complaints in the course of deciding, with the patient, what class (code) to use from Component 1 of the classification. Substantial improvement in patient satisfaction and cooperation in management have been reported as a result.

It seems unfortunate that in publishing *ICPC* itself the authors did not bring forward the definitions found in *ICHPPC-2 Defined* and the added detail for the classification of process information found in *IC-Process-PC*. One wishing to use *ICPC* would have to obtain those volumes in order to take advantage of the work which went into these elaborations of the classification.

ICPC-2 contains, among other changes, a table giving about 70 changes from *ICPC-1*, changes which destroy continuity between the editions as to the meanings and contents of the categories. For example, "anorexia nervosa w/wo bulimia," which was T06, became P86, in order to change it from an endocrine disorder to a psychogenic problem. A new rubric, X21, was provided for "concern about body image in pregnancy."

Results of the desire to relate *ICPC-2* with *ICD-10*, noted above as a prime motivation for its publication, are found in two places: the tabular list and a new "conversion" table.

ICPC-2 to ICD-10

In the tabular list of *ICPC-2*, each *ICPC* category is accompanied by the *ICD-10* category code or codes to which it is related. For example:

X73, genital trichomoniasis, corresponds to *ICD-10* code A59.0

S16, bruise/contusion, may correspond to a long list of *ICD-10* codes, including S00.0, S00.7 to S00.9, Y14.0, and others

R89, congenital anomaly, respiratory, could relate to *ICD-10* codes Q30 to Q34

ICD-10 to ICPC-2

A table is included, "Conversion codes from *ICD-10*." This table is the reverse of the presentation in the tabular list — where *ICPC-2* coded cases might fit into *ICD-10*. "Conversion" hardly seems the appropriate term for this table, though, which contains a great many approximations. The authors are aware of the difficulties in relating *ICPC-2* and *ICD-10*:

> The relationship between *ICPC* and *ICD-10* is complex. There are some concepts in both which are not exactly represented in the other. However, for most rubrics in each classification one or more corresponding rubrics in the other can be mapped. This has been done in both directions in this book.

> Because of these complexities, quite often conversion of a code from one classification to the other and then re-conversion back again will not necessarily lead back to the same original code, because in each direction there may be several codes to choose from ... the point of having the code conversions in this book is only to indicate where the contents of the rubrics in each classification overlap.

Norway since 1995 has required the use of *ICPC* as a coded classification for payment of primary care encounters and recording clinical content of records. Also in the Netherlands, *ICPC* is used by general practitioners for data collection and reporting as a government recommendation. Australia now has several networks associated with universities which are using *ICPC* in routine data collection.

H

Index for Radiological Diagnoses

IN 1992, the American College of Radiology published the 4th Edition of the *Index for Radiological Diagnoses (IRD)*, which is now available in both hard copy and an electronic version.

To some extent, the name *Index for Radiological Diagnoses* is misleading, since the volume indexes not only diagnoses but also sites of examination, examination modalities, and etiologies. The result is a code system which is somewhat confusing, and sometimes results in unnecessary duplication of information. For example, an examination of one site with one modality, resulting in three diagnoses, requires duplication of the site and modality for each diagnosis.

The system is a "transformation system," resulting in fairly specific transformed terms, but losing the actual language of the physician.[1] Using the codes in the *IRD*, there is no way that a user could discover what a given diagnosis would have been as normally recorded by a radiologist.

Structure of the *IRD*

The Diagnostic Code (for which there is both a Tabular List and an Alphabetical Index) is a structured, strictly numerical code with 2 to 4 digits to the left of a decimal point denoting the site (Anatomy), and 2 to 5 digits to the right denoting the findings ("Pathology" — or lack of it, because "normal," meaning no pathology, is a common radiological diagnosis).

---

1. See "Transformation Coding," page 127.

Anatomy Codes

The *IRD* provides ten sections for the Anatomy codes:

Section	Rubrics[a]	Site
1	10-19	Skull and contents
2	20-29	Face, mastoids and neck
3	30-39	Spine and contents
4	40-49	Skeletal system
5	51-59	Heart and great vessels
6	60-69	Lung, mediastinum, and pleura
7	70-79	Gastrointestinal system
8	80-89	Genitourinary system
9	91-99	Vascular and lymphatic systems
10	00-09	Breast

a. "Rubric" is the label of a category in a classification (sometimes is used interchangeably with category). For example, "pickup trucks" might be the rubric for a category in a classification of motor vehicles.

The first of each of the ten rubrics in a section (e.g., "10" in Section 1, "Skull and contents") represents "Location not known or unspecified," except there are no codes "50" (Heart section) or "90" (Vascular section), because all locations (sites) in these two sections must be specified. The last of the numbers in all sections (e.g., "19", "29", etc.) represent "Other" (except "99" where it means "Lymphatic vessels, lymph nodes"). Most sections have exclusions and inclusions, e.g., Section 5, "Heart and great vessels," excludes abdominal and cervical vessels, which are directed to Section 9, "Vascular and lymphatic systems."

Within each of the rubrics, there are two remaining two digits available for providing greater detail depending on the part of the body involved. Users are expected to provide at least the first two digits of anatomy, with the remaining two digits optional.

Pathology Codes

Pathology codes are found to the right of the decimal point. All except digits 7 and 8 have the same headings across the ten anatomy sections:

Code	Finding
.1	Normal, technique, anomaly
.2	Inflammation
.3	Neoplasm, neoplastic-like condition
.4	Effect of trauma
.5	Metabolic, endocrine, toxic
.6	Other generalized systemic disorder
.7	Miscellaneous (in many of the anatomical fields, the subjects are specified in this section)
.8	Miscellaneous (this section is devoted to disorders of the lymphatic system in anatomic Section 9)
.9	Other

Instructions for use of the *IRD* are that a minimum of 2 digits of Pathology codes should be supplied, although in the Anatomy Section 7, Gastrointestinal System, no subdivisions are given for .5, "Metabolic, endocrine, toxic."

Procedure Designators

Pathology codes also include an option to identify the procedure used. For example, in Section 5, "Heart and Great Vessels," pathology code .12 is devoted to "Special Technique, Procedure, Projection," with code .121 entitled "Digital radiographic techniques, tomography, MR, nuclear medicine."

Box Codes

In various areas of the IRD, added detail is offered by "box codes," codes which may be added to specific pathology codes. The name "box codes" comes from the way they are presented, that is, in boxes inserted in the code book, for example:

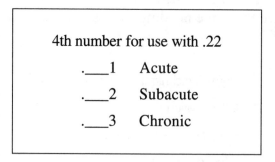

In the case of the box codes, the location of the digit is critical, and the user is instructed that blanks "_" must be inserted in front of the digit if necessary in order to keep it in the correct position and thus preserve its meaning.

Procedure Codes

An optional method of specifying the procedure employed is provided by prefixes. One can indicate procedures by prefixing the diagnosis code with one of ten possible procedure codes, separated from the diagnosis code by a hyphen:

Prefix	Procedure
0-	Ultrasonic examination
1-	Plain film examination
2-	Fluoroscopic, cinefluoroscopic, or videotape examination
3-	Tomographic technique, including computed tomography
4-	Digital techniques
5-	Examination using barium as a contrast agent
6-	Organ examination using an intravenous contrast agent
7-	Angiographic examination, excluding digital radiographic techniques
8-	Other examination using iodinated contrast agent, including bronchogram, oral cholecystogram

9-   Other, including special radiographic projection, lymphangiography, examination using air as a contrast agent, NMR

Users are encouraged to add a second digit to the procedure code where they wish to show greater detail.

This procedure code prefix option creates redundancy, because in many areas of the pathology codes the type of procedure has already been indicated, and in greater detail than offered by the prefixes.

Special Instructions

The authors of the *IRD* recognize that special situations will be encountered, and so provide special instructions under the headings of:

- Normal Examinations (for example, "normal plain films, normal ultrasound procedures, and normal special procedures, special techniques, and special radiological projections with normal results")
- Special procedures and special radiological projections and techniques demonstrating abnormalities
- Situations that require more than one code number
- Multiple bone lesions
- Infections
- Angiography

There are also suggestions made as to how to use the code if the purpose is to index and file radiological studies, reprints, teaching notes, or other teaching materials.

"Customizing" the Code

The *IRD* includes a page entitled, "How to Change the Diagnostic Code" in order to meet local needs and preferences. The final note here reads "When you change the code, you should also (a) change the index [Alphabetical Index] and (b) change all copies of the ACR *Index* in your department."

Problems with Coding "Options"

It is clear from the permissiveness, in fact the encouragement, given to tailoring and using the *IRD* as the radiologist sees fit, that the *Index* has been devised for the individual imaging department, with no intention that the codes provided be used to collect or compare information from more than one site for clinical or other research. This is unfortunate, because it limits the usefulness of the classification. It also makes using the system more difficult and time-consuming, even within a single department.

Complexity

The *Index*, permitting different coding combinations for a single procedure/finding, can result in multiple and sometimes redundant codes. In the *IRD*, if the user wants to show both the procedure and its findings, and elects not to use the procedural prefix codes, the solution is to "double code" within the anatomical section. So a code for the procedure would read:

[anatomy].[procedure]

while the code for the finding would read

[anatomy].[pathology]

and thus two entire codes would be required, with the site duplicated in each. Several significant findings at the same site compounds the problem, because for each significant finding, the site must be repeated.

If the user decides instead to use prefix codes to show the procedure and its findings, the result would be:

[procedure]-[anatomy].[pathology]

This approach permits far less detail as to procedure.

As mentioned above, pathology code .12 in Section 5 ("Heart and Great Vessels") is dedicated to "Special Technique, Procedure, Projection." There are under .12 predefined codes for about 50 possible digital techniques, tomography, MR, and nuclear medicine. But if the prefix codes are used, the two digits (4-) allowed for "digital techniques" permits a breakdown of only 10 possibilities, the two digits (3-) allowed for tomography (including computed tomography) another 10, and the two digits (9-) for "Other," which includes MR, must be shared with several other modalities.

Provinciality

The person doing the coding would have to know the local coding conventions, which would have to be easily available, in writing, and be slavishly followed by everyone doing coding. The procedures to insure this discipline are extremely difficult to establish and enforce.

The system gives freedom for the coder to create codes locally (in fact, the user is encouraged to create codes virtually anywhere in the system). This makes case retrieval very difficult — a researcher would have to find some local record of code meanings before a search could begin. For example, a user seeking to retrieve all cases with a given modality has to know, and search for, every code someone could possibly have used to record the modality. The pathology code .121, for example, does not have an uniform meaning across all of the anatomy sections.

Accuracy

Since codes can be created "on the fly," verification of their validity may be impossible. The system also permits conflicting entries in the "procedural code" and "pathology code" sections of the same diagnosis code.

Index for Radiological Diagnoses, Computer Version 4.1

The Computer Version of the *IRD* is a database application developed with Foxpro™. It consists of two facilities:[2]

- a coding "submenu" called the ACR Coding Index
- a Teaching File

The Coding Index

The Coding Index has two functions:

- to code a given diagnosis
- to look up a code and present its meaning

Coding is a menu-driven process. The coder uses a keyboard or a mouse to walk through each digit of the anatomy and pathology sections of the *Index*. If the user enters more digits in either anatomy or pathology than are found in the codes offered by the *Index*, the extra digits are ignored, and the code is shown to be "completed." Literal translation from the *Index* is shown on the screen at that point in the process, complete with "excludes," "includes," and other modifying or explanatory information. In other words, the "English language diagnosis," as the

---

2. The version described here is 4.1, released in 1998.

program refers to this display, is not a diagnosis which the radiologist would record in the usual radiology report.

No provision is made for use of the "box codes," nor can the user introduce local codes into the system — coding is strictly "by the book."

When the coding is complete, the user can return to the menu or, by a single keystroke, transfer the diagnosis to the Teaching File. This opens the entry screen for the Teaching File and the user is prompted to provide the patient's name and other relevant information.

Looking up a code permits the user to enter up to four digits of anatomy and six digits of pathology. When the program looks up the code, however, it recognizes only the codes provided in the *Index*, which may be as few as one of anatomy and one of pathology, if for that particular set of leading digits, no second or greater digits are offered. Code lookup doesn't permit use of the box codes, either.

The Teaching File

The Teaching File is a database in which each record is a report of an individual examination. A form is displayed for data entry. Completion of the form assigns the report a serial number in the file, asks for the patient's name and basic demographic information, and records the physician and the modalities employed. Two diagnoses, the primary and secondary, are allowed, as well as "comments." For the diagnoses, fields are provided for the codes. The program intercepts "illegal" codes, i.e., those not in the *Index*, and presents the message "Incorrect ACR Code." If the Teaching File record is initiated by transfer of the ACR code from the coding module, of course, this message is never displayed.

After ACR codes are in place, the user has two options for filling in the narrative boxes accompanying each code. The computer will, on demand, display the "English language diagnosis," which is a literal printout of the entries in the *Index* for each digit of the code number, or the user can type the entry. It is at this point in the system that ordinary radiology diagnostic descriptions could be entered. The narrative fields are generous in size, permitting a fairly lengthy dictation. The comments field also is available for further narrative.

A limited number of standard reports are predefined, and there is some ability to create custom reports. Of course, individual case records can be printed out and could be used as radiology reports.

I

Mortality Medical Data System

Death certificates throughout the United States are completed and submitted in narrative rather than coded form, i.e., the diagnoses are in natural language. In 1967, the United States National Center for Health Statistics (NCHS) embarked on a program called the Mortality Medical Data System (MMDS) to automate the entry, classification, and retrieval of cause-of-death information reported on these death certificates.

The cause-of-death information is first written or typed on the death certificate in narrative form. The relevant section of the U.S. Standard Certificate of Death is reproduced below.

Figure I.1 Cause of Death Information

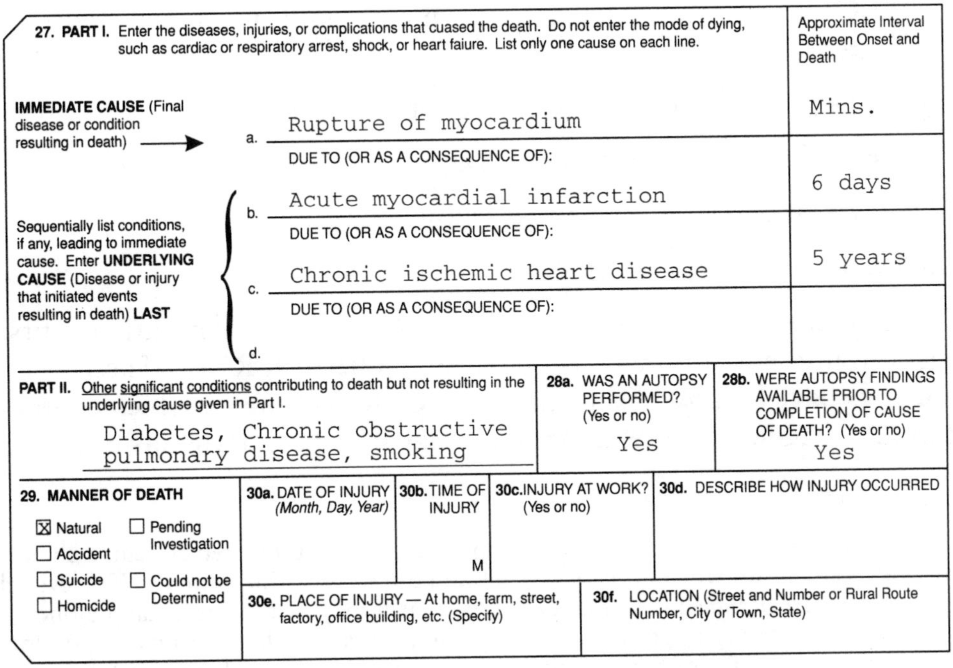

27. PART I. Enter the diseases, injuries, or complications that cuased the death. Do not enter the mode of dying, such as cardiac or respiratory arrest, shock, or heart faiure. List only one cause on each line.

		Approximate Interval Between Onset and Death
IMMEDIATE CAUSE (Final disease or condition resulting in death) →	a. Rupture of myocardium	Mins.
	DUE TO (OR AS A CONSEQUENCE OF):	
Sequentially list conditions, if any, leading to immediate cause. Enter **UNDERLYING CAUSE** (Disease or injury that initiated events resulting in death) **LAST**	b. Acute myocardial infarction	6 days
	DUE TO (OR AS A CONSEQUENCE OF):	
	c. Chronic ischemic heart disease	5 years
	DUE TO (OR AS A CONSEQUENCE OF):	
	d.	

PART II. Other significant conditions contributing to death but not resulting in the underlyiing cause given in Part I.
Diabetes, Chronic obstructive pulmonary disease, smoking

28a. WAS AN AUTOPSY PERFORMED? (Yes or no) Yes

28b. WERE AUTOPSY FINDINGS AVAILABLE PRIOR TO COMPLETION OF CAUSE OF DEATH? (Yes or no) Yes

29. MANNER OF DEATH
☒ Natural ☐ Pending Investigation
☐ Accident
☐ Suicide ☐ Could not be Determined
☐ Homicide

30a. DATE OF INJURY *(Month, Day, Year)*

30b. TIME OF INJURY M

30c. INJURY AT WORK? (Yes or no)

30d. DESCRIBE HOW INJURY OCCURRED

30e. PLACE OF INJURY — At home, farm, street, factory, office building, etc. (Specify)

30f. LOCATION (Street and Number or Rural Route Number, City or Town, State)

Sample "Cause of Death" portion of a U.S. Standard Certificate of Death PHS-T-003. Department of Health and Human Services, Public Health Service, National Center for Health Statistics – 1989 Revision.

Process

The Mortality Medical Data System (MMDS) process involves four basic steps:

1. Encoding the original information with numeric "entity reference numbers" (ERNs).

2. Assigning *ICD* codes to the ERNs.

3. Using the *ICD* codes to select the underlying cause of death.

4. Converting the output into a specific statistical format (i.e., following the rules promulgated by WHO for assignment of cases to the categories of *ICD-9* and *ICD-10*).

These steps are accomplished with the help of software developed for the MMDS. There are now five basic programs:[1]

- PC-MICAR Data Entry System

- Super-MICAR

- MICAR (Mortality Medical Indexing, Classification, and Retrieval System)

- ACME (Automated Classification of Medical Entities)

- TRANSAX (TRANSlation of Axis)

These will be described in context below.

Entity Reference Numbers (ERNs)

To automate the data processing, the cause of death information is first encoded into numeric "entity reference numbers" (ERNs). These numbers have been published in the MICAR Dictionary, which contains 145,223 diagnostic terms in natural language. Each term has been

---

1. "Currently there are interrelated components of the automated system, a choice between one of two data entry systems and three processing systems. However, the systems are designed such that each component may be used as a stand-alone package. Description of the software components as well as documentation for system managers and users explaining installation and use of the software is included on the screens under medical software. The installation software will be made available for downloading in the future." More information about MICAR is available at the NHCS website, http://www.cdc.gov/nchs.

assigned to an ERN. There are presently 28,964 entity reference numbers, in the range from 000001 to 190031 (gaps have been left in the series). Code 999999 represents "term not in dictionary."

There is almost always more than one way to state or abbreviate a given diagnostic term. These alternative expressions are assigned to the same ERN; in fact, no ERN represents less than two terms. The diagnosis "alcoholism," for example, has two entries, but one ERN:

```
000007 = ALC
000007 = ALCOHOLISM
```

Typically, a diagnosis has more entries:

```
000012 = ARTERIOSCLEROTIC CORHD
000012 = ARTERIOSCLEROTIC CORONARY HEART D
000012 = ARTERIOSCLEROTIC CORONARY HEART DISEASE
000012 = ASCHD
000012 = CORONARY AHD
000012 = CORONARY ARTERIOSCLEROTIC HEART D
000012 = CORONARY ARTERIOSCLEROTIC HEART DISEASE
000012 = CORONARY ASHD
```

The largest ERN — 115749 — represents 60 alternative ways to state "acute bronchial pneumonia of the left upper lobe":

```
115748 = ACUTE IDIOPATHIC  CEREBRITIS

115749 = A IMMEDIATE LEFT UL BRONCH PN
115749 = A IMMEDIATE LT UL BRONCH PN
... 58 other expressions of the pneumonia, ending with
115749 = ACUTE IMMEDIATE LUL BRONCHUS PNEUMONIA

115750 = A  INCIPIENT MYELOCYTIC LEUKEMIA
```

The terms which transform into each of these illustrations are obviously alternative methods of expressing the same concept. It does not appear that there is a portion of the system which, given an ERN as a query, will translate it back into a single term. Instead, asking for the meaning of code 115749 will retrieve all 60 expressions, without telling which one was used. So the original diagnoses are never retrievable verbatim, as entered, from the ERNs.

Two software programs were created to assist in the encoding process:

PC-MICAR Data Entry System Assists MICAR data entry operators in encoding the diagnoses on the death certificate into the numeric entity reference numbers.

Super-MICAR Performs the same task by allowing the data entry operator to type the diagnoses exactly as they appear on the death certificate. It then "processes the data, dividing terms, replacing words with synonyms, dropping unnecessary words, and arranging words in proper order to be found in the NCHS MICAR Dictionary. The result is a file that can be processed through MICAR software to produce ACME input files."

ERNs to ICD Codes

This step is performed entirely by the MICAR software.

MICAR (Mortality Medical Indexing, Classification, and Retrieval System)
Automates the multiple cause coding rules and assigns *ICD* codes to each numeric entity reference number.

"MICAR 100" takes the output of PC-MICAR or Super-MICAR and assigns ENRs to any unassigned text.

"MICAR 200" takes the output of MICAR 100 and assigns the ERNs to the appropriate *ICD* categories (there are programs for both *ICD-9* and *ICD-10*).

ICD Codes to Cause of Death

A fourth software application is used to determine the underlying cause of death.

ACME (Automated Classification of Medical Entities) Automates the underlying cause of death coding rules. ACME uses the multiple *ICD* codes assigned to each entity (e.g., disease condition, accident, or injury), preserving the location and order as reported by the certifier. ACME then applies the World Health Organization (WHO) rules to the *ICD* codes and selects an underlying cause of death.

Cause of Death to Statistical Format

A fifth program provides output in the specific format required by the National Center for Health Statistics (NCHS) for mortality statistics.

TRANSAX (TRANSlation of Axis) Converts the ACME output data into a fixed format and translates the data into a more desirable statistical form using the linkage provisions of the *ICD*. TRANSAX creates the data necessary for person-based tabulations by translating the axis of classification from an entity basis to a record basis.

Example

The MMDS process

The Mortality Medical Data System process is, of course, a bit more complicated than the brief descriptions given here. An inquiry to NCHS elicited the following illustration:

An infant's death certificate reported "gram negative sepsis."

MICAR assigns ERN as 000347.

In the MICAR Dictionary, one finds:

- 000347 SEPTICEMIC EMBOLI
- 000347 SEPTICEMIC EMBOLISM
- 000347 SEPTICEMIC EMBOLUS

When MICAR200, the "rules application program," deals with the certificate, it converts 000347 to the interim ERN code 202981. This code is used internally en route to the final *ICD* assignment ("original" ERNs presently extend only through code 190031).

Code 000347 is retained permanently with the death record and the case can be retrieved as a case in which MICAR had placed code 000347. It is not clear which of the three versions of the term "sepsis" would be displayed.

MICAR as Prototype

The MMDS system has many of the elements of a prototype for a system which could one day replace the current methods of classifying clinical diagnostic information. It takes free text as input and encodes it with entity codes. These entity codes serve as input for computer systems which classify the information to multiple classifications, using algorithms written specifically for each classification (currently *ICD-9* and *ICD-10*). This is the model suggested in this book for capturing and preserving clinical detail by using entity coded information.

MICAR's chief difference from the entity coding proposed in this volume is that MICAR, by the uniform application of rules, transforms the exact diagnostic language on the death certificate to its own set of terms. Clinical entity coding, as proposed by the authors of *The Endangered Medical Record*, preserves and codes the original clinical language verbatim, with any desired transformations done in a subsequent step (a classification step).

The MICAR Dictionary has, over the more than 20 years of its development, dealt with virtually all of the terms which have been used on death certificates. It is prepared, however, to accept new diagnoses as new entities appear, and to deal with them as exceptions (code 999999). For clinical purposes, it is, of course, incomplete, because there are a great many diagnoses which are needed in medical records and for morbidity purposes but which do not result in death.

The counterpart system for clinical use in medical care would need only to expand the entity term and code list to permit verbatim coding (and decoding) of the diagnoses used in actual, day-to-day, care, and to develop the algorithms for their classification.

J

Medcin

MEDCIN™ appeared in the public eye in early 1997 with the publication by Springer-Verlag of a book entitled *Medcin — A New Nomenclature for Clinical Medicine*, authored by Peter Goltra, President and Founder of Medicomp Systems, Inc., of Chantilly, Virginia. Medcin had been developed by Medicomp Systems for use in the electronic medical record system, MedTrac™, offered by that company, and in Medcin Expert™, another Medicomp product, described as a system "used to analyze the patient's chart ... and prompt ... the physician ... " Goltra states that

> ... a Medcin nomenclature license is available for any size site, unlimited number of users, for $25.00 per year. A Medcin Expert license is available for $15.00 per user per year. These prices have been published as valid for ten years starting February 15, 1997.

Medcin was published as a 744-page volume and is also available in electronic form. The published volume consists of brief introductory material, the nomenclature in hierarchical form (occupying 706 of the pages, no alphabetical index), and three appendices.

- Appendix A: Additional Data Components Used with Medcin

- Appendix B: Using Medcin to Build Applications

- Appendix C: Supplemental Files and Tools for Medcin

The publication of Medcin put the nomenclature itself in its hierarchical form (in its present state of development) into public view. From the Preface:

> Through MediComp Systems, interested readers can also obtain the Medcin nomenclature as a computer file. This is currently available for a nominal license fee in keeping with the pro bono intent for this project.

> I [the author] hope very much that users of Medcin will contribute to future updates of the nomenclature.

Medcin's introductory material states that it was created over a period of nearly 20 years in the development of an electronic medical record, following the thought process of the clinician in the patient-physician encounter, and thus, the author contends, it is more acceptable to clinicians than other nomenclatures. As a result of this point of view, the data elements (findings of the clinician) are placed in six categories, which form the Parts of the book.

Figure J.1 Medcin Schema

Hierarchical List of Terms in Medcin		
Part	Title	Approximate Number of Terms[a]
I	Symptoms	2,800
II	History	2,100
III	Physical Findings	10,500
IV	Tests	27,100
V	Diagnoses, Syndromes, and Conditions	10,100
VI	Therapy and Management	16,100
	Total Terms	68,700

a. Using an average of 100 terms per page to estimate the counts.

A panel of twenty-four consulting editors is listed, essentially all of them medical school faculty members, the largest number, eleven, at Cornell. No information is available about the use of the system in non-academic clinical settings or the influence of and input from such settings reflected in the current version of Medcin.

The structure of the nomenclature is hierarchical in such a fashion that each element inherits the characteristics of the higher levels of that hierarchy; between each two levels there is a parent-child relationship; elements of equal level within a given hierarchy are called siblings. The example given in the introduction to the volume is that

> ... "numbness" is a fairly common symptom, and can be present almost anywhere in the body ... Medcin has more than eighty findings [symptoms] for numbness, starting with the general finding and proceeding in a structured hierarchy through all areas of the body, increasing in detail at each level.

... This structure presents two distinct advantages. First, a finding need only be recorded as a specific clinical observation. The clinician records information with only the degree of specificity needed to support diagnosis and treatment.[1]

Second, the nomenclature hierarchy automatically passes these findings up the hierarchy by reverse inheritance to meet the needs of the researcher. Using "numbness of the first two fingers of the right hand" as an example, Medcin knows this includes the characteristics of "numbness of the right hand," "numbness of the extremities," and "numbness." Therefore any future searches using Medcin will locate the detailed finding from the more general terms in the hierarchy above it.

The rationale above is the author's argument for advantages in data entry for the clinician and data retrieval for the researcher. These advantages would be dependent upon the ease with which a given term could be found.

To find any term in the Medcin volume, as in any hierarchical or tabular list without an alphabetical index, it is necessary to know not only the organization of the list, but also something of the thinking which went into its development. The problem of using Medcin's hierarchical list without such information (which is not supplied in the book) can be illustrated by reporting the problem of looking up "numbness," which the introduction to the book uses (above) to illustrate the hierarchical nature of the nomenclature.

Numbness first has to be recognized as a symptom, which would place it in Part I of the book.

Because of the absence of an alphabetic index, "numbness" could only be located by scanning the printed pages until it was found. Back-tracking then placed numbness within the hierarchy group called "focal disturbances."[2] The levels of the hierarchy are shown in the volume by indentation. Further backtracking disclosed the hierarchical trail as shown below. The "numbness trail" is in bold type. Terms in each

---

1. It would appear that this limitation, "for the convenience of the clinician," might keep out of the record information which other users of that information, an epidemiologist or health services researcher, for example, might find useful.

2. The hierarchical list in the browser is not an exact replica of the same list in the book. In the example tested, "numbness" was not found in the browser as a child of "focal disturbances" as it is in the book, but rather as a "sensory disturbance," which is perhaps more logical.

hierarchy level immediately adjacent to numbness in the trail are shown here to illustrate the apparently random organization of the list.

The numbers to the left of the terms are called "finding identification numbers." They accompany each finding, although here are shown only those in the "numbness" trail. The numbers vary from one to six digits in length.

> The Medcin finding identification number has no inherent meaning, structure, order, or hierarchy. It is merely a computer-assigned number which never changes, and is used to record each piece of medical information as a single data element, rather than as free-text or as a composite code structure.

The facing illustration shows the structure.

"Numbness", a symptom in Medcin[a]

Part I – Symptoms

 . . .

endocrine symptoms

skin symptoms

hematalogic symptoms

musculoskeletal symptoms

1885[a] **neurological symptoms**

psychological symptoms

 . . .

 . . .

repeated questioning about recent events

683 **focal disturbances**

difficulty with starting and stopping movements

 . . .

 . . .

tingling

burning sensation

1647 **numbness (hypesthesia)**[b]

increased sensitivity to pain

 . . .

 . . .

one entire side

839 **of the extremities**

in the perianal region

 . . .

 . . .

of both arms

849 **just the right hand**

just the left hand

 . . .

 . . .

just the right thumb

[a] The indentation in this table has been exaggerated to show the parent-child relationship. In the printed volume, the indentation is so small (about 1/8 inch) as to be virtually impossible to see.

Other illustrations showing the apparently random entry of findings are:

Part I — Symptoms

...

| 2902 | otolaryngeal symptoms |

...

...

179	dryness of the nose
180	nasal lump or mass
181	pain in the jaw
1793	right side
1794	left side
182	jaw spasms (trismus)
184	jaw stiffness
185	jaw click
186	lump in the jaw
187	pain in the teeth
1840	teeth chip easily
188	recent tooth loss

...

and,

Part V — Diagnoses, Syndromes, and Conditions

...

34165	Gastroenterology
90242	Gastrointestinal Infections
90241	Esophagus

...

| 90246 | Gallbladder and Biliary Tree |

...

37301	Laceration of Gallbladder
37302	Gunshot Wound of Gallbladder
30050	Adenomyosis of the Gallbladder
34177	Gallbladder Obstruction
34178	Cholosterolosis of Gallbladder

...

The principles behind the sequences within hierarchies, as illustrated above, are not apparent. They clearly are not alphabetical, nor is the logic used explained in the volume.

Other examples of the need to know the thinking of the author are numerous throughout the various Parts. For example:

- Skull fracture is found in the diagnostic section as an orthopedic term. Another natural location for skull fracture would appear to be neurology.

- Bronchoscopy for diagnostic purposes might logically be sought under "Pulmonary Procedures." A somewhat arduous search found it as a child under "Fiberoptic Procedures" in the electronic version. In the printed volume, Pulmonary Procedures has no children.

- "Sigmoidoscopy (fiberoptic)" is found under "Digestive System Services" in the printed version but under "Fiberoptic Procedures" in the electronic browser.

Diagnoses, syndromes, and conditions are placed in 22 categories:

Ophthalmology
Otorhinolaryngology
Cardiology
Pulmonary Medicine
Gastroenterology
Nephrology
Urology
Gynecology
Obstetrics
Pediatrics [includes "Genetic disorders"]
Metabolic Disorders
Endocrinology
Dermatology
Rheumatology
Orthopedics
Neurology
Psychiatry
Infectious Disease
Hematology

Immunology
Oncology
Environmental Disorders

The phrasing as shown in the hierarchical illustration is called by the author "hierarchical phrasing," while the symptom description given by the clinician, "numbness of the right thumb and index finger," is called "standalone phrasing." A search tool provided by MediComp uses the standalone phrasing. In the MediComp systems where the nomenclature is used, each finding identification number is accompanied by the two sets of terms, hierarchical phrasing and standalone phrasing, and presumably the tool to be used in the output is at the discretion of the user.

Medcin is designed, apparently, for pick-list data entry, which is perhaps the data entry method most easily accepted by the physician, since she is unlikely to type in the term. However, if the hierarchical arrangement in the printed volume and in the Demonstration Copy, the "browser," represents the pick-list sequence, then locating a "finding" via the pick list must present a great mystery to the user unless that user's clinical thought process exactly matches that of the author. Recall the procedure which had to be followed to track down the "numbness" illustration.

If data entry is to be by other than the physician, e.g., by someone else at a keyboard, then a word wheel[3] would be a preferable technique, and the entries would be the standalone terms, which are more likely to be those used by a clinician, rather than the hierarchical terms. It would still be necessary to enter the terms exactly as they are stated in the nomenclature, however, and these statements naturally reflect the language usage of the author and the advisory panel which developed the list.

Numbers of terms It is impossible to predict what proportion of the numbers of terms, "medical findings," which will be encountered in a widespread application of the electronic medical record would be found in today's Medcin. A table in the Discussion estimates the numbers under each heading. Roughly 10,000 physical findings are listed, and this may be enough. But just three segments of the hierarchy for physical findings account for two-thirds of the total: the eyes (1,200),

---

3.   See ""Click and Enter" Technologies," page 238.

cardiovascular system (1,800, of which 1,100 refer to murmurs), and the musculoskeletal system (3,400, of which 1,600 refer to the fingers).

Diagnoses The marked differences in the numbers of diagnostic terms from several common coding sources is a mystery. Although some lists of "diagnoses" contain more synonyms than others, that can't be the entire answer.

Figure J.2 Comparison of Numbers of Diagnostic Terms

Approximate numbers of diagnostic terms in various sources		
ICD-9-CM	SNOMED	Medcin
Alphabetic Index directs its entries to the 12,000 group codes (some entries pertain to external causes, etc.)	Module D, Diseases/ Diagnoses — number of "Records," each presumably a preferred term	Part V Diagnoses, Syndromes, Conditions — estimate from page count in volume
100,000	37,000 (human)	10,000

It should be noted that there is no accepted definition with which to standardize such counts as those of diagnoses, physical findings, tests, and so on.

Adding terms There is no information as to how terms can be added to the list. The author stated on inquiry that a utility is provided with which, at the local site, a user can put in a new term, which will be given a unique temporary or local number and be added to the local list. Such local numbers must be greater than the number 1,000,000 (the official numbers in Medcin are below that threshold). It is not clear whether the addition is only to the hierarchical list or to the search engine, or both. MediComp states that it is ready to accept such input from the local user and to have the term evaluated by its staff. If it is found acceptable, it will become an official term in the next quarterly (?) version of Medcin. It is not clear how the local user can easily replace the temporary number with the new official one in the affected records.

Navigation The question must be raised as to whether a typical physician is willing to learn the structure of the hierarchy in Medcin. Such knowledge is essential in order to find the desired terms, unless there is some adequate navigational device in the electronic medical record systems. The problem exists in both the printed book and the electronic version. The organization of the hierarchy in Medcin is not apparent (except for the highest — six group — level). The search engine in the browser doesn't help unless one knows exactly the term for the "finding" as it is expressed in Medcin.

Unique codes The insistence of the author that once used, a code (number) will be unique to its term as well as that it will never be reused states a principle which is essential to a satisfactory electronic medical record system.

It is to be hoped that this would be slavishly enforced. But apparently a restatement of the concept does not necessarily result in a different code. In the Introduction to the book, the phrase used as an illustration is:

"numbness of the first two fingers of the right hand"

In the text, however, the (slightly different) concept is stated quite differently:

"numbness only of the right thumb and index finger."

A preferable coding system would be one in which such shifts in the meanings of the codes could never occur.

Findings numbers Using the findings numbers as purely accession numbers with no inherent meanings is highly desirable. This eliminates any temptation for a user to try to create a code number, and thus protects the integrity of the system. However, a given accession number should be forever locked verbatim to the term which it represents.

Printed volume The printed volume, Medcin, has several shortcomings:

- There is no alphabetic index.

- There is no users' guide.

- The typography with its minimal indentations to show the parent-child relations (1/8") makes detection of these relationships extremely difficult, especially when the positions are spread over several columns.

Electronic version The electronic version also needs the equivalent of an adequate alphabetical index and documentation as to its organization.

A true "Help" facility would be a great improvement.

System in which Medcin would be employed The usefulness of the nomenclature depends on the system or application in which it is employed. It cannot stand alone. For example, under physical findings, an entry in the list is "pupil size, right eye." The system would have to accommodate a way to put in the appropriate modifier such as "pinpoint," or a measurement, e.g., "1 mm."

"Terms of clinical interest" Goltra states that Medcin codes "terms of clinical interest" rather than using what he calls a "data dictionary" approach. Actually, "terms of clinical interest" is one of the variants of what is called "transformation coding." These variants are:

Modular language coding, what Goltra calls the "data dictionary approach," which is the process in which the meaning of ordinary natural language is forced into a structured set of coded components. In the process, the original language becomes irretrievable. The chief example of this approach is *SNOMED* when used as prescribed in its introductory material, i.e., when each concept is expressed by a concatenation of components from several *SNOMED* modules. Goltra points out that in such a system one can code the same thing different ways.

Concept coding, which is the process in which the preferred term for a concept, as defined by experts (or by "the system"), is used instead of any of its synonyms which might have been the original term used in the medical record. In concept coding the original language may be lost. Concept coding is used in UMLS (Unified Medical Language System), in Module D (Diseases/Diagnoses) of *SNOMED*, and in the Read Codes, and is the process used in Medcin.

In modular language coding the original language used by the clinician is never preserved, i.e., the original input is lost forever. In concept coding, which is the variant Goltra calls "terms of clinical interest," the system provides the term it will accept or retrieve, and thus the term retrieved by decoding may be the original language which the clinician (would have?) used, but it may not. If it is not, the meaning may be seriously distorted.

Mandating language There seems to be no evidence that anyone has been successful in requiring physicians to use "preferred terms" in their daily communications, yet Medcin seems to be based on the assumption that mandated language is practical. The early attempts by the American Medical Association failed, as apparently have all others.[4] The use of pick lists to get information into medical records could introduce such standardized language into the records, but it has the serious danger of forcing dishonesty on the part of the user:

- The list simply may not have a term that is applicable.

- The difficulty in finding the terms, either by pursuing the pick list hierarchy or using a search facility, encourages use of a term with which the user is familiar (hopefully one reasonably close to the correct term). In *CPT*, for example, this problem is behind the production of "specialty" versions of the classification.

- The method outlined above to add new terms even to the local list is burdensome; the user is likely to settle for some available term reasonably close in meaning (or which will not be challenged by the information system, human or electronic).

Appendices to Medcin

There are three appendices which seem to reflect the usage of Medcin in the electronic medical record and other products of MediComp Systems, Inc. A brief description of each follows.

Appendix A – Additional Data Components Used with Medcin

These are components which may be attached to any of the findings in Medcin. They cover:

History Status — which can be designated by a blank (absence of any other status code), one or two letters (or characters, e.g., "?"), or a number. Examples taken from the 29 status codes listed are:

O   Ordered

H   Personal History

RI   Risk of

?   Possible

---

4.   See "Uniformity in Clinical Language," page 77.

?+ Probable

W   Working diagnosis

RF Referred elsewhere for

AL Allergy to

D   Cause of death

1-9 Finding specified as part of a group

Modifier — an adjective used to further describe or modify the finding. The modifiers are single or double alphabetic characters, plus a blank (no modifier). Examples taken from the list of 29 shown are:

TI tiny, insignificant

T   tiny

S   small

SM small-moderate

M   moderate

SV severe

BO borderline

EP episodic

SE seasonal

RE recent

Course — an adjectival phrase showing the patient's progress. Six possibilities are offered:

I   improving

W   worsening

U   unchanged

E   expanding

L   louder

S   softer

Result of a Finding. "A result indicator may be linked to an item which is a measurable physical finding or a test." Five options are offered:

> blank (no entry)

A   abnormal or positive

B   high

N   normal or negative

L   low

Appendix B – Using Medcin to Build Applications

Supplemental files and tools are offered by MediComp Systems, Inc. to support clinical applications. Some of the files or tools are patented or patent pending. The appendix lists the following:

> EMR Database Components
>
> Status
>
> Result
>
> Modifier
>
> Course
>
> Value
>
> Additional Information for a Finding
>
> Use of Clinical Data for Reporting and Analysis
>
> Differential Diagnosis — An Example of Clinical Analysis
>
> Searching for Findings by Disease
>
> Searching for Findings by Vocabulary Words
>
> Searching for Findings for Intelligent Prompting
>
> Cohort Studies
>
> Reporting to External Systems

Appendix C – Supplemental Files and Tools for Medcin

These are available on computer media from MediComp Systems. They are listed as:

Medcin Nomenclature — this is stated to be comparable to the printed volume and to be accompanied by a browser and a Windows 95 program with a branching tree display format. The demonstration copy supplied for review does not match the printed volume exactly.

Medcin Search — which combines Medcin Nomenclature with vocabulary words, synonyms, and standalone phrasing for each finding.

Medcin Chart — which combines Medcin Search with other resources which are used in an electronic medical record application. One component is a "narrative engine" which can compose reports in both professional and lay language.

Medcin Expert — is an expert system with a multidimensional matrix of Medcin findings and 3,100 diagnoses, syndromes, and conditions. This can be used to create clinical protocols and for other purposes.[5]

Additional Tools — Mapping tables for allocating Medcin codes to classifications such as *ICD-9-CM*, *ICD-10*, *CPT*, and others. There are also certain "function-specific" tools available.

---

5. This expert system employs what the company calls "Intelligent prompting," a patent-pending system which provides diagnostic and other guidance within the electronic medical record. Placing guidance systems within the EMR is an important use of computer technology. At present the system is reported as available for something like 3,000 diagnoses. Plans for expanding it to cover additional diagnoses and perhaps therapies are not described. See the discussion above about the number of diagnoses in Medcin.

Section 5: Other Resource Materials

K

ICD-9-CM Classification of the Circulatory System

The following table was developed from the Official Version of *ICD-9-CM* (CDROM), 5th Edition, 1994, U. S. Department of Health and Human Services, Public Health Service, Health Care Financing Administration. It gives the numbers of references in the Alphabetic Index (Volume 2) to each of the categories in the Tabular List (Volume 1) for the Circulatory Disease Chapter of *ICD-9-CM* (390-459).

It was constructed to show several things:

1. The compression of terms in this chapter into categories is about 9 to 1 if the number of individual, discrete diagnoses (diagnosis entity terms) is represented by the number of references listed in column 1. Thus the first row shows that 21 terms were allocated to the one category, code 390. The last line in the table, a summary, shows that 3,550 terms were found in 395 categories.

2. The numbers of references in the Alphabetic Index to each of the available categories in Chapter 7 varies from 0 to over 70.

3. Column 3 shows the titles of the categories. Each of the 21 terms which contributed to the count in the first row would be retrieved with the single category term "Rheumatic fever without mention of heart involvement."

4. Scanning column 3 gives the "flavor" of the terms retrieved throughout the chapter.

5. Numerous combination categories can be seen, e.g., "Rheumatic fever with heart involvement."

6. The numbers of "other" categories is impressive. Such categories are sometimes useful for statistics, but for clinical purposes, the user must know what the categories were that were *not* "other," and the content of the "other" would still be a mystery.

7. A number of categories, those with "-" in the first column in the Table, were not referenced in Volume 2 of the CD-ROM version of *ICD-9-CM*. Some of these categories, e.g., 459.81, peripheral venous insufficiency, are, however, found in the printed version of Volume 2. Other categories, e.g., 405, Secondary hypertension, are the headings of subdivided categories, and presumably all relevant diagnoses were placed in the subdivisions.

Figure K.1 Chapter 7 of ICD-9-CM — Index References to Categories

Number of references in Alphabetic Index	Category Code (in Tabular List)	Rubric (Label) of Category in Tabular List
21	390	Rheumatic fever without mention of heart involvement
1	391	Rheumatic fever with heart involvement
5	391.0	Acute rheumatic pericarditis
16	391.1	Acute rheumatic endocarditis
11	391.2	Acute rheumatic myocarditis
13	391.8	Other acute rheumatic heart disease
9	391.9	Acute rheumatic heart disease, unspecified
-	392	Rheumatic chorea
32	392.0	With heart involvement
2	392.9	Without mention of heart involvement
14	393	Chronic rheumatic pericarditis
-	394	Diseases of mitral valve
2	394.0	Mitral stenosis
1	394.1	Rheumatic mitral insufficiency
3	394.2	Mitral stenosis with insufficiency
5	394.9	Other and unspecified mitral valve diseases
-	395	Diseases of aortic valve

Figure K.1 Chapter 7 of ICD-9-CM — Index References to Categories *(continued)*

2	395.0	Rheumatic aortic stenosis
1	395.1	Rheumatic aortic insufficiency
2	395.2	Rheumatic aortic stenosis with insufficiency
4	395.9	Other and unspecified rheumatic aortic diseases
-	396	Diseases of mitral and aortic valves
5	396.0	Mitral valve stenosis and aortic valve stenosis
6	396.1	Mitral valve stenosis and aortic valve insufficiency
4	396.2	Mitral valve insufficiency and aortic valve stenosis
6	396.3	Mitral valve insufficiency and aortic valve insufficiency
6	396.8	Multiple involvement of mitral and aortic valves
7	396.9	Mitral and aortic valve diseases, unspecified
-	397	Diseases of other endocardial structures
7	397.0	Diseases of tricuspid valve
3	397.1	Rheumatic diseases of pulmonary valve
4	397.9	Rheumatic diseases of endocardium, valve unspecified
-	398	Other rheumatic heart disease
15	398.0	Rheumatic myocarditis
24	398.9	Other and unspecified rheumatic heart diseases
-	398.90	Rheumatic heart disease, unspecified
-	398.91	Rheumatic heart failure (congestive)
-	398.99	Other
-	401	Essential hypertension
3	401.0	Malignant
1	401.1	Benign
-	401.9	Unspecified

Figure K.1 Chapter 7 of ICD-9-CM — Index References to Categories *(continued)*

3	402	Hypertensive heart disease
16	402.0	Malignant
-	402.00	Without congestive heart failure
-	402.01	With congestive heart failure
15	402.1	Benign
-	402.10	Without congestive heart failure
-	402.11	With congestive heart failure
27	402.9	Unspecified
-	402.90	Without congestive heart failure
-	402.91	With congestive heart failure
2	403	Hypertensive renal disease
11	403.0	Malignant
7	403.1	Benign
45	403.9	Unspecified
-	404	Hypertensive heart and renal disease
13	404.0	Malignant
14	404.1	Benign
40	404.9	Unspecified
-	405	Secondary hypertension
42	405.0	Malignant
-	405.01	Renovascular
-	405.09	Other
42	405.1	Benign
-	405.11	Renovascular
-	405.19	Other
43	405.9	Unspecified

Figure K.1 **Chapter 7 of ICD-9-CM — Index References to Categories** *(continued)*

-	405.91	Renovascular
-	405.99	Other
2	410	Acute myocardial infarction
1	410.0	Of anterolateral wall
4	410.1	Of other anterior wall
1	410.2	Of inferolateral wall
2	410.3	Of inferoposterior wall
2	410.4	Of other inferior wall
5	410.5	Of other lateral wall
3	410.6	True posterior wall infarction
4	410.7	Subendocardial infarction
8	410.8	Of other specified sites
43	410.9	Unspecified site
-	411	Other acute and subacute forms of ischemic heart disease
5	411.0	Postmyocardial infarction syndrome
13	411.1	Intermediate coronary syndrome
20	411.8	Other
17	412	Old myocardial infarction
-	413	Angina pectoris
2	413.0	Angina decubitus
3	413.1	Prinzmetal angina
13	413.9	Other and unspecified angina pectoris
-	414	Other forms of chronic ischemic heart disease
7	414.0	Coronary atherosclerosis
13	414.1	Aneurysm of heart
-	414.10	Of heart (wall)

Figure K.1 Chapter 7 of ICD-9-CM — Index References to Categories (continued)

-	414.11	Of coronary vessels
-	414.19	Other
8	414.8	Other specified forms of chronic ischemic heart disease
12	414.9	Chronic ischemic heart disease, unspecified
-	415	Acute pulmonary heart disease
3	415.0	Acute cor pulmonale
7	415.1	Pulmonary embolism and infarction
-	416	Chronic pulmonary heart disease
15	416.0	Chronic pulmonary heart disease
2	416.1	Primary pulmonary hypertension
4	416.8	Other chronic pulmonary heart diseases
7	416.9	Chronic pulmonary heart disease, unspecified
-	417	Other diseases of pulmonary circulation
5	417.0	Arteriovenous fistula of pulmonary vessels
2	417.1	Aneurysm of pulmonary artery
21	417.8	Other specified diseases of pulmonary circulation
2	417.9	Unspecified disease of pulmonary circulation
-	420	Acute pericarditis
15	420.0	Acute pericarditis in diseases of classified elsewhere
34	420.9	Other and unspecified acute pericarditis
-	420.90	Acute pericarditis, unspecified
-	420.91	Acute idiopathic pericarditis
-	420.99	Other
-	421	Acute and subacute endocarditis
32	421.0	Acute and subacute bacterial endocarditis

Figure K.1 Chapter 7 of ICD-9-CM — Index References to Categories *(continued)*

6	421.1	Acute and subacute infective endocarditis in diseases classified elsewhere
8	421.9	Acute endocarditis, unspecified
-	422	Acute myocarditis
14	422.0	Acute myocarditis in diseases classified elsewhere
29	422.9	Other and unspecified acute myocarditis
-	422.90	Acute myocarditis, unspecified
-	422.91	Idiopathic myocarditis
-	422.92	Septic myocarditis
-	422.93	Toxic myocarditis
-	422.99	Other
-	423	Other diseases of pericardium
3	423.0	Hemopericardium
14	423.1	Adhesive pericarditis
22	423.2	Constrictive pericarditis
10	423.8	Other specified diseases of pericardium
20	423.9	Unspecified disease of pericardium
-	424	Other diseases if endocardium
21	424.0	Mitral valve disorders
29	424.1	Aortic valve disorders
8	424.2	Tricuspid valve disorders, specified as nonrheumatic
21	424.3	Pulmonary valve disorders
39	424.9	Endocarditis, valve unspecified
-	424.90	Endocarditis, valve unspecified, unspecified cause
-	424.91	Endocarditis in diseases classified elsewhere
-	424.99	Other

Figure K.1 Chapter 7 of ICD-9-CM — Index References to Categories *(continued)*

-	425	Cardiomyopathy
4	425.0	Endomyocardial fibrosis
8	425.1	Hypertrophic obstructive cardiomyopathy
8	425.2	Obscure cardiomyopathy of Africa
7	425.3	Endocardial fibroelastosis
12	425.4	Other primary cardiomyopathies
7	425.5	Alcoholic cardiomyopathy
51	425.7	Nutritional and metabolic cardiomyopathy
22	425.8	Cardiomyopathy in other diseases classified elsewhere
4	425.9	Secondary cardiomyopathy, unspecified
1	426	Conduction disorders
15	426.0	Atrioventricular block, complete
19	426.1	Atrioventricular block, other and unspecified
-	426.10	Atrioventricular block, unspecified
-	426.11	First degree atrioventricular block
-	426.12	Mobitz (type) II atrioventricular block
-	426.13	Other second degree atrioventricular block
7	426.2	Left bundle branch hemiblock
8	426.3	Other left bundle branch block
7	426.4	Right bundle branch block
22	426.5	Bundle branch block, other and unspecified
-	426.50	Bundle branch block, unspecified
-	426.51	Right bundle branch block and left posterior fascicular block
-	426.52	Right bundle branch block and left anterior fascicular block

Figure K.1 Chapter 7 of ICD-9-CM — Index References to Categories *(continued)*

-	426.53	Other bilateral bundle branch block
-	426.54	Trifascicular block
19	426.6	Other heart block
11	426.7	Anomalous atrioventricular excitation
13	426.8	Other specified conduction disorders
-	426.81	Lown-Ganong-Levine syndrome
-	426.89	Other
20	426.9	Conduction disorder, unspecified
1	427	Cardiac dysrhythmias
11	427.0	Paroxysmal supraventricular tachycardia
5	427.1	Paroxysmal ventricular tachycardia
8	427.2	Paroxysmal tachycardia, unspecified
6	427.3	Atrial fibrillation and flutter
5	427.4	Ventricular fibrillation and flutter
-	427.41	Ventricular fibrillation
-	427.42	Ventricular flutter
8	427.5	Cardiac arrest
39	427.6	Premature beats
-	427.60	Premature beats, unspecified
-	427.61	Supraventicular premature beats
-	427.69	Other
62	427.8	Other specified cardiac dysrhythmias
-	427.81	Sinoatrial node dysfunction
-	427.89	Other
12	427.9	Cardiac dysrhythmia, unspecified
4	428	Heart failure

Figure K.1 Chapter 7 of ICD-9-CM — Index References to Categories *(continued)*

35	428.0	Congestive heart failure
18	428.1	Left heart failure
28	428.9	Heart failure, unspecified
-	429	Ill-defined descriptions and complications of heart disease
16	429.0	Myocarditis, unspecified
46	429.1	Myocardial degeneration
11	429.2	Cardiovascular disease, unspecified
11	429.3	Cardiomegaly
35	429.4	Functional disturbances following cardiac surgery
3	429.5	Rupture of chordae tendineae
2	429.6	Rupture of papillary muscle
14	429.7	Certain sequelae of myocardial infarction, not elsewhere classified
-	429.71	Acquired cardiac septal defect
-	429.79	Other
34	429.8	Other ill-defined heart diseases
-	429.81	Other disorders of papillary muscle
-	429.82	Hyperkinetic heart disease
-	429.89	Other
14	429.9	Heart disease, unspecified
42	430	Subarachnoid hemorrhage
33	431	Intracerebral hemorrhage
-	432	Other and unspecified intracranial hemorrhage
4	432.0	Nontraumatic extradural hemorrhage
5	432.1	Subdural hemorrhage
5	432.9	Unspecified intracranial hemorrhage

Figure K.1 Chapter 7 of ICD-9-CM — Index References to Categories *(continued)*

-	433	Occlusion and stenosis of precerebral arteries
9	433.0	Basilar artery
11	433.1	Carotid artery
7	433.2	Vertebral artery
18	433.3	Multiple and bilateral
47	433.8	Other specified precerebral artery
4	433.9	Unspecified precerebral artery
-	434	Occlusion of cerebral arteries
21	434.0	Cerebral thrombosis
20	434.1	Cerebral embolism
12	434.9	Cerebral artery occlusion, unspecified
1	435	Transient cerebral ischemia
5	435.0	Basilar artery syndrome
11	435.1	Vertebral artery syndrome
3	435.2	Subclavian steal syndrome
7	435.8	Other specified transient cerebral ischemias
29	435.9	Unspecified transient cerebral ischemia
71	436	Acute, but ill-defined, cerebrovascular disease
-	437	Other and ill-defined cerebrovascular disease
27	437.0	Cerebral atherosclerosis
11	437.1	Other generalized ischemic cerebrovascular disease
10	437.2	Hypertensive encephalopathy
11	437.3	Cerebral aneurysm, nonruptured
4	437.4	Cerebral arteritis
4	437.5	Moyamoya disease

Figure K.1 Chapter 7 of ICD-9-CM — Index References to Categories *(continued)*

7	437.6	Nonpyogenic thrombosis of intracranial venous sinus
2	437.7	Transient global amnesia
35	437.8	Other
15	437.9	Unspecified
64	438	Late effects of cerebrovascular disease
1	440	Atherosclerosis
10	440.0	Of aorta
10	440.1	Of renal artery
49	440.2	Of native arteries of the extremities
-	440.20	Atherosclerosis of the extremities, unspecified
-	440.21	Atherosclerosis of the extremities with intermittent claudication
-	440.22	Atherosclerosis of the extremities with rest pain
-	440.23	Atherosclerosis of the extremities with ulceration
-	440.24	Atherosclerosis of the extremities with gangrene
-	440.29	Other
9	440.3	Of bypass graft of the extremities
6	440.8	Of other specified arteries
3	440.9	Generalized and unspecified atherosclerosis
-	441	Aortic aneurysm
27	441.0	Dissecting aneurysm
-	441.00	Unspecified site
-	441.01	Thoracic
-	441.02	Abdominal
-	441.03	Thoracoabdominal
12	441.1	Thoracic aneurysm, ruptured

Figure K.1 Chapter 7 of ICD-9-CM — Index References to Categories *(continued)*

7	441.2	Thoracic aneurysm without mention of rupture
5	441.3	Abdominal aneurysm, ruptured
3	441.4	Abdominal aneurysm without mention of rupture
13	441.5	Aortic aneurysm of unspecified site, ruptured
3	441.6	Thoracoabdominal aneurysm, with mention of rupture
2	441.7	Thoracoabdominal aneurysm, without mention of rupture
14	441.9	Aortic aneurysm of unspecified site without mention of rupture
-	442	Other aneurysm
3	442.0	Of artery of upper extremity
1	442.1	Of renal artery
2	442.2	Of iliac artery
3	442.3	Of artery of lower extremity
17	442.8	Of other specified artery
-	442.81	Artery of neck
-	442.82	Subclavian artery
-	442.83	Splenic artery
-	442.84	Other visceral artery
-	442.89	Other
7	442.9	Of unspecified
-	443	Other peripheral vascular disease
10	443.0	Raynaud's syndrome
5	443.1	Thromboangiitis obliterans (Buerger's disease)
30	443.8	Other specified peripheral vascular diseases
-	443.81	Peripheral angiopathy in diseases classified elsewhere

Figure K.1 Chapter 7 of ICD-9-CM — Index References to Categories *(continued)*

-	443.89	Other
45	443.9	Peripheral vascular disease, unspecified
-	444	Arterial embolism and thrombosis
14	444.0	Of abdominal aorta
4	444.1	Of thoracic aorta
28	444.2	Of arteries of the extremities
-	444.21	Upper extremity
-	444.22	Lower extremity
15	444.8	Of other specified artery
-	444.81	Iliac artery
-	444.89	Other
12	444.9	Of unspecified artery
-	446	Polyarteritis nodosa and allied conditions
19	446.0	Polyarteritis nodosa
5	446.1	Acute febrile mucocutaneous lymph node syndrome [MCLS]
17	446.2	Hypersensitivity angiitis
-	446.20	Hypersensitivity angiitis, unspecified
-	446.21	Goodpasture's syndrome
6	446.3	Lethal midline granuloma
9	446.4	Wegener's granulomatosis
12	446.5	Giant cell arteritis
16	446.6	Thrombotic microangiopathy
22	446.7	Takayasu's disease
-	447	Other disorders of arteries and arterioles
3	447.0	Arteriovenous fistula, acquired
17	447.1	Stricture of artery

Figure K.1 **Chapter 7 of ICD-9-CM — Index References to Categories** *(continued)*

8	447.2	Rupture of artery
7	447.3	Hyperplasia of renal artery
12	447.4	Celiac artery compression syndrome
2	447.5	Necrosis of artery
9	447.6	Arteritis, unspecified
41	447.8	Other specified disorders of arteries and arterioles
7	447.9	Unspecified disorders of arteries and arterioles
-	448	Diseases of capillaries
22	448.0	Hereditary hemorrhagic telangiectasia
18	448.1	Nevus, non-neoplastic
16	448.9	Other and unspecified capillary diseases
-	451	Phlebitis and thrombophlebitis
14	451.0	Of superficial vessels of lower extremities
42	451.1	Of deep vessels of lower extremities
-	451.11	Femoral vein (deep) (superficial)
-	451.19	Other
10	451.2	Of lower extremities, unspecified
44	451.8	Of other sites
-	451.81	Iliac vein
-	451.82	Of superficial veins of upper extremities
-	451.83	Of deep veins of upper extremities
-	451.84	Of upper extremities, unspecified
-	451.89	Other
10	451.9	Of unspecified site
8	452	Portal vein thrombosis
-	453	Other venous embolism and thrombosis

Figure K.1 Chapter 7 of ICD-9-CM — Index References to Categories *(continued)*

10	453.0	Budd-Chiari syndrome
6	453.1	Thrombophlebitis migrans
3	453.2	Of vena cava
3	453.3	Of renal vein
18	453.8	Of other specified veins
7	453.9	Of unspecified site
-	454	Varicose veins of lower extremities
10	454.0	With ulcer
13	454.1	With inflammation
19	454.2	With ulcer and inflammation
6	454.9	Without mention of ulcer or inflammation
-	455	Hemorrhoids
1	455.0	Internal hemorrhoids without mention of complication
2	455.1	Internal thrombosed hemorrhoids
6	455.2	Internal hemorrhoids with other complication
1	455.3	External hemorrhoids without mention of complication
2	455.4	External thrombosed hemorrhoids
6	455.5	External hemorrhoids with other complication
1	455.6	Unspecified hemorrhoids without mention of complication
1	455.7	Unspecified thrombosed hemorrhoids
5	455.8	Unspecified hemorrhoids with other complication
8	455.9	Residual hemorrhoidal skin tags
-	456	Varicose veins of other sites
7	456.0	Esophageal varices with bleeding

Figure K.1 Chapter 7 of ICD-9-CM — Index References to Categories *(continued)*

6	456.1	Esophageal varices without mention of bleeding
6	456.2	Esophageal varices in diseased classified elsewhere
-	456.20	With bleeding
-	456.21	Without mention of bleeding
3	456.3	Sublingual varices
7	456.4	Scrotal varices
9	456.5	Pelvic varices
9	456.6	Vulval varices
19	456.8	Varices of other sites
-	457	Noninfectious disorders of lymphatic channels
11	457.0	Postmastectomy lymphedema syndrome
24	457.1	Other lymphedema
6	457.2	Lymphangitis
24	457.8	Other noninfectious disorders of lymphatic channels
2	457.9	Unspecified noninfectious disorder of lymphatic channels
-	458	Hypotension
2	458.0	Orthostatic hypotension
2	458.1	Chronic hypotension
7	458.9	Hypotension, unspecified
-	459	Other disorders of circulatory system
31	459.0	Hemorrhage, unspecified
2	459.1	Postphlebitic syndrome
18	459.2	Compression of vein
33	459.8	Other specified disorders of circulatory system

Figure K.1 Chapter 7 of ICD-9-CM — Index References to Categories *(continued)*

-	459.81	Venous (peripheral) insufficiency, unspecified
-	459.89	Other
33	459.9	Unspecified circulatory system disorder
3550		TOTAL REFERENCES (in 395 categories)

L

NCVHS – 1993 Annual Report

THE FULL TEXT of the 1993 Annual Report of the United States National Committee on Vital and Health Statistics is reproduced here because of its comprehensive discussion of procedure classification. It should be noted that the Report's authors make no clear distinction between "classification" and "coding," referring most frequently to a "procedure classification system," but also occasionally using "coding system" to refer to apparently the same thing. In the context of *The Endangered Medical Record*, the NCVHS is in fact recommending a "procedure *coding* system" as we have distinguished between coding and classification.[1]

The current product commissioned by the Health Care Financing Administration, the *ICD-10 Procedure Coding System* (*ICD-10-PCS*), is precisely such a coding system, not a classification (see page 191).

Executive Summary

During 1993 the National Committee on Vital and Health Statistics (NCVHS), in its advisory capacity to the Department of Health and Human Services (DHHS), accomplished the following activities through the work of the full Committee, seven subcommittees, a work group, and several monitors:

- Held a series of discussions with policymakers within the Department to consider information needs for health reform. Emphasized the importance of uniform data standards and policies in meeting these needs.

- Completed a major report recommending development and adoption of a single system for classification of healthcare services and procedures to be used in all settings in which healthcare is delivered in the United States. Preparation of the report included extensive consultation with a wide range of organizations and individuals who have a stake in procedure classification. The report, which was transmitted to the Secretary, is contained in appendix V.

---

1. See "Code or classification?," page 117.

- Presented its recommendations on procedure classification at a Symposium on Coding and Classification Issues sponsored by the American Health Information Management Association.

- Transmitted to the Assistant Secretary for Health a significant report related to State and local capacity to perform the core public health function of assessment and to use data for policy development and assurance. The report was the result of 2 years of study and deliberation and recommended that the Department develop and implement a strategy to establish a coordinated Federal, State, and community health statistics system to support the health policy process. The report can be found in appendix VI.

- Developed a detailed draft report on findings and recommendations concerning long-term care data gaps and issues, bringing to closure a series of meetings to review numerous national surveys and receive testimony from a wide array of experts in the field. Several recommendations concerning planned and proposed data collection efforts that require timely action by the Department were transmitted to the Assistant Secretary for Health. The full report will be finalized for submission to the Department in early 1994.

- Responded to the report and recommendations of the Interagency Task Force on the Uniform Hospital Discharge Data Set (UHDDS), reaffirming the major recommendations included in the NCVHS Proposed Revision to the UHDDS submitted to the Assistant Secretary for Health in 1992.

- Wrote to the Assistant Secretary for Health and the Administrator of the Health Care Financing Administration (HCFA) urging that the Department dedicate the necessary resources to determine the feasibility of implementing the 10th revision of the *International Classification of Diseases (ICD-10)* for morbidity application in the United States.

- Jointly sponsored with the National Center for Health Statistics (NCHS) a special meeting to obtain public comments on needed revisions of the World Health Organization's *International Classification of Impairments, Disabilities, and Handicaps (ICIDH)* for applications in the United States.

- Agreed to keep the ICIDH on the NCVHS agenda in order to be supportive of the revision process, facilitate sharing of information, and foster articulation of a U.S. approach.

- Initiated a process to receive input on possible revisions to the recommendations contained in the report on the Uniform Ambulatory Care Data Set submitted to the Department by the NCVHS and an Interagency Task Force in 1989.

- Continued efforts to encourage HCFA and the Social Security Administration to improve current and future racial and ethnic identifiers in the Medicare administrative data bases.

- Encouraged development by the NCHS Minority Health Statistics Grants Program of a summer institute on methods and materials related to minority health statistics and continued to monitor the implementation of the grants program.

- Reviewed plans by the National Institute of Mental Health (NIMH) for a child epidemiological catchment area project and provided NIMH with several recommendations concerning implementation of the project and related methodological research.

- Monitored efforts by NCHS to develop appropriate mental health status measures for the National Health Interview Survey.

- Received a briefing on issues of data access and privacy as they might impact on the ability to monitor and assess healthcare reform and appointed a Committee liaison for ongoing monitoring of these issues.

- Participated in a Conference on Health Records: Social Needs and Personal Privacy, sponsored by the DHHS Task Force on the Privacy of Private-Sector Health Records.

- Participated in an NCHS-sponsored Workshop on Family Data and Family Health Policy issues.

- Reviewed and provided comments on the 1992 and 1993 publications of Health, United States.

In 1994 the Committee will continue and expand efforts related to many of the above activities.

Appendix V. Recommendations for a Single Procedure Classification System, November 1993

Summary and Recommendations

In its capacity as advisor to the Secretary of Health and Human Services, the National Committee on Vital Health Statistics (NCVHS) has for years been concerned with the manner in which patient classification systems contribute to health data. The Medical Classification Subcommittee of NCVHS is charged with the responsibility of identifying circumstances when evolving health data needs create requirements for changes in classification systems or processes for system maintenance and updating. Classification systems play a crucial role in nearly all uses of health data, including reimbursement, outcomes research, and program evaluation. If such systems are deficient, the uses of health data are inevitably compromised.

This report concerns the systems used in the United States for classifying medical and related services and procedures. The Committee has evaluated substantial information over a long period indicating that existing systems are structurally flawed and wastefully redundant. Over the past year, the Subcommittee sought advice from a wide range of organizations and individuals who have a stake in procedure classification. Although there was considerable diversity of opinion on priorities and potential solutions to the current situation, there was also consistent support for the concept of moving as quickly as possible to a single, unified system. It is largely on the basis of this support that the Subcommittee advised the full Committee that the need for action was evident.

A combination of forces make movement to a single system timely. First, existing systems are increasingly limited in their ability to meet the evolving needs for procedure classification. The growing requirements to classify new procedures and to more fully describe preventive and primary care services, for example, have outstripped the capacities of existing systems. Specifically, we are running out of code numbers in each of the existing systems. Also, the two systems (*International Classification of Diseases, 9th edition, Clinical*

Modification and *Physicians' Current Procedural Terminology*) cannot be combined or crosswalked, and neither can be "fixed" without a complete overhaul (that is, creating a new classification).

Second, existing systems are incapable of permitting recent advances in information technology to create the data bases necessary to evaluate an increasingly complicated healthcare technology. The need to evaluate healthcare on the basis of health outcomes demands data that describe the full range of services provided for treatment of given illnesses and conditions. Continued use of existing procedure classification systems presents a serious obstacle to accomplishing this goal.

Third, and most important, the healthcare reform movement presents a window of opportunity and an intensified need to consolidate procedure classification. Healthcare reform will require substantial retooling of healthcare data systems. Reform of procedure classification can be accomplished as part of this retooling effort, rather than as a completely separate endeavor. New healthcare financing and delivery systems that are created through healthcare reform will require monitoring to evaluate their effects and data to design improvements. This need is evident regardless of whether the significant reforms are enacted at the Federal, State, or private sector level.

For these reasons, as explained in greater detail below, the NCVHS is recommending to the Secretary of Health and Human Services that immediate steps be taken to create a single procedure classification system for multiple purposes in the United States. The Committee believes that the social benefits of this action would outweigh the social costs, and that the time is right to implement a change of this magnitude. Despite our conviction that this is the proper course, however, the Committee recognizes that important questions remain about how to proceed to a unified system and what precisely the system should look like. The Committee, therefore, intends to continue its deliberations on this issue and provide more concrete recommendations and consultations with components of Department of Health and Human Services (DHHS) and the private sector over the coming months.

Recommendations

- The National Committee on Vital and Health Statistics recommends development and adoption of a single system for classification of healthcare services and procedures to be used in all settings in which healthcare is delivered in the United States.

- The Secretary of the Department of Health and Human Services should assume the responsibility for the development and maintenance of a single classification system as a collaborative effort involving those who have an interest or stake in a new system.

- Development of the single procedure classification system should be given immediate priority, and implementation should be coordinated with national health reform.

- The Secretary should ensure that the system is easy to use, comprehensive, hierarchical, flexible, and serves present and future needs in the public and private sectors of healthcare.

- Adequate resources must be provided to support all aspects of development, implementation, evaluation, education, and maintenance.

Background

Two major classification systems are used to code medical procedures in the United States. Volume 3 of the *International Classification of Diseases, 9th edition, Clinical Modification (ICD-9-CM)* was developed in the United States to classify procedures performed during inpatient hospital stays. The *Physicians' Current Procedural Terminology (CPT)* system was developed by the American Medical Association (AMA) to classify procedures performed by physicians in inpatient and ambulatory settings. The two classifications have widely differing conceptual foundations, maintenance and updating systems, advantages, and limitations. Payment and other considerations require both classifications to be coded when the patient is hospitalized. The two systems are sufficiently different that they cannot be "crosswalked" on a code to code basis.

Both systems are used for multiple purposes, including research and payment. The *ICD-9-CM* system, for example, is integral to the creation of Diagnosis Related Groups (DRG's), which are used for payment under the Medicare Prospective Payment System. The CPT system is the core of the Health Care Financing Administration (HCFA) Common Procedure Coding System (HCPCS), which is used for Medicare reimbursement of noninstitutional providers of health services. Non-CPT components of HCPCS are used for many nonphysician-provided services.

Having two systems for coding procedures is costly for providers of care, who frequently must code both systems for the same services. It is also unproductive for research and administrative purposes to have two systems because care delivered for episodes of illness cannot always be tracked across different provider settings. However, it is costly to change; the two systems are widely used and replacement with a consolidated single system would be disruptive and expensive. Even though few would agree that the present dual system is ideal, there will be considerable resistance to movement to a single system, because of transitional costs and other factors.

Despite these costs, interest in a unified classification system is widespread. Congressman Fortney "Pete" Stark, for example, introduced a bill (H.R. 1255) in the 103rd Congress that would require the development of a "single uniform coding system for diagnostic and procedure codes." Although this provision is part of a program to reduce fraud and abuse in the Medicare program, and the bill apparently has been tabled in favor of incorporation into the larger healthcare reform legislative initiative, it is indicative of congressional interest in rationalizing procedure classification.

NCVHS has monitored medical procedure classification for over a decade. The Committee recommended moving to a single procedure classification system in 1986. In 1993 the Committee believes that the need to consolidate procedure classification is even more compelling. The NCVHS Subcommittee on Medical Classification Systems undertook anew a review of procedure classification beginning in 1992. The Subcommittee sought advice from a wide range of organizations and individuals who have a stake in procedure classification.

Initially, we sought information on the attributes and deficiencies of existing procedure classification systems. Second, we solicited feedback on the Subcommittee's provisional recommendations for the development and implementation of a single system. Information on persons and organizations responding to the Subcommittee's inquiries appears on pp. 71-75 [not reproduced here].

Most of the individuals who provided detailed information to the Subcommittee, particularly those who use procedure classification systems or represent system users, expressed frustration at the current state of procedure classification in the United States. They were frustrated by the deficiencies of each system and by the necessity of coding both systems, sometimes on the same cases. Although it is not possible to provide an exhaustive list of system deficiencies, some of the frequently cited problems with *ICD-9-CM* (volume 3) and CPT are shown in exhibit 1. These problems were culled from correspondence and from minutes of Subcommittee meetings.

The *ICD-9-CM* system is seen by many respondents as the better one of the two at meeting criteria for a "good" classification, such as a hierarchical structure, but woefully lacking in specificity and detail. The CPT system is more detailed, but narrowly oriented to physicians' services and poorly structured as a classification system. Both systems share many deficiencies, such as lack of space for expansion, overlapping codes, and inconsistent use of terminology. Most of the system critics did not believe that either system is "fixable" for the long term, and therefore neither system should be viewed as a potential candidate for becoming the single classification for all-purpose usage in the United States.

Certain advantages of the two systems were also pointed out. The structure established by the American Medical Association to update the CPT represents a serious effort to maintain currency with technological advancement. The broad-based foundation of the *ICD-9-CM* system in the international disease classification community was also seen as a positive attribute. None of these advantages, however, emerged as a sufficient justification to prefer one system over the other.

In the summer of 1993 a draft of the Subcommittee's report and recommendations was sent to a mailing list of organizations and individuals having a stake in procedure classification and its potential reform. Twenty-eight written responses from individuals representing themselves or constituent organizations were received. Respondent positions on the need for moving toward a single system of procedure classification, as articulated by the Subcommittee in its draft report, are summarized in exhibit 2.

The results of this inquiry are striking because positions adopted by respondents tend to be determined by their discipline or the type of organization they represent. All of the health information management respondents, including coders in the field, were in favor of moving to a single system. In contrast, nearly all physicians or representatives of medical organizations oppose this position. Allied (nonphysician) health occupations favored moving to a unified system, provided that their constituents were represented in system design and implementation issues. Responses of other organizations, such as government agencies and insurance organizations, were mixed.

These responses do not constitute a representative sample of all who might be affected by procedure classification or its overhaul. Nevertheless, the responses appear to provide a consistent message that should be recognized when procedure classification reform proceeds further. Medical organizations, probably because of their control of the CPT updating process through the auspices of the American Medical Association, tend not to see a need for change.

Other types of organizations do see this need because of the deficiencies in the current systems and because of the perceived lack of representation in the maintenance and control of procedure classification. Careful planning of the participation of stakeholders in the design, implementation, and maintenance of a new system will be required.

Exhibit 1: Commonly Cited Flaws of ICD-9-CM and CPT-4 Procedure Classification Systems

Both Classifications

- lack of space for expansion
- overlapping and duplicative codes
- inconsistent and noncurrent use of terminology
- lack of codes for preventive services

ICD-9-CM (volume 3)

- insufficient specificity and detail
- insufficient structure to capture new technology

CPT-4

- nonhierarchical structure
- physician service orientation (not multidisciplinary)
- poorly defined, nondiscrete coding categories, with variable coding detail

Exhibit 2: Position on Moving to a Single Procedure Classification System by Respondent Type[2]

Type of Respondent	Pro	Con	Neutral[a]	Total
Health Information Management	7	0	0	7
Medical Organizations and Clinicians	1	8	0	9
Allied Health Professionals	4	0	0	4
Others	4	1	3	8
Total	16	9	3	28

a. No position stated.

2. Based on written responses to the Subcommittee's second mailing soliciting comments on the draft report and recommendations.

Benefits and Costs of a Single Procedure Classification System

The Subcommittee discussed the pros and cons of recommending a single procedure classification system, continuation of the present situation with multiple classification systems, or some third alternative. After reviewing feedback from the field, the Subcommittee decided that a single procedure classification system is by far the preferred option.

Pursuing the development of a single procedure classification system will provide a unique opportunity to develop a refined system by retaining strengths and eliminating weaknesses of existing and tested systems. The Subcommittee recognizes that the cost of developing a single classification system is significant, but it also believes that the cost of NOT developing a single system would ultimately be more costly and harmful to the healthcare industry and to patients.

In the United States medical procedure classification is used for reimbursement and is also used for outcome evaluation. Adoption of a single coding scheme will facilitate development of integrated systems for procedure reimbursement in managed care and other settings. Better integration of data from inpatient and outpatient settings will improve the ability of researchers to develop diagnosis and procedure relationship studies, epidemiological studies, and statistical evaluation.

Conversion to a new system is ultimately less costly than maintenance and training on dual systems, which significantly add to the administrative burden. Current emphasis on streamlining administrative processes to reduce healthcare costs provides an opportunity for leadership directed to widespread adoption of automated patient records, hastening the abandonment of primitive computer systems, software, and paper forms.

In attempting to identify the benefits and costs of a single procedure classification system, the Subcommittee looked at potential effects on patients, providers, payers, and the research community.

Effect on Industry

The introduction of a new classification system will affect all levels of the healthcare industry. Long-term effects of a single procedure classification system can be categorized into the following areas: reimbursement, automation, and administrative and regulatory costs.

Reimbursement — A single procedure classification system will improve payment processing because reimbursement will be simplified by reducing the need to use dual systems for insurers who reimburse for services using CPT and *ICD-9-CM* volume 3 for physician procedures and hospital-based services. However, claims histories will have to be developed if no cross reference is available.

Intangible benefits would include less frustration on the part of coders and billers trying to use two systems. If the procedure classification system is tied to reimbursement, inpatient coding and documentation would be enhanced. Coders and billers could work together to improve the quality of their data instead of experiencing the competitiveness and fragmentation of different healthcare groups using different coding systems.

Automation — There is no doubt that the initial costs of converting to a new coding system will be significant. The largest cost will be in converting computer software used in the healthcare industry, especially if the new system differs dramatically from the currently used coding schemes. Industry costs for upgrading or altering computer systems (hardware and software) will be substantial. But it will be a one-time conversion of the coding system.

There will be a need to translate existing codes to the new system and a need for increased computer processing and storage. Validity of codes, data retrieval, crosswalks, and transition validity checks will be necessary. Sites where data are collected, processed, and analyzed will have to undergo modifications and behavioral changes by providers, payers, and researchers.

In the long run, however, it is reasonable to assume that it will be less costly to convert to a single coding system than it would be to continue indefinitely absorbing the costs to maintain training and education in *ICD-9-CM* and CPT. Automation might slow the reimbursement process initially but, once established, will facilitate reporting and paying.

Administrative and regulatory costs — For providers and insurers, a single system will reduce administrative costs of providing and maintaining data in two different systems. It will eliminate the need for multiple documentation, thereby reducing the amount of paper work needed to support different systems and improving claims processing. By providing a standardized vocabulary, a single procedure classification system will permit uniform communication among health professionals across healthcare settings and will facilitate utilization review.

Proponents of the present dual classification systems feel that increased administrative costs to initiate the system do not justify the problems incurred when other systems are already in place and could be improved to work better. For instance, maintenance mechanisms are in place in the CPT system for a physician consensus process. Timeliness with HCFA statutory regulatory requirements are in place. To meet the demands of allied health professionals who used the HCFA HCPCS based on the CPT, the AMA has organized a second Advisory Committee with representatives from major limited licensed practitioner groups. Major reservations have been expressed by others about the proprietary nature of the CPT and the role of the AMA in the maintenance of a system that is widely used for public purposes.

A new classification system will require a revision of all DRG's, Resource-Based Relative Value Scale (RBRVS) relative value units, and Ambulatory Patient Groups (APG's). Additional revisions of Uniform Bill-92 (UB-92) and HCFA 1500 forms, tumor registry abstracts, Medicare code editors, DRG groupers, and all automated encoders will be necessary. State Medicaid programs will require major changes and the Federal share of State costs would probably be significant. Many forms will have to be redesigned and printed and coding manuals revised.

Effect on Healthcare Delivery

A single procedure classification system will expedite development of treatment profiles associated with various configuration of demographic profiles and medical conditions across healthcare settings. A single system would aid in the development of needed improvements in medical record keeping, especially when combined with automation of medical records. Current physician documentation is often incomplete and abbreviated. An explicit structure will improve terminology and provide clarity and accuracy. This would facilitate understanding by entry level coders as well. Ultimately, complete documentation will help in the provision of improved healthcare to the patient.

Comparability of Data Across All Settings and Over Time

A single system for all healthcare settings will improve retrospective analysis and projections of cost and utilization and enhance analytic capability regarding episodes of care and provider practice habits. It will also allow better integration of data from inpatient and outpatient settings and the eventual merging of coding of all systems.

The Subcommittee recommends that the new coding structure be hierarchical, that is, data coded with the new system may be aggregated according to a predetermined structure. The Subcommittee feels such a structure will permit aggregation of clinical data for small area analysis to:

- detect patterns of over or under use,
- monitor outcomes,
- detect fraud,
- monitor archaic or ineffective procedures,
- distinguish clinical objectives of diagnostic, preventive, and therapeutic interventions,
- detect excessive device failure rates, and
- provide early warning of unacceptable procedural risks.

Coding is only as good as the patient source data available to coders who have to use the system. Initially, all parties will need cross reference data from the old to new system, including major software conversion. There could be an interruption of longitudinal data trends and comparability of longitudinal studies may be affected. There will be a need to develop a conversion system to cross-reference between pre- and post-crossover periods so that researchers can understand the new system and how it correlates to data already collected from existing systems.

Record Keeping and Data Retrieval

A single procedure classification system would facilitate the standardization of data collection and processing systems and reduce redundancy in data bases. The integrity of the data bank will improve with less complexity of computer applications. It would improve the environment for developing a standard electronic data collection system, thus, accelerating movement toward electronic patient records. With an automated system, data elements independent of classification can be collected easily for research and administrative purposes.

Most users do not need a complex detailed system. Office-based physicians may find new training costs especially burdensome in smaller practices but eventually the cost of data reporting would decrease and accuracy will improve with increasing familiarity of classification. Finally, a single procedure classification system will foster cooperation between coders and billers to improve the quality of data.

Maintenance and Training

Development and maintenance of the data processing system will be simplified, owing to the ease of a single system for reference. Revisions will be easier to maintain. A coordination and maintenance mechanism representing the public and private sectors needs to be established to oversee revisions to the classification system. It will be necessary to establish and staff a clearinghouse to provide end users with technical advice on the use of the system, validation of proper code assignments, and a forum to address common complaints.

Initial training costs will be high for health information managers, physicians and other health practitioners, payers, and researchers. Major industry investment in training and hiring more personnel will be required. But it is unrealistic to expect hospitals to bear all the costs for training and implementation. A federally mandated system should include a provision for a national training initiative. Overall, less training time will be needed once the new system is in place and users' familiarity with the new system improves. A single system will simplify ongoing training at facilities.

An additional side benefit could be the provision of career paths and ladders for experienced coding personnel, encouraging more people into the profession.

Characteristics of a Procedure Classification

The Subcommittee observed that the new system should be centered on the patient rather than on the needs of the institution. A procedure classification system should have the capability of capturing a procedure that can be used with other data elements for other purposes. Inherent in the recommendation is the need to agree upon a common definition of procedure classification boundaries.

Potential uses of data from procedure classification include:

- patient care evaluation
- program or systems management
- reimbursement
- effectiveness or outcome assessment
- health services and epidemiological research and trends
- policy development
- ability to make national or international comparisons

A single procedure classification system should facilitate data retrieval and analysis (see exhibit 3). The organization of the classification must be systematic and meaningful and should relieve users of the burden of assigning meanings and associations imposed by entity coding. Insignificant procedures should not be included ("omit code" notes in index).

A procedure classification system should have a hierarchical structure so that data from individual codes may be aggregated into increasingly larger groups of procedures. Each code number should have a unique definition that does not change over time. The system must be flexible enough to incorporate new techniques, technologies, and types of procedures. It must be comprehensive enough to include a place for every type of procedure used in all settings and by all provider groups. The categories must be discrete (that is, no overlap is permitted).

The system should be easy to use. This can be accomplished through standardization of definitions and terminology, and by adequate annotations in the tabular list and extensive and consistent indexing. The same procedure should be coded the same way regardless of the site or provider of care.

The system must be multi-axial in order to accommodate procedures performed on different body systems, using different techniques and technologies. It should be limited to the classification of procedures and should not attempt to incorporate diagnoses or other elements found elsewhere in the medical record.

Process to Establish a Single Procedure Classification System

The process of implementing a classification system should enunciate global issues concerning the applicability of a procedure classification system. Further, in highlighting these issues, it is necessary to identify the entities or major players responsible for addressing them. The global issues are as follows:

- clarity of the purpose(s) of the classification;
- criteria for its design components, auditable evaluation mechanisms, flexibility, and ability to incorporate new techniques;
- long range ramifications of implementation;
- maintenance mechanisms to update periodically;
- the need for cross-walks from *ICD-9-CM* (volume 3) and CPT to the new system for comparability of data over time, ease of implementation, etc.;
- multiple applications of a new procedure classification system, which distinguish between financial and reimbursement issues and statistical and epidemiological research issues; and,
- if feasible, tandem implementation with *ICD-10* to minimize impact upon users of the classification.

Figure L.1 NCVHS Exhibit 3

Exhibit 3: An Outline of the Characteristics of a Procedure Classification System

I.   Hierarchical structure
  A.   ability to aggregate data from individual codes into larger categories
  B.   each code has unique definition forever—not reused
II. Expandability
  A.   flexibility to incorporate new procedures and technologies ("empty" code numbers)
  B.   mechanisms for periodic updating
  C.   code expansion must not disrupt systematic code structures
III. Comprehensive
  A.   provides not otherwise specified (NOS) and not elsewhere classified (NEC) categories so that all possible procedures can be classified somewhere.
  B.   includes all types of procedures
    1.   diagnostic, therapeutic, and preventive procedures
    2.   invasive, noninvasive (including counseling, evaluation, and management)
  C.   applicability to all settings and types of providers
IV. Nonoverlapping
  A.   each procedure (or component of a procedure) is assigned to only one code
V.   Ease of use
  A.   standardization of definitions and terminology
  B.   adequate indexing and annotation for all users (physicians and nonphysicians)
VI. Setting and provider neutrality
  A.   same code regardless of who or where procedure is performed
  B.   discourage "turf battles"
VII. Multi-axial
  A.   body system(s) affected
  B.   technology used
  C.   techniques or approaches used
  D.   physiological effect or pharmacologic properties
  E.   characteristics or composition of implant
VIII.   Limited to classification of procedures
  A.   should not include diagnostic information
  B.   other data elements (such as age) should be elsewhere in the record

Development

The fundamental needs of a system that can serve multiple users (providers, payers, and researchers) across settings must be considered by assessing, as thoroughly as possible, benefits and costs of moving to a single classification system. Early on the components for a single classification system, including the political feasibility of the components, should be identified. Consideration of the necessary level of coding specificity, computer requirements, capacity and support for data collection, quality of data, and uses of information in all systems must also be made.

A major concern is the effect a new classification system would have on the human infrastructure (that is, the impact on health information managers, physicians and other providers, hospital administrators, third party payers, and researchers). There is a large range of abilities among coders (health information managers) and, depending upon its complexity, a new classification system may require sophistication that exceeds the abilities of health information managers accustomed to the current systems. Providers of services, especially physicians, may have to change the way they document procedures. This may require increased interaction between physicians and coders, particularly during the implementation phase.

Hospital administrators and third party payers will be affected because reimbursement mechanisms such as DRG's, relative value units, APG's, etc., will have to be revised to account for coding changes. Simple crosswalks between the old and new systems probably will not suffice or be possible.

A determination of the type of information necessary for a national database to conduct trend analyses should be made. For instance, researchers may have to develop new groups of old codes to allow analyses of groups of procedures rather than individual procedure codes. Translations will be necessary for certain key procedures to continue longitudinal trends.

Careful consideration should be given to ensure that the classification system does not inadvertently create incentives for the performance of one type of procedure over another (for example, by providing more detailed classification for invasive procedures than for noninvasive procedures). The new procedure classification system must also provide interspecialty balance. Procedures performed by specialists and providers other than physicians should be coded in a similar fashion to avoid reimbursement and evaluation discrepancies.

A single procedure classification system must be comprehensive and include all types of diagnostic, therapeutic, and preventive procedures across healthcare settings and for different types of providers. Accommodation must be made to include invasive procedures and noninvasive types of procedures, such as counseling, evaluation, and management of patients. This implies a need to reevaluate what is meant by "procedure."

Implementation

Natural and future constraints in implementing the new system should be recognized. Adequate lead time to implement the new system is paramount.

Field testing — It will be necessary to set up several demonstration projects to evaluate the costs, benefits, and impact of a new procedure coding system. The classification should be rigorously tested for validity and reliability by an independent agency employing real users with various levels of skill and experience in all settings in which the classification will be used. Results from the testing should be used to modify the classification and guidelines as necessary.

Training needs — Training needs for health information managers, physicians, third party payers, researchers, and others who will have to learn to use the new system must be accommodated. Training should be coordinated so that the same information is provided uniformly across sites and regions. Involving potential users in the development process will allow provider associations to assure that on-the-job training is accomplished.

Organizations such as the AMA, AHA (American Hospital Association), and AHIMA (American Health Information Management Association) as well as the Federal Government must identify resources to provide training for end users. The Federal Government should support the development and preparation of training packages.

A major "Train the Trainer" program should be developed and supported by the Federal Government and the healthcare industry. Training can be accomplished by training representatives of professional associations and societies. These members will train members of their profession at national, regional, State, and local meetings to develop informational networks and continuity of training efforts. Specialty societies can provide training to physicians as part of their continuing medical education program during their national membership meetings. Time should also be allocated to train key personnel in each healthcare setting who will be responsible for training others in their facilities.

Transition — Crosswalks between *ICD-9-CM* (volume 3) and the new system and CPT and the new system need to be developed. The feasibility of this must be investigated given the impossibility of developing a crosswalk between *ICD* and CPT. Software conversion programs will be needed, as well as increased computer processing and storage capacities.

An official source of crosswalk information should be in place before any change is implemented, and the identification of this source should be well publicized to all users. Responses to inquiries must be timely to ensure the integrity of the new classification coding system. Quality controls should be established to monitor the systems during the transition period and periodically to ensure conformity to the new system.

Maintenance

The implementation process must provide for a public forum to discuss maintenance issues and changes to the system similar to the role played by the *ICD-9-CM* Coordination and Maintenance Committee. As a central source, the functions of such a coordination and maintenance entity will be to:

- serve as a formal mechanism for maintenance of the system,
- serve as an official organ to inform users of revisions and updates,
- receive recommendations for revisions,
- make decisions about the grey areas ("appropriate exclusions"), and

- widely disseminate information on how the maintenance system operates and how to gain access to it

Evaluation

The ability to code procedures accurately and consistently is paramount in evaluating a new system. If providers are to code accurately, clarity of procedure definitions is essential. The quality of the data will be high and statistics retrieved from them will accurately reflect the care that was provided.

Evaluating a new system will require extensive testing and revision. At a minimum, the new system will have to be able to provide the types of data provided by the current systems. Intensive initial auditing will be required to determine how coding and data entry quality might have changed. Data analyzed under the new coding scheme will need to be compared with previous analysis to determine if any changes were attributable to the coding change itself or to actual systemic changes. Pilot auditing with automated medical records systems would be an efficient means of analyzing the data under both systems.

Ongoing monitoring in areas of quality assurance and utilization review by peer groups, third party payers, and other purchasers of care need to be established. Other monitoring mechanisms include: software edits, reabstraction, peer review organization (PRO) studies and audits to ensure coding data quality and quality of medical records documentation, and linking computerized medical records into on-line quality or utilization review.

Maintaining the validity of the system needs to be a cooperative effort involving those who perform the procedures reflected in the data, those who use the system to collect the data, and those who use the data to analyze healthcare issues and trends.

Conclusion

By virtue of being able to respond to changes in the clinical environment, the single procedure classification system should possess utility as a statistical classification and an administrative tool. There is a general resistance to altering the existing systems except where changes are considered necessary to reflect current clinical trends. Because of multiple deficiencies, however, the current systems are badly in need of overhaul and consolidation. Pressure for change derives not only from end users who must contend with these deficiencies, but also from political forces that must address major healthcare reform. As the healthcare reform movement progresses, reliance on administrative data sets will increase. The Committee notes, however, that these data sets currently do not permit the ability to track patients through the system as they enter and leave various care settings over the course of an illness or over a longer time. Reform measures adopted at all levels will require this tracking ability to evaluate the appropriateness and effectiveness of care received.

The scope of services covered by a single procedure classification system is not specified in this report. It seems clear that it should be broader than hospital and physician office-based provider services, the focus of current coding systems. On the other hand, there is a broad range of services, such as social services, housing, and some public health functions, that contribute to the health and well-being of the population but may not be appropriate to include in a classification system. Therefore, defining what is meant by "procedure" is a crucial initial task of developing a unified system.

The Committee realizes that recognition of the necessity for the development and implementation of a single procedure classification system is only the first step in a difficult and time consuming process of reform. Public and private sector resources will be required to achieve a successful and timely solution to the issues enumerated above. The Committee will continue its work in this area to provide more specific advice in system design and implementation alternatives and a forum where the stakeholders in procedure classification reform may present information and express their views.

M

Coding Resources

HEALTHCARE CODING in the United States today requires considerable training, plus additional reference and cross-reference materials. Below is an example of the extensiveness of this: a list of coding resources available in 1996 from the American Health Information Management Association (AHIMA).

Figure M.1 AHIMA Coding Resources

Author	Title[a]	Price	Comments
Graham	DRG Optimization	$56.00	
Rogers	Total Data Quality for the Coding Manager	$48.50	
Rogers	ICD-9-CM: Focus on Pediatrics	$48.50	
Albaum-Feinstein	DSM-IV to ICD-9-CM Crosswalk	$30.50	
Lee	Using the DSM-IV to ICD-9-CM Crosswalk	$30.50	
Nicholas	Basic ICD-9-CM Coding Handbook	$56.00	
Anderson	ICD-9-CM (self-study)	$185.00	Instructional materials only, no CE credit, no grading.
Anderson	ICD-9-CM: Beyond the Basics (self-study)	$225.00	Instructional materials only, no CE credit, no grading.

Figure M.1 AHIMA Coding Resources *(continued)*

Anderson	CPT: Beyond the Basics (self-study)	$225.00	Instructional materials only, no CE credit, no grading.
McGraw-Hill	ICD-9-CM 1996, Vol. 1, 2, & 3	$44.95	Two grades are offered.
McGraw-Hill	HCPCS 12996	$29.95	
Medicode	ICD-9-CM 1996 Standard, Vol. 1, 2, & 3	$49.95	Three grades are offered.
Medicode	CPT 1996, softbound	$44.95	Four grades are offered.
Medicode	HCPCS 1996	$39.95	
St. Anthony's	St. Anthony's Color Coded ICD-9-CM Code Book, Softbound Edition	$69.95	Three grades are offered, the second, illustrated is $89.95, the third is $139.
St. Anthony's	AMA CPT 1996 Code Book	$59.95	
St. Anthony's	HCPCS Level II 1996	$39.95	
Unicoder	Easy Coder ICD-9-CM 1996	$49.00	
Nicholas	CPT/HCPCS Basic Coding Handbook	$40.50	
Brown	ICD-9-CM Coding Handbook, revised edition (with answers)	$47.00	
Rowell	Understanding Medical Insurance: A Step-by-Step Guide, 3rd edition	$35.95	
Rogers	Intermediate ICD-9-CM Coding Handbook for Hospitals	$56.70	
HMA	Coding for Quality™ Introduction to APGs on Audiocassette	$89.00	Audiocassette.

Figure M.1 AHIMA Coding Resources *(continued)*

HMA	CPT Coding for Outpatient Surgery: A Comprehensive Guide	$149.00	
Finnegan	EduCode® Solo Courseware: Basic ICD-9-CM and Ambulatory Coding	$375.00	Software; each course is 12 CE credits.
"	" Intermediate Coding — I	$375.00	
"	" Intermediate Coding — II	$375.00	
"	" Intermediate Coding — III	$375.00	
"	" Intermediate Coding - IV	$375.00	
"	" Advanced Coding for Reimbursement	$375.00	
"	" HCPCS/CPT Coding — I	$375.00	
"	" HCPCS/CPT Coding — II	$375.00	
McGraw-Hill	The McGraw-Hill Complete RBRVS: The Resource Based Relative Value Scale	$89.95	
Graham	Advanced Clinical Topics for ICD-9-CM	$64.00	
Morin-Spatz	CP "Teach" Expert Coding Made Easy	$44.95	
Morin-Spatz	CP "Teach" Student Workbook	$29.95	With answers.
MedBooks	CP "Teach" Case Study Workbook	$34.95	
Medical Learning	Chargemaster Coding and Optimization: An Instructional Guide to Coding and Reimbursement for Radiology, Laboratory, and other Diagnostic Services	$149.00	Annual updates $69.

Figure M.1 AHIMA Coding Resources *(continued)*

Medical Learning	Coding for Ambulatory Surgery Procedures: An Instructional Guide to Coding and Reimbursement for Hospital-Based …	$149.00	Annual updates $69.
Medical Learning	Emergency Services Reimbursement: An Instructional Guide to Effectively Managing Coding and Reimbursement …	$149.00	Annual updates $69.
Medicode	Coder's Desk Reference	$79.95	
Rogers	Ambulatory Surgery Coding	$64.00	
Medicode	Coding Illustrated: Eye	$99.95	
"	" Face: Soft Tissue	$99.95	
"	" Face: Skeletal Structures and Definition	$99.95	
"	" Female Reproductive System	$99.95	
"	" Hip and Knee	$99.95	
"	" Male Reproductive System	$99.95	
"	" Nose, Throat, and Ear	$99.95	
"	" Spine	$99.95	
"	" Urinary System	$99.95	
HMA	Coding for Quality™ ICD-9-CM Videotape Series, Level 1	$2,495.00	Videotape. These tapes can be purchased in some 14 separate sets which add up to $6,700. CE credits for the series: 56.
HMA	Coding for Quality™ Introduction to CPT Coding Videotape Series	$349.00	CE credits: 10.

Figure M.1 AHIMA Coding Resources *(continued)*

Medicode	Code It Right	$49.95	
Cummins	A Guide to Coding in Long Term Care	$32.00	
Adams	Adams' Guide to Coding and Reimbursement	$31.95	
Insurance Career Development Center	Guide to Medical Billing and Exercises for coding and Reimbursement	$54.95	
St. Anthony's	St. Anthony's APG Guidebook	$79.00	
"	St. Anthony's APG Sourcebook: A Comprehensive Guide to the Outpatient Prospective Payment System	$269.00	Updated year-round; first year's updates free.
"	St. Anthony's DRG Guidebook	$69.00	
"	St. Anthony's DRG Optimizer	$129.00	
AHIMA	Coding Curriculum Guide[b]	$20.00	
	Total:	$10,085.00	

a. The order of entries is that of the sequence in the catalog under the heading, "Clinical Data Management: Coding." All are print publications unless otherwise specified. The prices are non-member prices; member prices are slightly lower. Where more than one grade of a product is listed, the lower-priced version is shown in the table.

b. AHIMA also offers a home-study course in coding for $1,200 and several Independent Study Modules at about $200 each.

ICD-9-CM is available direct from the Federal Government, Superintendent of Documents, on CD-ROM as set up in Folio Views® software (which provides hypertext indexing of the entire document, codes as well as words) for about $20.00. An *ICD-9-CM* "subscription" is also available from the Superintendent of Documents for $65.00, postpaid. It includes the 4th Edition, Volumes 1-2 and the procedures volume, and automatic shipment of all addenda issued to this edition. Full text of *ICD-9-CM* is also available for download direct off the Internet.

Bibliography

1. Albaum-Feinstein, Andrea. *DSM-IV to ICD-9-CM Crosswalk*. Chicago, IL: American Health Information Management Association, 1995.

2. Alschuler, Liora. "Introducing HL7's Patient Record Architecture." *HL7 News* (2000).

3. Amatayakul, Margaret. "CPR Definition Becoming Clearer." *Health Management Technology* (1995): 66-76.

4. ———. "The State of the Computer-Based Patient Record." *Journal of AHIMA* 69, no. 9 (1998): 34-40.

5. American Association of Medical Record Librarians. "Efficiency in Hospital Indexing of the Coding Systems of the *International Statistical Classification* and *Standard Nomenclature of Diseases and Operations*." *Journal of the American Association of Medical Record Librarians (JAMRA)* 30 (1959): 95-110, 111, 129.

6. ———. "ICD-9-CM Notes." *Journal of the American Association of Medical Record Librarians (JAMRA)* (1982): 87-88.

7. American College of Radiology. *Index for Radiological Diagnoses (IDR), 4th Edition*. Reston VA: American College of Radiology, 1992.

8. ———. *Index for Radiological Diagnoses (IDR), Computerized 4th Edition, Version 4.1*. Reston VA: American College of Radiology, 1994.

9. ———. *Index for Radiological Diagnoses (IDR), Revised 3rd Edition*. Reston VA: American College of Radiology, 1986.

10. American Health Information Management Association. *1996 Professional Resource Directory Catalog*. Chicago: American Health Information Management Association (AHIMA), 1996.

11. ———. "Certified Coding Specialist Examinations." *CodeWrite* 7, no. 1 (1998): 1-2.

12. ———. "Preparing Your Organization for a New Coding System." *Journal of AHIMA* 69, no. 8 (1998).

13. American Medical Association. *CPT 1993, Physician's Current Procedural Terminology*. Chicago, IL: American Medical Association, 1993.

14. ———. *CPT 1993, Physician's Current Procedural Terminology, Clinical Examples Supplement*. Chicago, IL: American Medical Association, 1993.

15. ———. *CPT 1993, Physician's Current Procedural Terminology, Medical Specialties*. Chicago, IL: American Medical Association, 1993.

16. ———. "CPT 1995 Code Update." *CPT Assistant* 4, no. 4 (1994): 1-11.

17. ———. "CPT 1996 Code Update." *CPT Assistant* 5, no. 4 (1995): 1-29.

18. ———. *CPT 95: Medical Specialties.* Chicago, IL: American Medical Association, 1994.

19. ———. *CPT '95: Physicians' Current Procedural Terminology.* Chicago, IL: American Medical Association, 1994.

20. ———. *CPT '96: Physicians' Current Procedural Terminology, Professional Edition.* Chicago, IL: American Medical Association, 1995.

21. ———. *Current Medical Information and Terminology, Fourth Edition.* Chicago: American Medical Association, 1971.

22. ———. *Current Medical Terminology 1963.* Chicago IL: American Medical Association, 1962.

23. ———. *Current Medical Terminology, 1964.* Chicago IL: American Medical Association, 1963.

24. ———. *Current Medical Terminology, Third Edition.* Chicago IL: American Medical Association, 1966.

25. ———. *Current Procedural Terminology, First Edition.* Chicago: American Medical Association, 1966.

26. ———. *Current Procedural Terminology, Second Edition.* Chicago IL: American Medical Association, 1970.

27. ———. *Future of Physicians' Current Procedural Terminology (CPT): A Statement to the United States National Committee on Vital and Health Statistics, Subcommittee on Medical Classification Systems.* Chicago: American Medical Association, 1995.

28. ———. *Physician's Current Procedural Terminology, Fourth Edition, CPT.* Chicago, IL: American Medical Association, 1977.

29. ———. *Physician's Current Procedural Terminology, Fourth Edition, CPT 1987.* Chicago, IL: American Medical Association, 1986.

30. ———. *Physicians' Current Procedural Terminology (CPT), 3rd Edition.* Chicago: American Medical Association, 1973.

31. ———. "Preventive Medicine Services." *CPT Assistant* 4, no. 4 (1994): 21-23.

32. ———. "Review of Hernia Repair Codes." *CPT Assistant* 4, no. 4 (1994): 12-17.

33. ———. *Standard Nomenclature of Athletic Injuries.* Chicago, IL: American Medical Association, 1966.

34. ———. *Standard Nomenclature of Disease and Standard Nomenclature of Operations, 3rd Edition (SNDO).* Chicago IL: American Medical Association, 1942.

35. ———. *Standard Nomenclature of Diseases and Operations, 4th Edition (SNDO).* New York: Blakiston, 1952.

36. ———. *Standard Nomenclature of Diseases and Operations, 5th Edition (SNDO)*. New York: McGraw Hill (Blakiston), 1961.

37. American Psychiatric Association. *Diagnostic and Statistical Manual, Mental Disorders*. Washington DC: American Psychiatric Association, 1952.

38. ———. *Diagnostic and Statistical Manual of Mental Disorders: 2nd Edition (DSM-II)*. Washington DC: American Psychiatric Association, 1968.

39. ———. *Diagnostic and Statistical Manual of Mental Disorders: 3rd Edition (DSM-III)*. Washington DC: American Psychiatric Association, 1980.

40. ———. *Diagnostic and Statistical Manual of Mental Disorders: 3rd Edition Revised (DSM-III-R)*. Washington DC: American Psychiatric Association, 1987.

41. ———. *Diagnostic and Statistical Manual of Mental Disorders: 4th Edition (DSM-IV)*. Washington DC: American Psychiatric Association, 1994.

42. Andrew, William, and Richard Dick. "On the Road to the CPR: Where Are We Now?" *Healthcare Informatics* 13, no. 5 (1996): 48-62.

43. ———. "Where We'Ve Been and Where We'Re Headed." *Healthcare Informatics* (1997): 52-56.

44. Association of Sleep Disorders Centers. *Diagnostic Classification of Sleep and Arousal Disorders, First Edition*. New York, NY: Raven Press Books, Ltd., 1979.

45. ASTM. "Guide Addressing Security of Health Record Dictation and Transcription Approved." *ASTM Standardization News* 25, no. 11 (1997): 10.

46. ———. "Guide for a View of Emergency Medical Care in the Computerized Patient Record—E 1744-95.", 785-95. Vol. 14.01. American Society for Testing and Materials, 1996.

47. ———. "Guide for Content and Structure of the Computer-Based Patient Record—E 1384-96.", 265-379. Vol. 14.01. 1996.

48. ———. "Guide for Properties of Electronic Health Records and Record Systems—E 1769-05.", 825-30. Vol. 14.01. 1996.

49. ———. "Nine Provisional Standards on Privacy and Confidentiality of Computer Health Records Under Development." *ASTM Standardization News* 25, no. 11 (1997): 8-10.

50. ———. "Specification for Defining and Sharing Modular Health Knowledge Bases (Arden Syntax for Medical Logic Systems)—E-1460-92.", 403-51. Vol. 14.01. 1996.

51. ———. "Standard E 1284 - 89: Standard Guide for Nosologic Standards and Guides for Construction of New Biomedical Nomenclature." *1997 Annual Book of ASTM Standards* Section 14 (1997): 207-11.

52. ———. "Standard E 1384 - 96: Standard Guide for Content and Structure of the Computer-Based Patient Record." *1997 Annual Book of ASTM Standards* Section 14 (1997): 260-373.

53. ———. "Standard E 1460 - 92: Standard Specifications for Defining and Sharing Modular Health Knowledge Bases (Arden Syntax for Medical Logic Modules)." *1997 Annual Book of ASTM Standards* Section 14 (1997): 398-446.

54. ———. "Standard E 1578 - 93: Standard Guide for Laboratory Information Management Systems (LIMS)." *1997 Annual Book of ASTM Standards* Section 14 (1997): 600-628.

55. ———. "Standard E 1633 - 96: Standard Specification for Coded Values Used in the Computer-Based Patient Record." *1997 Annual Book of ASTM Standards* Section 14 (1997): 629-58.

56. ———. "Standard E 1712 - 96: Standard Specification for Representing Clinical Laboratory Test and Analyte Names." *1997 Annual Book of ASTM Standards* Section 14 (1997): 687-714.

57. ———. "Standard E 1714 - 95: Standard Guide for Properties of a Universal Healthcare Identifier (UHID)." *1997 Annual Book of ASTM Standards* Section 14 (1997): 728-39.

58. ———. "Standard E 1744 - 95: Standard Guide for View of Emergency Medical Care in the Computerized Patient Record." *1997 Annual Book of ASTM Standards* Section 14 (1997): 780-790.

59. ———. "Standard E 1769 - 95: Standard Guide for Properties of Electronic Health Records and Record Systems." *1997 Annual Book of ASTM Standards* Section 14 (1997): 820-825.

60. ———. "Standard E 1869 - 97: Standard Guide for Confidentiality, Privacy, Access, and Data Security Principles for Health Information Including Computer-Based Patient Records." *1997 Annual Book of ASTM Standards* Section 14 (1997): 826-34.

61. Averill, Richard F. *Ambulatory Patient Groups Definitions Manual, Version 2.0.* Internet: 1996.

62. Baldwin, Gary. "Doctors' Bible Updated to Reflect Clinical and Medical Advances." *American Medical News* (1998): 20,22.

63. Barer, David. *Comment on Medical Records.* Internet: 1996.

64. Beckett, Ronald S. "History of Coding Nomenclature in a General Hospital Medical Records Department." *Pathologist* (1977).

65. Benesch, C., D. M. Witter Jr, A. L. Wilder, and and others. "Inaccuracy of the International Classification of Diseases (ICD-9-CM) in Identifying the Diagnosis of Ischemic Cerebrovascular Disease." *Neurology* 49 (1997): 660-664.

66. Benson, Tim. *Application of the Standard Generalized Markup Language (SGML) in Electronic Patient Records, Version 2.0.* Internet: The NHS Executive's EPR Project Board, 1996.

67. Berg, Marc. *Rationalizing Medical Work: Decision-Support Techniques and Medical Practices.* Cambridge, MA: MIT Press, 1997.

68. Berg, Marc, and Geoffrey Bowker. *The Multiple Bodies of the Medical Record: Towards a Sociology of an Artifact.* Internet: 1997.

69. Berg, Marc, Chris Langenberg, Ignas van de Berg, and Jan Kwakkernaat. *Experiences With an Electronic Patient Record in a Clinical Context: Considerations for Design.* Internet: 1997.

70. Berkenwald, Alan D. "In the Name of Medicine." *Annals of Internal Medicine* 128, no. 3 (1998): 246-50.

71. Berkow, Robert, and Andrew J. Fletcher. *Merck Manual of Diagnosis and Therapy, 17th Edition.* Rahway NJ: Merck Research Laboratories, 1992.

72. Bero, Lisa, and Drummond Rennie. "The Cochrane Collaboration—Preparing, Maintaining, and Disseminating Reviews of the Effects of Health Care." *Journal of the American Medical Association* 274, no. 24 (1995): 1935-38.

73. Borzo, Greg. "Breaking the E-Code." *American Medical News* 39, no. 14 (1996): 1, 27.

74. ———. "Coding Confusion." *American Medical News* (1994).

75. ———. "HCFA Rejects Push for New Uniform Coding System." *American Medical News* (1994): 1, 7.

76. ———. "Pulling the Plug on Paper." *American Medical News* 40, no. 12 (1997): 13-15.

77. Brömer, G. R. "Tenth Revision of the International Classification of Diseases—in Progress." *British Journal of Psychiatry* 152, no. Supplement 1 (1988): 29-32.

78. Brand, Christopher. *GALEN, Generalized Architecture for Language, Encyclopaedias, and Nomenclatures in Medicine.* Internet: University of Manchester, 1996.

79. Brett, Allan S. "New Guidelines for Coding Physicians' Services—a Step Backward." *New England Journal of Medicine (NEJM)* 339, no. 23 (1998): 1705-8.

80. British National Formulary. *British National Formulary.* Pharmaceutical Press, 1998.

81. Brown, Faye. *ICD-9-CM Coding Handbook, With Answers, 1996 Revised Edition.* Chicago, IL: American Hospital Publishing Company, 1966.

82. California Medical Association. *1960 Relative Value Studies.* San Francisco, CA: California Medical Association, 1960.

83. ———. *1964 Relative Value Studies (Fourth Edition).* San Francisco, CA: California Medical Association, 1964.

84. ———. *1969 California Relative Value Studies (Fifth Edition)*. San Francisco, CA: California Medical Association, 1969.

85. ———. *1974 Revision, California Relative Value Studies (Fifth Edition (Revised)*. San Francisco, CA: California Medical Association, 1975.

86. ———. *Relative Value Schedule*. San Francisco, CA: California Medical Association, 1956.

87. ———. *Relative Value Study, Second Edition*. San Francisco, CA: California Medical Association, 1957.

88. Cassel, Christine K., and Bruce C. Vladeck. "ICD-9 Code for Palliative or Terminal Care." *New England Journal of Medicine (NEJM)* 335, no. 16 (1996): 1232-33.

89. Cavert, Winston. "Preventing and Treating Major Opportunistic Infections in AIDS." *Postgraduate Medicine* 102, no. 4 (1997).

90. Central Office on ICD-9-CM. "Ask the Editor: Coding Gulf War Syndrome." *Coding Clinic* 15, no. 1 (1998): 4-9.

91. ———. "Ask the Editor: 'What Is the Correct Code for AIDS?'." *Coding Clinic for ICD-9-CM* 2, no. 2 (1985): 6.

92. ———. "Classification of AIDS." *Coding Clinic for ICD-9-CM* 9, no. 1 (1992): 3-4.

93. ———. "Conversion Table of New *ICD-9-CM* Codes." *Coding Clinic* (1989): 7-13.

94. ———. "Conversion Table of New ICD-9-CM Codes." *Coding Clinic for ICD-9-CM* 8, no. 4 (1991): 3-13.

95. ———. "Human Immunodeficiency Virus (HIV) Infection Codes. Official Authorized Addendum, *ICD-9-CM*, (Revision No.1), Effective 1-1-88." *Morbidity and Mortality Weekly Report (MMWR) Supplement* 36, no. S-7 (1997): 4-24.

96. ———. "Introducing Coding Clinic for ICD-9-CM." *Coding Clinic for ICD-9-CM* 1, no. 1 (1984): 1.

97. ———. "Principal Diagnoses and Other Diagnoses." *Coding Clinic for ICD-9-CM* 2, no. 2 (1985): 1.

98. Chidley, Elise. "Coding and Classification: Window on the Future." *For the Record* (1999).

99. Chute, Christopher. "Comments on the Framework for Clinical Terminology Development." *Meeting Minutes, Public Health Service, National Committee on Vital and Health Statistics* (1997): 24.

100. Chute, Christopher G., Simon P. Cohn, Keith E. Campbell, Diane E. Oliver, and James R. Campbell. "The Content Coverage of Clinical Classifications." *Journal of the American Medical Informatics Association* 3, no. 3 (1996): 224-33.

101. Cimino, James. "Comments on the Needs for Coding and Classification Systems." *Meeting Minutes, Public Health Service, National Committee on Vital and Health Statistics* (1997): 22.

102. CIOMS. *International Nomenclature of Diseases: Diseases of the Lower Respiratory Tract, Volume III.* Geneva, Switzerland: WHO, 1979.

103. ———. *International Nomenclature of Diseases: Infectious Diseases, Volume II, Part 1: Bacterial Diseases.* Geneva, Switzerland: WHO, 1985.

104. ———. *International Nomenclature of Diseases: Infectious Diseases, Volume II, Part 2: Mycoses.* Geneva, Switzerland: WHO, 1982.

105. ———. *International Nomenclature of Diseases: Infectious Diseases, Volume II, Part 3: Viral Diseases.* Geneva, Switzerland: WHO, 1983.

106. CIOMS/WHO. *International Nomenclature of Diseases: Cardiac and Vascular Diseases, Volume V.* Geneva, Switzerland: WHO, 1989.

107. ———. *International Nomenclature of Diseases: Diseases of the Digestive System, Volume IV.* Geneva, Switzerland: WHO, 1990.

108. ———. *International Nomenclature of Diseases: Diseases of the Female Genital System, Volume VIII.* Geneva, Switzerland: CIOMS/WHO, 1992.

109. ———. *International Nomenclature of Diseases: Diseases of the Kidney, the Lower Urinary Tract, and the Male Genital System, Volume VII.* Geneva, Switzerland: CIOMS/WHO, 1992.

110. ———. *International Nomenclature of Diseases: Infectious Diseases, Volume II: Parasitic Diseases.* Geneva, Switzerland: WHO, 1987.

111. ———. *International Nomenclature of Diseases: Metabolic, Nutritional, and Endocrine Disorders, Volume VI.* Geneva, Switzerland: CIOMS/WHO, 1991.

112. Clark, Holly. "Continuous Speech Recognition: What You Should Know." *Journal of AHIMA* 69, no. 9 (1998): 68-69.

113. Cohen, B. B., R. Pokeas, M. S. Meads, and et al. "How Will Diagnosis-Related Groups Affect Epidemiologic Research?" *American Journal of Epidemiology* 126 (1987): 1-9.

114. Colenbrander, August. "Thoughts About Medical Languages, Nomenclatures, Coding Systems, and Classifications." *Personal Communication.*

115. College of American Pathologists, Committee on Nomenclature and Classification of Disease, and American Cancer Society. *Systematized Nomenclature of Pathology (SNOP).* College of American Pathologists, 1965.

116. College of American Pathologists, Roger A. Côté, David J. Rothwell, Palotay, Ronald S. Beckett, and Louise Brochu. *The Systematized Nomenclature of Human and Veterinary Medicine—SNOMED International—4 Volumes.* Waukegan IL: College of American Pathologists, 1993.

117. Collen, Morris Frank. *A History of Medical Informatics in the United States.* Bethesda, Maryland: American Medical Informatics Association, 1995.

118. Commission on Professional and Hospital Activities. *Hospital Adaptation of ICDA, (HICDA), 2 Volume Set.* Ann Arbor, MI: Commission on Professional and Hospital Activities, 1968.

119. ———. *Hospital Adaptation of ICDA, (HICDA), 2nd Edition, 2 Volume Set.* Ann Arbor, MI: Commission on Professional and Hospital Activities, 1973.

120. ———. "*ICD-9-CM* List A: Hospital Diagnosis Groups, and *ICD-9-CM* List B: Hospital Procedure Groups." (1979).

121. ———. *International Classification of Diseases, 9th Revision, Clinical Modification, 3-Volume Set.* Ann Arbor, MI: Commission on Professional and Hospital Activities, 1978.

122. ———. *International Classification of Diseases, 9th Revision, Clinical Modification, Annotated Edition, 3 Volume Set.* Ann Arbor, MI: Commission on Professional and Hospital Activities, 1986.

123. Committee on Quality of Health Care In America. *To Err Is Human: Building a Safer Health System.* Washington, DC: National Academy Press, 1999.

124. Computer Aided Medical Systems Limited. *Read Clinical Classification (Read Codes).* Loughborough, Leicestershire, England: Computer Aided Medical Systems Limited, 1996.

125. Connolly, H. M., J. L. Crary, M. D. McGoon, D. D. Hensrud, B. S. Edwards, W. D. Edwards, and Schaff. H. V. "Valvular Heart Disease Associated With Fenfluramine-Phentermine." *New England Journal of Medicine (NEJM)* 337, no. 9 (1997): 581-88.

126. Context Software Systems Inc. *HCPCS 1995: Medicare Level 2 National Codes.* New York, NY: McGraw-Hill, Inc., 1995.

127. Cook, Deborah J., Nancy L. Greengold, Gray Ellrodt, and Scott R. Weingarten. "The Relation Between Systematic Reviews and Practice Guidelines." *Annals of Internal Medicine* 127, no. 3 (1997): 208-16.

128. Cook, Deborah J., Cynthia D. Mulrow, and R. Brian Harnes. "Systematic Reviews: Synthesis of Best Evidence for Clinical Decisions." *Annals of Internal Medicine* 126, no. 5 (1997): 376-88.

129. Côté, Roger A. "The SNOP-SNOMED Concept: Evolution Towards a Common Medical Nomenclature and Classification." *Pathologist* (1977).

130. Côté, Roger A., and David J. Rothwell. "The Systematized Nomenclature of Human and Veterinary Medicine: SNOMED International." *Canadian Medical Informatics* 1, no. 4 (1994).

131. D'Amato, Cheryl. "Roundtable Survey Results." *CodeWrite* 6, no. 2 (1997): 8-9.

132. Dansky, Kathryn H., Larry D. Gamm, Joseph J. Vasey, and Camille K. Barsukiewicz. "Electronic Medical Records: Are Physicians Ready." *Journal of Healthcare Management* 44, no. 6 (1999): 440-455.

133. Davis, Neil M. *Medical Abbreviations: 12,000 Conveniences at the Expense of Communications and Safety, Eighth Edition.* Huntingdon Valley, PA: Neil M. Davis Associates, 1997.

134. ———. *Medical Abbreviations: 14,000 Conveniences at the Expense of Communications and Safety, Ninth Edition.* Huntingdon Valley, PA: Neil M. Davis Associates, 1999.

135. ———. *Medical Abbreviations: 4200 Conveniences at the Expense of Communications and Safety, Third Edition.* Huntingdon Valley, PA: Neil M. Davis Associates, 1987.

136. de Maeseneer, Jan. "The ICPC Classification of Drugs." *The International Classification of Primary Care in the European Community—With a Multi-Language Layer.* Henk Lamberts, Maurice Wood, and Inge Hofmans-Okkes, 163-70. Oxford: Oxford University Press, 1993.

137. Dean, Julia. "Medicare's Outpatient Prospective Payment System—APCs." *Footprints* 20, no. 4 (1998): 3-4.

138. DeBakey, Michael. "The National Library of Medicine: Evolution of a Premier Information Center." *Journal of the American Medical Association* 266, no. 9 (1991): 1252-58.

139. Delbanco, Thomas L. "Enriching the Doctor-Patient Relationship by Inviting the Patient's Perspective." *Annals of Internal Medicine* 116 (1992): 414-18.

140. Delong, Marilyn Fuller. *Medical Acronyms & Abbreviations, Second Edition.* Oradell NJ: Medical Economics Books, 1989.

141. Dick, Richard S., and William F. Andrew. "Explosive Growth in CPRs: Evaluation Criteria Needed." *Healthcare Informatics* (1995): 110-114.

142. ———. "Point of Care: an Essential Technology for the CPR." *Healthcare Informatics* (1995): 64-78.

143. Dick, Richard S., and James M. Gabler. "Still Searching for the "Holy Grail"." *Health Management Technology* (1995): 30-35, 80.

144. Dick, Richard S., and Elaine B. Steen. *The Computer-Based Patient Record: An Essential Technology for Health Care.* Washington DC: National Academy Press for the Institute of Medicine, 1991.

145. ———. *The Computer-Based Patient Record: An Essential Technology for Health Care—Revised Edition.* Washington DC: National Academy Press for the Institute of Medicine, 1997.

146. Doenges, Marilynn E., Mary F. Jeffries, and Mary Frances Moorhouse. *Nursing Care Plans—Nursing Diagnoses in Planning Patient Care.* Philadelphia PA: F. A. Davis Company, 1984.

147. Douglas, R. M. "The Read Codes: Towards a Common Language of Health." *Informatics in Health Care, Australia* 1, no. 1 (1993).

148. Dubendorfer, Christine, and CIOMS Secretariat. Letter to Vergil Slee, 15 June 1999.

149. Duke University. *Informatics Standards of Interest to Nurses.* Internet: Healthcare Informatics Standards, Duke University, 1998.

150. Dun and Bradstreet. *MOD 10 Calculation (Check Digits).* Internet: 1996.

151. Eisele, C. Wesley, Vergil N. Slee, and Robert G. Hoffmann. "Can the Practice of Internal Medicine Be Evaluated?" *Annals of Internal Medicine* 44, no. 1 (1956): 144-61.

152. Elliott, Jeff. "HL7 Announces Its Limitations." *Healthcare Informatics* (1997): 14,16.

153. Elson, Robert B. "Uniting Practice Management and the CPR." *Healthcare Informatics* (1997): SS3-SS7.

154. Erkinjuntti, Timo, Truls ÿstbye, Runa Steenhuis, and Vladimir Hachinski. "The Effect of Different Diagnostic Criteria on the Prevalence of Dementia." *New England Journal of Medicine (NEJM)* 337, no. 23 (1997): 1667-74.

155. Evidence-based medicine working group. "Evidence-Based Medicine—a New Approach to Teaching the Practice of Medicine." *Journal of the American Medical Association* 268, no. 17 (1992): 2420-2425.

156. Farseth, Paul H. "Changing Diagnosis Codes." *New England Journal of Medicine (NEJM)* 299, no. 21 (1978): 1187-90.

157. Federal Register. "Coding Clinic for ICD-9-CM." *Federal Register* 54, no. 139 (1989): 30561.

158. Fetter, Robert B., David A. Brand, and Dianne Gamache. *DRGs—Their Design and Development.* Ann Arbor, Michigan: Health Administration Press, 1991.

159. Fitzmaurice, J. Michael. "Computer-Based Patient Records." *The Biomedical Engineering Handbook.* 1995 ed., Editor Joseph D. Bronzino, 2623-34. Boca Raton, Florida: CRC Press, 1995.

160. Frances, Allen, Michael B. First, and Harold Alan Pincus. *DSM-IV Guidebook.* Washington DC: American Psychatric Press, 1995.

161. Frawley, Kathleen A. "Update on Healthcare Informatics Standards Development in the United States." *Journal of AHIMA* 67, no. 8 (1996): 68-69.

162. Friedman, Rick. "Comment Re Medicaid/Medicare Common Data Initiative (McData)." *Meeting Minutes, Public Health Service, National Committee on Vital and Health Statistics* (1995): 20.

163. Froom, Jack. "Issues in Primary Care Classification." *Personal Communication.*

164. Furfaros, Carmen, Kristen Muchoney, and Patti Anania-Firouzan. "CPR by the Year 2000—A Myth?" *Healthcare Informatics* (1996): 45,47.

165. Gabrieli, Elmer R. "Aspects of a Computer-Based Patient Record." *Journal of AHIMA* 64, no. 7 (1993): 70-82.

166. ———. "Professional Society Group #14, Report to American Association for Medical Systems and Informatics (AAMSI)." *Journal of Clinical Computing* 12, no. 4 (1984): 102-22.

167. Gantner, George E. "History of Coding." *Pathologist* (1977).

168. ———. "SNOMED and the Pathologist." *Pathologist* (1977).

169. Garner, Rochelle. "A Medical Moon." *InfoWorld* (1995).

170. Gibbs, W. Wayt. "Taking Computers to Task." *Scientific American* 277, no. 1 (1997): 82-90.

171. Goldman, Janlori. "Protecting Privacy to Improve Health Care." *Annals of Internal Medicine* 129, no. 12 (1998): 47-60.

172. Goltra, Peter S. *MEDCIN A New Nomenclature for Clinical Medicine.* New York: Springer-Verlag, 1997.

173. Gray, J. A. Muir. *Evidence-Based Healthcare—How to Make Health Policy and Management Decisions.* New York NY: Churchill Livingstone, 1997.

174. Grimaldi, Paul L., and Julie A. Micheletti. *DRGs: Diagnosis Related Groups—a Practitioner's Guide, Second Edition.* Chicago IL: Pluribus Press, 1983.

175. ———. *Medicare's Prospective Payment Plan—DRG Update.* Chicago IL: Pluribus Press, 1983.

176. Gupta, Garesh. "Diagnosis-Related Groups: a Twentieth-Century Nosology." *The Pharos* (1990): 12-17.

177. Gustafson, David H., Robert P. Hawkins, Suzanne Pingree, Eric W. Boberg, Earl Bricker, Fiona McTavish, and Meg Wise. *CHESS: a Computer-Based System for Empowering Health Care Consumers Through Education and Social Support.* Madison WI: University of Wisconsin, Center for Health Systems Research and Analysis, 1994.

178. Hadley, Linda. "Developing *ICD-10*: An American Advisor's Experience." *For the Record: A Weekly Newsmagazine for Medical Record Administrators and Technicians* 1, no. 3 (1989): 1, 4-5, 8-9.

179. Hammond, W. Ed, and Mark McDougall. "Health Level Seven: the Clinical Data Interchange Standard." *Journal of AHIMA* 67, no. 8 (1996): 42-45.

180. Hanzlick, Randy. "National Autopsy Data Dropped From the National Center for Health Statistics Database." *Journal of the American Medical Association* 280, no. 10 (1998): 886.

181. Harding, Ann, and Charlie Stuart-Buttle. "The Development and Role of the Read Codes." *Journal of AHIMA* 69, no. 5 (1998): 34-38.

182. Hartge, Patricia. "Abortion, Breast Cancer, and Epidemiology." *New England Journal of Medicine (NEJM)* 336, no. 2 (1996): 127-28.

183. Hassard, Howard. *Fifty Years in Law and Medicine: Reminiscences.* San Francisco CA: Hassard, Bonnington, Rogers & Huber, 1985.

184. Helbig, Susan. "Online Coding Using an Imaging System." *Journal of AHIMA* 67, no. 9 (1996): 44-45.

185. Held, Robert F. "ASTM Launches Web-Based Interactive Standards Development Forums." *ASTM Standardization News* 25, no. 12 (1997): 20-23.

186. Hellerstein, David. "A New Object of Component-Object Computing." *Healthcare Informatics* (1997): 128-40.

187. Henry, Suzanne Bakken, Judith J. Warren, and Rita D. Zielstorff. "Nursing Data, Classification Systems, and Quality Indicators: What Every HIM Professional Needs to Know." *Journal of AHIMA* 69, no. 5 (1998): 48-53.

188. Hirschi, Nancy. "A Closer Look at Ambulatory Patient Groups: APG Version 2.0 Update." *Journal of AHIMA* 67, no. 2 (1996): 22-25.

189. Hofmans-Okkes, Inge. "An International Study into the Concept and Validity of the "Reason for Encounter"." *The International Classification of Primary Care in the European Community—With a Multi-Language Layer.*, 34-42. Oxford: Oxford University Press, 1993.

190. Hofmans-Okkes, Inge, and Henk Lamberts. "The International Classification of Primary Care (ICPC): New Applications in Research and Computer-Based Patient Records in Family Practice." *Family Practice* 13, no. 3 (1996): 294-302.

191. ———. *Episodes of Care and the Large Majority of Personal Health Care Needs: Is the New IOM Definition Reflected in Primary Care Data Available in the US?* Amsterdam: Academic Medical Centre, Department of Family Medicine, University of Amerstdam, 1995.

192. Hripcsak, George, Carol Friedman, Philip O. Alderson, William DuMouchel, Stephen B. Johnson, and Paul D. Clayton. "Unlocking Clinical Data From Narrative Reports: a Study of Natural Language Processing." *Annals of Internal Medicine* 122, no. 9 (1995): 682-88.

193. Hsia, David C., W. Mark Krushat, Ann B. Fagan, Jane A. Tebbutt, and Richard P. Kusserow. "Accuracy of Diagnostic Coding for Medicare Patients Under the Prospective-Payment System (PPS)." *New England Journal of Medicine (NEJM)* 318, no. 6 (1988): 352-55.

194. Hudson, Terese. "Computerized Patient Records Goal of New Group." *Hospitals* (1991): 48-52.

195. Hughes, Edward C. *Obstetric-Gynecologic Terminology.* Philadelphia PA: F. A. Davis, 1972.

196. Humphreys, Betsy L. "Do Existing Controlled Vocabularies Contain Terminology Needed for Patient Records?" *Journal of AHIMA* 69, no. 5 (1998): 30-33.

197. Humphreys, Betsy L., and Donald A. B. Lindberg. "Building the Unified Medical Language System (UMLS)." *Proceedings of the Thirteenth Annual Symposium on Computer Applications in Medical Care* (1989): 475-80.

198. Iezzoni, Lisa I. "Comments Re Diagnosis Recording in Capitated Payment Systems for Managed Care." *Meeting Minutes, Public Health Service, National Committee on Vital and Health Statistics* (1996): 20.

199. ———. "The Demand for Documentation for Medicare Payment." *New England Journal of Medicine (NEJM)* 341, no. 5 (1999): 365-67.

200. ———. "How Much Are We Willing to Pay for Information About Quality of Care?" *Annals of Internal Medicine* 126, no. 5 (1997): 391-93.

201. ———. *Risk Adjustment for Measuring Health Outcomes, Second Edition.* Chicago IL: Health Administration Press, 1997.

202. ———. "Using Administrative Diagnostic Data to Assess the Quality of Hospital Care: Pitfalls and Potential of *ICD-9-CM.*" *International Journal of Technology Assessment in Health Care* 6 (1990): 272-81.

203. Iezzoni, Lisa I., Susan Burnside, Laurie Sickles, Mark A. Moskowitz, Eric Sawitz, and Paul A. Levine. "Coding of Acute Myocardial Infarction: Clinical and Policy Implications." *Annals of Internal Medicine* (1988): 745-51.

204. Inmon, W. H. *Building the Data Warehouse.* Boston: QED Technical Publishing Group, 1992.

205. Institute for the Future. *A Forecast of Health and Health Care in America.* Palo Alto, CA: Institute for the Future, 1998.

206. Institute of Medicine. *Reliability of Hospital Discharge Abstracts.* Washington DC: National Academy of Sciences, 1977.

207. International ISBN Agency. *The ISBN System Users Manual.* Berlin: International ISBN Agency, 1986.

208. IRP, Inc. *Refinement of the Medicare Diagnosis-Related Groups (DRGs) to Incorporate a Measure of Severity.* Internet: Information Research Products, Inc., 1996.

209. Israel, Robert A. "A Conceptual Framework for Future Revisions of the International Classification of Diseases." *ICD/C* 78, no. 11.

210. ———. "The International Classification of Diseases: Two Hundred Years of Development." *Public Health Reports* 93 (1978): 150-152.

211. Jablonski, Stanley. *Dictionary of Medical Acronyms and Abbreviations.* St Louis, MO: C. V. Mosby Company, 1987.

212. Johnson, Gary. "Computer-Based Patient Record Systems: A Planned Revolution." *Healthcare Informatics* (1994): 42-52.

213. Johnson, R. L. "Today's CDRs—the Elusive "Complete" Solution." *Healthcare Informatics* (1997): 57-60.

214. Joint Commission on Accreditation of Healthcare Organizations. *1995 Comprehensive Accreditation Manual for Hospitals.* Oakbrook Terrace IL: Joint Commission on Accreditation of Healthcare Organizations, 1994.

215. Journal of AHIMA. "1998 Coding Guide." *Journal of AHIMA* (1998).

216. ———. "Software and Systems 1997 Guide." *Journal of AHIMA* 68, no. 8 (1997).

217. Juran, J. M., Frank M. Gryna, and R. S. Bingham Jr. *Quality Control Handbook.* New York: McGraw Hill Book Company, 1974.

218. Kassirer, Jerome P., and Marcia Angell. "Evaluation and Management Guidelines—Fatally Flawed." *New England Journal of Medicine (NEJM)* 339, no. 23 (1998): 1697-98.

219. Kelly, John T. "'After the Chaos': Expected Benefits of Health Information Management." *Health Affairs* 17, no. 6 (1998): 39-40.

220. Kendall, David B., and S. Robert Levine. "Pursuing the Promise of an Information-Age Health Care System." *Health Affairs* 17, no. 6 (1998): 41-42.

221. Kleinke, J. D. "Release 0.0: Clinical Information Technology in the Real World." *Health Affairs* 17, no. 6 (1998): 23-38.

222. Kloss, Linda. "The CPR: a Watershed Issue for HIM." *Journal of AHIMA* 69, no. 9 (1998): 30-32.

223. Kramer, Caroline F. Barancik Jerome I. Thode Hendy C. Jr. "Improving the Sensitivity and Specificity of the Abbreviated Injury Scale Coding System." *Public Health Reports* 105, no. 4 (1990): 334-40.

224. Kudla, Karen M., and Marjorie Rallins. "SNOMED: A Controlled Vocabulary for Computer-Based Patient Records." *Journal of AHIMA* 69, no. 5 (1998): 40-44.

225. Kupka, Karel. "International Classification of Diseases, Ninth Revision." *WHO Chronicle* 32 (1978): 219-25.

226. Kurtz, Dorothy. "The Use of the International Statistical Classification for Indexing Purposes." Personal communication (1954).

227. L'Hours, André G. P. *An Overview of the Tenth Revision of the International Statistical Classification of Diseases and Related Health Problems (ICD-10).* Geneva Switzerland: World Health Organization, 1990.

228. Lamberts, Henk. "International Classification of Primary Care (ICPC) in the European Community." *Health Services Research.* G. N. Fracchia, and M. Theofilatou, 145-62. IOS Press, 1993.

229. Lamberts, Henk, and Inge Hofmans-Okkes. "The Generic Patient Record: an Alliance Between Patient Documentation and Medical Informatics." *Methods of Information in Medicine* 35 (1996): 5-7.

230. Lamberts, Henk, Maurice Wood, and Inge Hofmans-Okkes. *The International Classification of Primary Care in the European Community With a Multi-Language Layer.* Oxford: Oxford University Press, 1993.

231. Landro, Laura. *Survivor.* Simon and Schuster, 1998.

232. Langlois, Jean A., Jay S. Buechner, Elizabeth A. O'Connor, Elizabeth Q. Nacar, and Gordon S. Smith. "Improving E Coding of Hospitalizations for Injury: Do Hospital Records Contain Adequate Documentation?" *American Journal of Public Health* 85, no. 9 (1995): 1261-65.

233. Lanham, Richard A. *Style, an Anti-Textbook.* Yale University Press, 1974.

234. Lasker, Roz, and M. Susan Marquis. "The Intensity of Physicians' Work in Patient Visits: Implications for the Coding of Patient Evaluation and Management Services." *New England Journal of Medicine (NEJM)* 341, no. 5 (1999): 337-41.

235. Last, John M. *A Dictionary of Epidemiology.* New York: Oxford University Press, 1983.

236. ———. *Dictionary of Epidemiology, Third Edition.* New York: Oxford University Press, 1995.

237. Last, John M, and Robert B. Wallace. *Maxcy-Rosenow-Last—Public Health and Preventive Medicine—13th Edition.* Norwalk, CT: Appleton & Lange, 1992.

238. Lenfant, Claude, Lawrence Friedman, and Thomas Thom. "Fifty Years of Death Certificates: the Framingham Heart Study." *Annals of Internal Medicine* 129, no. 12 (1998): 1066-67.

239. Lindberg, Donald A. B., B. L. Humphreys, and A. T. McCray. "The Unified Medical Language System." *Methods of Information in Medicine* 32, no. 4 (1993): 281-91.

240. Lindberg, Donald A. B., and Betsy L. Humphreys. "The UMLS Knowledge Sources: Tools for Building Better User Interfaces." *Proceedings of the Fourteenth Annual Symposium on Computer Applications in Medical Care* (1990): 121-25.

241. Lloyd-Jones, Donald M., David O. Martin, Martin G Larson, and Daniel Levy. "Accuracy of Death Certificates for Coding Coronary Heart Disease As the Cause of Death." *Annals of Internal Medicine* 129, no. 12 (1998): 1020-1026.

242. Lloyd, S. S., and J. P. Rissing. "Physician and Coding Errors in Patient Records." *Journal of the American Medical Association* 254 (1985): 1330-36.

243. Lorenzini, Jean A. *Medical Phrase Index—a One-Step Reference to the Terminology of Medicine.* Oradell NJ: Medical Economics Books, 1989.

244. MacEachern, Malcolm T. *Hospital Organization and Management.* Chicago: Physicians' Record Company, 1935.

245. ———. *Hospital Organization and Management, Revised Third Edition.* Chicago: Physicians' Record Company, 1957.

246. Malet, Gary. "Toward a Global Patient Case Repository." *Medicine on the Net* (1997): 24-25.

247. Marietti, Charlene. "Doing the Right Thing—HIPAA." *Healthcare Informatics* (1998): 51-64.

248. ———. "Extensibility Sensibility—Is XML the Solution for Electronic Medical Records Data Exchange?" *Healthcare Informatics* (1998): 23-26.

249. ———. "Will the Real CPR EMR EHR Please Stand Up." *Healthcare Informatics* (1998): 76-81.

250. ———. "Writing to the Rules—If You'Re Looking at a Clinical Decision Support System, It Had Better Be Arden Syntax Compliant." *Healthcare Informatics* (1998): 17.

251. Martin, Sean. "Revamp of AMA's Coding System Under Way." *American Medical News* (1998): 5-6.

252. Martin, Tom, and Sandra Fuller. "Components of the CPR: an Overview." *Journal of AHIMA* 69, no. 9 (1998): 58-64.

253. McCray, Alexa T. "The UMLS Semantic Network." *National Library of Medicine*: 503-7.

254. McCray, Alexa T., and William T. Hole. "The Scope and Structure of the First Version of the UMLS Semantic Network." *Proceedings of the Fourteenth Annual Symposium on Computer Applications in Medical Care* (1990): 126-30.

255. McDonald, Clement J. "The Barriers to Electronic Medical Record Systems and How to Overcome Them." *Journal of the American Medical Informatics Association* 4, no. 3 (1997): 213-21.

256. ———. "Need for Standards in Health Information." *Health Affairs* 17, no. 6 (1998): 44-56.

257. McDonald, Clement J., P. R. Dexter, B. Takesue, and J. M. Overhage. "Health Informatics Standards: a View From Mid-America." *Yearbook of Medical Informatics, 1997.* 67-74. 1997.

258. McDonald, Clement J., Marc Overhage, Paul Dexter, Blaine Y. Takesue, and Diane M. Dwyer. "A Framework for Capturing Clinical Data Sets From Computerized Sources." *Annals of Internal Medicine* 127, no. 8 (1997): 675-82.

259. McMahon, Laurence F. Jr., and Helen L. Smits. "Can Medicare Prospective Payment Survive the *ICD-9-CM* Disease Classsification System?" *Annals of Internal Medicine* 104 (1986): 562-66.

260. Melton III, L. Joseph. "The Threat to Medical Records Research." *New England Journal of Medicine (NEJM)* 337, no. 20 (1997): 1466-70.

261. Mengelkoch, Angie. "Toward a CPR Solution—Survey of CPR Vendors Reflects Industry Growth." *Healthcare Informatics* (1999): 73-101.

262. Millenson, Michael L. *Demanding Medical Excellence: Doctors and Accountability in the Information Age.* Chicago IL: University of Chicago Press, 1997.

263. Moher, David, and Ingram Olkin. "Meta-Analysis of Randomized Controlled Trials—a Concern for Standards." *Journal of the American Medical Association* 274, no. 24 (1995): 1962-64.

264. Moran, Donald W. "Health Information Policy: on Preparing for the Next War." *Health Affairs* 17, no. 6 (1998): 9-22.

265. Moriyama, I. M. *Current Disease Classifications and Implications for the Future.* Geneva, Switzerland: World Health Organization, 1975.

266. Muir Gray, JA. *Evidence-Based Healthcare: How to Make Health Policy and Management Decisions*. United Kingdom: Churchill Livingstone, 1997.

267. Mulley, Albert G. "Supporting the Patient's Role in Decision Making." *Journal of Occupational Medicine* 32 (1990): 1227-28.

268. Mulrow, Cynthia D., and Deborah Cook. *Systematic Reviews—Synthesis of Best Evidence for Health Care Decisions*. Philadelphia PA: American College of Physicians, 1998.

269. Mulrow, Cynthis D., Deborah J. Cook, and Frank Davidoff. "Systematic Reviews: Critical Links in the Great Chain of Evidence." *Annals of Internal Medicine* 126, no. 5 (1997): 389-91.

270. Myers, Robert S., Vergil N. Slee, and Robert G. Hoffmann. "The Medical Audit: Protects the Patient, Helps the Physician, and Serves the Hospital." *The Modern Hospital* (1955).

271. National conference on nomenclature of disease, and H. R. Logie. *Standard Classified Nomenclature of Disease*. New York: The Commonwealth Fund, 1935.

272. National Library of Medicine, and Agency for Health Care Policy and Research. *Vocabularies for Computer-Based Patient Records: Identifying Candidates for Large Scale Testing. Minutes of a Meeting December 5-6, 1994, Lister Hill Auditorium, NLM, Bethesda, MD*. NLM, AHCPR, 1995.

273. Nelson, Eugene C., Mark E. Splaine, Paul B. Batalden, and Stephen K. Plume. "Building Measurement and Data Collection into Medical Practice." *Annals of Internal Medicine* 128, no. 6 (1998): 460-466.

274. Neumann, Peter J., Stephen T. Parente, and L. Clark Paramore. "Potential Savings From Using Information Technology Applications in Health Care in the United States." *International Journal of Technology Assessment in Health Care* 12, no. 3 (1996): 425-35.

275. NHS Centre for Coding and Classification. *General Information*. Loughborough, England: NHS Centre for Coding and Classification, 1994.

276. ———. *NHS CCC Communications: Index to Published Material*. Loughborough, England: NHS Centre for Coding and Classification, 1994.

277. ———. *Read Codes and the Terms Projects: a Brief Guide*. Loughborough, England: NHS Centre for Coding and Classification, 1994.

278. O'Leary, Margaret R., and et al. *LEXICON Dictionary of Health Care Terms, Organizations, and Acronyms for the Era of Reform*. Oakbrook Terrace, Illinois: Joint Commission on Accreditation of Healthcare Organizations, 1994.

279. Office of Inspector General, Department of Health and Human Services. "Using Software to Detect Upcoding of Hospital Bills." (1998).

280. Office of Technology Assessment. *Bringing Health Care Online*. Washington DC: U. S. Government Printing Office, 1995.

281. Omaha System. *The Use of a Standardized Language With the Nightingale Tracker*. Internet: Internet, 1998.

282. Oppenheimer, Todd. "The Computer Delusion." *Atlantic Monthly* 280, no. 1 (1997): 45-62.

283. ORION. *About APGs*. Internet: ORION, 1996.

284. Osheroff, Jeroma A. *Computers in Clinical Practice—Managing Patients, Information, and Communication*. Philadelphia: American College of Physicians, 1995.

285. Oskam, SK, HJ Brouwer, and J. Mohrs. "TRANS—an Interactive Program to Retrieve Information From a Large Dutch General Practice Database." *Journal of Informatics in Primary Care*: 14-18.

286. Ozbolt, Judy G. "From Minimum Data to Maximum Impact: Using Clinical Data to Strengthen Patient Care." *MD Computing* 14, no. 4 (1997): 295-301.

287. Pachter, Lee M. "Culture and Clinical Care: Folk Illness Beliefs and Behaviors and Their Implications for Health Care Delivery." *Journal of the American Medical Association* 271, no. 9 (1994): 690-694.

288. Percy, Constance, Donald Henson, Louis B. Thomas, and Peter Graepel. "International Classification of Diseases for Oncology." *Pathologist* (1977).

289. Petralia, J. W. "Information Technology (I/T) Can Save $159 Billion Per Year." *Health Management Technology* 16, no. 7 (1995): 62.

290. Physician Practice Coder. "You've Got 81 New ICD-9 Codes to Choose From, Including 30 V Codes, Starting Oct. 1." *Physician Practice Coder* 3, no. 9 (1997): 1,6.

291. Practice Management Information Corporation (PMI). *HCPCS (Health Care Financing Administration Common Procedure Coding System) Procedure Codes 1990: Medicare National Level 2 Codes With CPT Cross-Reference*. Los Angeles, CA: Practice Management Information Corporation (PMI), 1990.

292. ———. *Reimbursement Manual for the Medical Office: A Comprehensive Guide to Coding and Billing*. Los Angeles, CA: Practice Management Information Corporation (PMI), 1990.

293. ———. *Reimbursement Manual for the Medical Office—a Comprehensive Guide to Coding and Billing*. Los Angeles CA: PMI (Practice Management Information Corporation), 1990.

294. Prophet, Sue. "1996 CPT Revisions." *Journal of AHIMA* 67, no. 2 (1996): 16-20.

295. ———. "Classification Systems: Taking a Broader Look." *Journal of AHIMA* 68, no. 5 (1997): 46-50.

296. ———. "Code Assignments for Bone Marrow and Stem Cell Transplants; Liver Cell Transplants." *Journal of AHIMA* 67, no. 1 (1996): 16-18.

297. ———. "ICD-9-CM and CPT Maintenance and Guideline Development Processes." *CodeWrite* 6, no. 4 (1997): 1,3-4.

298. ———. "ICD-9-CM Revisions—Effective October 1, 1996." *Journal of AHIMA* 67, no. 9 (1996): 20-30.

299. ———. "Summary of ICD-9-CM Coordination and Maintenance Committee Meeting." *Journal of AHIMA* 67, no. 8 (1996): 20-27.

300. Public Health Reports. "New Diagnosis Guide Could Add Two Million to Diabetes Roster." *Public Health Reports* 112 (1997): 359.

301. Remington, Richard D. *Letter Re Entity Coding.* 1991.

302. Rempel, David, Bradley Evanoff, Peter C. Amadio, Marc deKrom, Gary Franklin, Alfred Franzblau, Ron Gray, Fredric Gerr, Mats Hagberg, Thomas Hales, Jeffrey N. Katz, and Glenn Pransky. "Concensus Criteria for the Classification of Carpal Tunnel Syndrome in Epidemiological Studies." *American Journal of Public Health* 88, no. 10 (1998): 1447-51.

303. Roberts, John, Sheila R. Decter, and Denise Nagel. "Confidentiality and Electronic Medical Records." *Annals of Internal Medicine* 128, no. 6 (1998): 510-511.

304. Rockefeller, Richard. "Informed Shared Decision Making: Is This the Future of Health Care?" *Health Forum Journal* 42, no. 3 (1999): 54-56.

305. Roper, William L. "The Resource-Based Relative Value Scale: a Methodological and Policy Evaluation." *Journal of the American Medical Association* 260, no. 16 (1988): 2444-46.

306. Rose, Geoffrey, and D. J. P. Barker. *Epidemiology for the Uninitiated.* London: British Medical Journal, 1986.

307. Rothwell, D. J. "SNOMED-Based Knowledge Representation." *Methods of Information in Medicine* 34 (1995): 209-13.

308. Roundtable. "Survey Results." *CodeWrite* 7, no. 1 (1998): 15-16.

309. Royal College of General Practitioners. *The Classification and Analysis of General Practice Data: 2nd Edition.* Royal College of General Practitioners, 1986.

310. Sackett, David L., WS Richardson, W Rosenberg, and RB Haynes. *Evidence-Based Medicine: How to Practice and Teach EBM.* New York: Churchill Livingstone, 1997.

311. Sackett, David L., William M. C. Rosenberg, J. A. Muir Gray, R. Brian Haynes, and W. Scott Richardson. "Evidence-Based Medicine: What It Is and What It Isn't." *British Medical Journal* 312 (1996): 71-2.

312. Sattler, Arlene R. "Software Reference Guide: Encoding, DRG Assignment, and Refined DRGs—Part II." *Journal of the American Association of Medical Record Librarians (JAMRA)* 61, no. 2 (1990): 38-51.

313. Scherertz, D. D., N. E. Olson, M. S. Tuttle, and M. S Erlbaum. "Source Inversion and Matching in the UMLS Metatheraurus." *Proceedings of the Fourteenth Annual Symposium on Computer Applications in Medical Care* (1990): 141-45.

314. Serb, Chris. "Just Say the Word—and New Software Will Make Quick Work of Tedious Reporting Systems." *Hospitals & Health Networks* 72, no. 5 (1998): 40.

315. Shakno, Robert J. *Physician's Guide to DRGs*. Chicago IL: Pluribus Press, 1984.

316. Simborg, D. W. "DRG Creep: A New Hospital-Acquired Disease." *New England Journal of Medicine (NEJM)* 304 (1981): 1602-4.

317. Slack, Warner V. *Cybermedicine: How Computing Empowers Doctors and Patients for Better Health Care*. San Francisco: Jossey-Bass Publishers, 1997.

318. Slater, Carl H. *Severity of Illness Measurement*. Internet: Carl H. Slater, 1996.

319. Slee, Vergil N. "Disease Classification: *ICD-9* and Beyond." *PAS Reporter* 16, no. 11 (1978): 1-9.

320. ———. "Entity Coding of Diagnoses." *Tringa Press Monograph Series* 1 (1992).

321. ———. *An Entity Coding System for Diagnoses*. Brevard NC: The Tringa Group, 1989.

322. ———. *The International Classification*. St. Paul, MN: Tringa Press, 1990.

323. ———. "The International Classification, Its Evolution and Implementation." *Tringa Press Monograph Series* 2 (1992).

324. ———. "The *International Classification of Diseases*: Ninth Revision (ICD-9)." *Annals of Internal Medicine* 88, no. 3 (1978): 424-26.

325. ———. "Remarks." *Journal of Clinical Computing* 12, no. 4 (1984): 124-28.

326. Slee, Vergil N., and Debora A. Slee. *Health Care Terms, Second Edition*. St. Paul MN: Tringa Press, 1991.

327. ———. *Slee's Health Care Reform Terms, January 1994 Supplement*. St. Paul MN: Tringa Press, 1994.

328. Slee, Vergil N., Debora A. Slee, and HJ Schmidt. *Slee's Health Care Terms: Third Comprehensive Edition*. St. Paul MN: Tringa Press, 1996.

329. Soderstrom, Naomi S. "Are Reporting Errors Under PPS Random or Systematic?" *Inquiry* 27, no. Fall (1990): 234-41.

330. Sperzel, David, Mark Erlbaum, Lloyd Fuller, David Sherertz, Nels Olson, Peri Schuyler, William Hole, Allan Savage, Philip Passarelli, and Mark Tuttle. "Editing the UMLS Metathesaurus: Review and Enhancement of a Computed Knowledge Source." *Proceedings of the Fourteenth Annual Symposium on Computer Applications in Medical Care* (1990): 136-40.

331. Stedman. *Stedman's Electronic Medical Dictionary*. Baltimore Maryland: Williams and Wilkins, 1998.

332. Sumkin, Joan. "The Coding Audit." *Annals of Internal Medicine* 128, no. 6 (1998): 502.

333. Taber. *Taber's Cyclopedic Medical Dictionary, 17th Edition*. Philadelphia: F. A. Davis Company, 1993.

334. Thomas, James. "What Is an International Standard?" *ASTM Standardization News* 25, no. 12 (1997): 11.

335. Thompson, Barbara J. *Implications of an Interactive Encoding System for ICD-9-CM*. Ann Arbor, MI: Commission on Professional and Hospital Activities, 1981.

336. Thompson, Barbara J., and Vergil N. Slee. "Accuracy of Diagnosis and Operation Coding." *Medical Record News* 49, no. 5 (1978).

337. Thompson, Edward T., and Adaline C. Hayden. *Handbook on Standard Nomenclature of Diseases and Operations*. New York: Blakiston Division, McGraw Hill Book Company, 1959.

338. Tierney, William M., J. Marc Overhage, and Clement J. McDonald. "Toward Electronic Medical Records That Improve Care." *Annals of Internal Medicine* 122, no. 9 (1995): 725-26.

339. Tolleson-Rinehart, Sue. "Clinical Practice Guidelines and Evidence-Based Practice." *CePOR* 3, no. 1 (1997): 1-4.

340. Tuttle, Mark, David Scherertz, Mark Erlbaum, Nels Olson, and Stuart Nelson. "Implementing Meta-1: The First Version of the UMLS Metatheraurus." *Proceedings of the Thirteenth Annual Symposium on Computer Applications in Medical Care* (1989): 483-87.

341. Tuttle, Mark, David Scherertz, Nels Olson, Mark Erlbaum, David Sperzel, Lloyd Fuller, and Stuart Nelson. "Using Meta-1—the First Version of the UMLS Metathesaurus." *Proceedings of the Fourteenth Annual Symposium on Computer Applications in Medical Care* (1990): 131-35.

342. U. S. Department of Commerce, Bureau of the Census. *Manual of Joint Causes of Death—Showing Assignment to the Preferred Title of the International List of Causes of Death When Two Causes Are Simultaneously Reported*. Washington   DC: United States Government Printing Office, 1933.

343. ———. *Manual of the International List of Causes of Death, 4th Decennial Revision, 1929*. Washington   DC: United States Government Printing Office, 1931.

344. ———. *Manual of the International List of Causes of Death, As Adopted for Use in the United States—Fifth Revision*. Washington   DC: United States Government Printing Office, 1940.

345. ———. *Physicians' Handbook of Birth and Death Registration, 9th Edition*. Washington   DC: United States Government Printing Office, 1939.

346. U. S. Department of Health and Human Services, Public Health Service Health Care Financing Administration. "ICD-9-CM: International

Classification of Diseases, 9th Revision, Clinical Modification, Fourth Edition, Volumes 1,2, and 3: Official Authorized Addendum, Effective October 1, 1992." *Coding Clinic for ICD-9-CM* 9, no. Special Edition (1992): 1-63.

347. U. S. Health Care Financing Administration. *Final Draft of ICD-10 Procedure Coding System (ICD-10-PCS) Introduction, Training Manual, Tabular List, and Alphabetic Index.* Internet HCFA Website: Health Care Financing Administration, 1998.

348. U. S. Health Care Financing Administration (HCFA). *UB-92 HCFA-1450.*

349. U. S. National Center for Health Statistics. *Eighth Revision International Classification of Diseases, Adapted for Use in the United States (ICDA-8), 2 Volume Set.* Washington, DC: U. S. National Center for Health Statistics, 1968.

350. ———. *ICD-9-CM to ICD-10-CM Conversion.* Internet: U. S. National Center for Health Statistics, 1997.

351. ———. *International Classification of Diseases, 10th Revision, Clinical Modification (ICD-10-CM).* Internet: U. S. National Center for Health Statistics, 1997.

352. ———. "Report of the National Committee on Vital and Health Statistics Concerning Issues Related to the Coding and Classification Systems." *U. S. National Center for Health Statistics, Working Paper Series*, no. 37 (1990).

353. ———. "Report of the Need to Collect External Cause-of-Injury Codes in Hospital Discharge Data." *U. S. National Center for Health Statistics, Working Paper Series*, no. 37 (1991).

354. ———. *Report of the United States Delegation to the International Conference for the Eighth Revision of the International Classification of Diseases, Geneva, Switzerland, July 6-12, 1965.* Washington DC: U. S. Government printing office, 1966.

355. U. S. National Committee on Vital and Health Statistics. *1989 Annual Report.* Washington, DC: U. S. Department of Health and Human Services, 1989.

356. ———. *1990 Annual Report.* Washington, DC: U. S. Department of Health and Human Services, 1990.

357. ———. *1991 Annual Report.* Washington, DC: U. S. Department of Health and Human Services, 1991.

358. ———. *1992 Annual Report.* Washington, DC: U. S. Department of Health and Human Services, 1992.

359. ———. *1993 Annual Report.* Washington, DC: U. S. Department of Health and Human Services, 1993.

360. ———. *1994 Annual Report.* Washington, DC: U. S. Department of Health and Human Services, 1994.

361. ———. *1995 Annual Report.* Washington, DC: U. S. Department of Health and Human Services, 1995.

362. ———. "Appendix V: Recommendations for a Single Procedure Classification System, November 1993." *1993 Annual Report* (1993): 54-68.

363. U. S. National Library of Medicine. *The Coach Metathesaurus Browser Fact Sheet.* Washington DC: National Library of Medicine, 1994.

364. ———. *Medical Subject Headings® (MeSH®) Annotated Alphabetic Index 1997.* Bethesda MD: United States National Library of Medicine, 1996.

365. ———. *Medical Subject Headings® (MeSH®) Permuted Medical Subject Headings.* Bethesda MD: United States National Library of Medicine, 1996.

366. ———. *Medical Subject Headings® (MeSH®) Tree Structures.* Bethesda MD: United States National Library of Medicine, 1996.

367. ———. *National Library of Medicine Classification—a Scheme for the Shelf Arrangement of Library Materials in the Field of Medicine and Its Related Sciences—Fifth Edition, 1994.* Bethesda MD: National Library of Medicine, 1994.

368. ———. *Natural Language Systems Program.* Washington DC: National Library of Medicine, 1995.

369. ———. *NLM Online Databases and Databanks.* Washington DC: National Library of Medicine, 1994.

370. ———. *UMLS® Bibliography* . Washington DC: National Library of Medicine, 1993.

371. ———. *UMLS® Information Sources Map (ISM)—Fact Sheet.* Washington DC: National Library of Medicine, 1996.

372. ———. *UMLS® Metathesaurus® Fact Sheet.* Washington DC: National Library of Medicine, 2000.

373. ———. *UMLS® Semantic Network® Fact Sheet.* Washington DC: National Library of Medicine, 2000.

374. ———. *UMLS® Specialist Lexicon® Fact Sheet.* Washington DC: National Library of Medicine, 2000.

375. ———. *Unified Medical Language System® (UMLS®)—Fact Sheet.* Washington DC: National Library of Medicine, 2000.

376. U. S. Public Health Service. *International Classification of Diseases Adapted for Indexing of Hospital Records and Operation Classification (ICDA) (PHS Publication 719).* Washington DC: U. S. Department of Health, Education, and Welfare, Public Health Service, 1959.

377. ———. *International Classification of Diseases Adapted for Indexing of Hospital Records by Diseases and Operations (ICDA) (PHS Publication 719 Revised 1962), 2 Volume Set.* Washington DC: U. S. Department of Health, Education, and Welfare, Public Health Service, 1962.

378. U. S. Treasury Department, Public Health Service. *Nomenclature of Diseases and Conditions.* Washington DC: United States Government Printing Office, 1935.

379. van Bemmel, Jan H., and Alexa T. McCray. *99 Yearbook of Medical Informatics.* Stuttgart, Germany: Schattauer Verlagsgesellschaft mbH, 1999.

380. Waegemann, C. Peter. "The Five Levels of Electronic Health Records." *MD Computing* 13, no. 3 (1996): 199-203.

381. ———. "Information Technology and Electronic Patient Records." *Toward an Electronic Patient Record* 5, no. 7 (1997): 1-8.

382. ———. "The Market for Electronic Patient Record Systems." *Toward an Electronic Patient Record* 5, no. 1 (1996): 1,3, 12-16.

383. ———. "Object Technology in Health Care." *Toward an Electronic Patient Record* 6, no. 7 (1998): 1-11.

384. ———. "Standards for Computer-Based Patient Records—Testimony Presented to the National Committee on Vital and Health Statistics, March 4, 1998." *Toward an Electronic Patient Record* 6, no. 8 (1998): 1-9.

385. Walden, Victoria. "Defining the UMLS® Metathesaurus®." *Journal of AHIMA* 68, no. 1 (1997): 38.

386. Walker, DC, RF Walters, JJ Cimino, P Dujols, Li Ensheng, W Giere, T Kiuchi, H Lamberts, WG Moore, FH Roger, Y Satomura, and FW Stitt. "Internationalization of Health Care Terminology." *MEDINFO 92.* K. C. Lun, 1444-51. Elsevier Science Publishers BV, 1992.

387. Wallace, Eleanor Z., and Rosanne M. Leipzig. "Doing the Right Thing Right: Is Evidence-Based Medicine the Answer?" *Annals of Internal Medicine* 127, no. 1 (1997): 91-94.

388. Wann, Marilyn. "Record-Keepers: Demand Grows, Supply Shrinks." *Health Week,* 30 July 1990, sec. 1, col. 2.

389. Weaver, Robert R. *Computers and Medical Knowledge—the Diffusion of Decision Support Software.* Boulder CO: Westview Press, 1991.

390. Weed, Lawrence L. *Knowledge Coupling.* New York: Springer-Verlag, 1991.

391. ———. *Medical Records, Medical Education, and Patient Care.* Chicago: Year Bood Medical Publishers, 1969.

392. Weigel, Karel M. "Comments From the Panel on Conceptual Framework for Coding and Classification." *Meeting Minutes, Public Health Service, National Committee on Vital and Health Statistics* (1997): 22.

393. Weigel, Karel M., Meryl Bloomrosen, Faye Brown, Diana Callen, Mary Converse, Kay Gooding, Linda Hyde, Cassandra Bissen, and Rita Finnegan. *Report of the AMRA Task Force on ICD-10.* Chicago IL: American Medical Record Association (AMRA), 1987.

394. Weigel, Karel M., and Carol A. Lewis. "In Sickness and in Health—the Role of the ICD in the United States Health Care Data and ICD-10." *Topics in Health Record Management* 12, no. 1 (1991): 70-82.

395. White, Kerr L. "Foreword." *ICD-9-CM: International Classification of Diseases, 9th Revision, Clinical Modification, Volumes 1* (1978).

396. ———. "Information for Health Care: an Epidemiological Perspective." *Inquiry* 17 (1980): 296-312.

397. ———. "Restructuring the International Classification of Diseases: Need for a New Paradigm." *The Journal of Family Practice* 21 (1985): 17-20.

398. Wible, Scott. "CPR Definition Up for Debate." *Healthcare Informatics* (1997): 20-21.

399. Wieners, Walter. "Quality Measurement and Severity Systems: an Overview." *Computers in Healthcare* (1988): 27-32.

400. Wilkerson, Gary, Chris Chute, and Simon Cohn. "Codes and Structures." *CPRI-Mail* 5, no. 2 (1996): 3.

401. Willard, Dianne. "HCFA Requires Use of Modifiers for Hospital Outpatient Services." *Journal of AHIMA* 69, no. 6 (1998): 75-78.

402. Williams, Kenneth J., and Paul R. Donnelly. *Medical Care Quality and the Public Trust*. Chicago IL: Pluribus Press, 1982.

403. Woloshin, Steven, Nina A. Bickell, Lisa M. Schwartz, Francesca Gany, and H. Gilbert Welch. "Language Barriers in Medicine in the United States." *Journal of the American Medical Association* 273, no. 9 (1995): 724-28.

404. WONCA. *ICPC International Classification of Primary Care*. New York: Oxford University Press, 1987.

405. ———. *International Classification of Health Problems in Primary Care (ICHPPC)*. Chicago: World Organization of National Colleges, Academies and Academic Associations of General Practitioners/Family Physicians (WONCA)/American Hospital Association, 1975.

406. ———. *International Classification of Health Problems in Primary Care (ICHPPC-2)*. Oxford: Oxford University Press, 1979.

407. ———. *International Classification of Health Problems in Primary Care (ICHPPC-2-Defined). Inclusion Criteria for the Use of the Rubrics of the International Classification of Health Problems in Primary Care*. Oxford: Oxford University Press, 1983.

408. ———. *International Classification of Primary Care, Second Edition (ICPC-2)—Second Edition*. New York: Oxford University Press, 1998.

409. ———. *International Classification of Process in Primary Care (IC-Process-PC)*. Oxford: Oxford University Press, 1986.

410. Wood, M., H. Lamberts, J. S. Meijer, and I. M. Hofmans-Okkes. "The Conversion Between ICPC and ICD-10. Requirements for a Family of Classification Systems in the Next Decade." *The International*

Classification of Primary Care in the European Community—With a Multi-Language Layer. Henk Lamberts, Maurice Wood, and Inge Hofmans-Okkes, 18-33. Oxford: Oxford University Press, 1993.

411. Workshop on Alternative Medicine. *Alternative Medicine: Expanding Medical Horizons*. Washington DC: National Institutes of Health, 1994.

412. World Health Organization. *The ICD-10 Classification of Mental and Behavioral Disorders: Clinical Descriptions and Diagnostic Guidelines*. Geneva, Switzerland: WHO, 1992.

413. ———. *The ICD-10 Classification of Mental and Behavioral Disorders: Diagnostic Criteria for Research*. Geneva, Switzerland: WHO, 1993.

414. ———. *International Classification of Diseases and Related Health Problems (ICD-10), 3 Volume Set*. Geneva, Switzerland: World Health Organization, 1992.

415. ———. *International Classification of Diseases for Oncology, Second Edition*. Geneva Switzerland: World Health Organization (WHO), 1990.

416. ———. *International Classification of Procedures in Medicine, Volume 1*. Geneva, Switzerland: World Health Organization, 1978.

417. ———. *International Statistical Classification of Diseases, Injuries, and Causes of Death. 6th Revision of the International Lists of Diseases and Causes of Death, 2 Volume Set*. Geneva, Switzerland: World Health Organization, 1949.

418. ———. *International Statistical Classification of Diseases, Injuries, and Causes of Death, 7th Revision, 1955, 2 Volume Set*. Geneva, Switzerland: World Health Organization, 1957.

419. ———. *International Statistical Classification of Diseases, Injuries, and Causes of Death, 8th Revision (1965), 2 Volume Set*. Geneva, Switzerland: World Health Organization, 1967.

420. ———. *International Statistical Classification of Diseases, Injuries, and Causes of Death, 9th Revision 2 Volume Set*. Geneva, Switzerland: World Health Organization, 1977.

421. ———. *Lexicon of Alcohol and Drug Terms*. Geneva, Switzerland: WHO, 1994.

422. ———. *Lexicon of Cross-Cultural Terms in Mental Health*. Geneva, Switzerland: WHO, 1997.

423. ———. *Lexicon of Psychiatric and Mental Health Terms, Volume 1, Second Edition*. Geneva, Switzerland: WHO, 1994.

424. ———. *Standard Acupuncture Nomenclature, Second Edition*. Manila, Phillipines: World Health Organization, Regional Office for the Western Pacific, 1993.

425. World Health Organization Collaborating Center for Classification of Diseases for North America. "Human T-Cell Lymphotropic Virus-III/Lymphadenopathy-Associated Virus (HTLV-III/LAV) Infection Classification." *Coding Clinic* (1986): 16-23.

426. World Health Organization Collaborating Centre for Drug Statistics Methodology. *Anatomic Therapeutic Chemical (ATC) Classification Index*. WHO Collaborating Centre for Drug Statistics Methodology, 1992.

427. Wos, Midge. *MESHin' Around—or I Got It From the Horse's Mouth*. Milwaukee WI: Midge Wos, 1984.

428. Wunderlich, Gooloo W. *Toward a National Health Care Survey—a Data System for the 21st Century*. Washington DC: National Academy Press, 1992.

429. Zintel, Harold A. "The Family of Classifications for Reporting Data in Health Care." *Role of Informatics in Health Data Coding and Classification Systems. Proceedings of the IFIP-IMIA WG6 International Working Conference, Ottawa, Canada, 26-28 September 1984* (1985): 259-70.

About the Authors

VERGIL SLEE received his BA in 1937 from Albion College, Michigan, and his MD in 1941 from Washington University School of Medicine, St. Louis, Missouri. Following service as a flight surgeon with the United States 14th Air Force in China in World War II, he obtained his MPH in 1947 from the University of Michigan School of Public Health. He then served as a county health officer and hospital administrator in southwestern Michigan. In carrying out his duties there, he soon encountered the difficulty of determining the wellness of the people in that community, and whether their healthcare needs were being met. This difficulty was due to lack of information: the only way to obtain data on patient care was to go to each hospital and pull individual patient records, then review each one for the specific information wanted. "There must be a better way," he thought.

In 1954, Dr. Slee obtained a grant from the W. K. Kellogg Foundation for the Southwest Michigan Hospital Council to pilot a program systematically to collect statistical information from patient records, in order to study each hospital's own clinical care, and to compare statistics with other area hospitals. This was the Professional Activity Study (PAS). The program was popular among the 13 hospitals, but it was frustrating because the statistics, compiled manually, were not the result of uniform definitions and tabulations. His proposal to use punch cards, each with a brief summary of an individual medical record, and with one punch card for every case, was tested with the help of the School of Public Health of the University of Michigan, and found feasible.

In 1955 he coauthored with C. Wesley Eisele, MD, and Robert G. Hoffmann, PhD, the first paper on evaluation of the quality of practice of internal medicine, a paper presented at the annual session of the American College of Physicians.[1]

In 1956 the Commission on Professional and Hospital Activities (CPHA) was established jointly by the American College of Physicians, the American College of Surgeons, the American Hospital Association, the

American Medical Association, and the Southwestern Michigan Hospital Council to expand PAS nationwide. Dr. Slee was its director and then its president. By 1969, over 2,000 hospitals subscribed to PAS and most of them also to is companion program, MAP (the Medical Audit Program), and using summarized patient data as one tool to evaluate the quality of patient care had become a way of life.

Over the years Dr. Slee has lectured nationally and internationally on quality management and hospital discharge abstract systems, has written numerous articles on these subjects, and is the senior author of *Health Care Terms, Fourth Edition (forthcoming, 2000)* a dictionary of multidisciplinary terminology used in healthcare. He is a Fellow of the American College of Physicians, a Fellow of the American Public Health Association, and an Honorary Fellow of the American College of Healthcare Executives.

Dr. Slee has worked extensively to improve the methods of coding clinical information to get it into the data system. He was a member of the United States delegation to the World Health Organization for the Ninth Revision Conference on the International Classification (1975). Upon being convinced of the Ninth Revision's lack of suitability for clinical use in the United States, unless it was given greater detail and certain other modifications, he formed and became the president of the Council on Clinical Classifications (CCC) with the official sponsorship and participation of the American Academy of Pediatrics, the American College of Obstetricians and Gynecologists, the American College of Physicians, the American College of Surgeons, the American Psychiatric Association, and the Commission on Professional and Hospital Activities. In collaboration with the United States National Center for Health Statistics, and using the facilities and resources of CPHA, CCC modified the then-new *International Classification of Diseases, Ninth Revision, (ICD-9)* creating and publishing the *International Classification of Diseases, Ninth Revision, Clinical Modification (ICD-9-CM)*. This is still the diagnosis and procedure classification in use today throughout the United States.

---

1. Eisele, C. Wesley, Vergil N. Slee, Robert G. Hoffmann. "Can the Practice of Internal Medicine be Evaluated?" *Annals of Internal Medicine*, 44, No. 1 (1956): 144-61.

Pioneering patient data systems taught Dr. Slee a great deal about the design and implementation, success and failure of information management systems. He has seen — and been involved in — the evolution of information management from paper records and carbon copies, through card punch systems (first McBee Keysort manual systems, then Hollerith machines), and the first computers in the early 1960's.[2]

Since retirement from CPHA in the early 1980's, Dr. Slee has continued as a consultant in healthcare quality management and electronic data management systems. He lectures regularly on healthcare informatics at the national conferences of Estes Park Institute.

In 1998, CPHA established the "Vergil N. Slee Distinguished Professor of Healthcare Quality Management" in the Department of Health Policy and Administration in the School of Public Health of the University of North Carolina in Chapel Hill.

In 1991, Dr. Slee became interested in the increasing — and promising — role of the personal computer and information systems in direct patient care, especially in providing the knowledge-support base required by the physician, along with empowering the patient to participate in his or her own medical care. This interest led him to found, along with Richard Rockefeller, MD, the Health Commons Institute (HCI), of which he is Chairman of the Board. HCI is a nonprofit corporation dedicated to applying modern information technology (IT) at the point of care (the primary such interface is the patient-physician encounter and relationship). Such information support is essential to informed shared decision making (ISDM). The name of the organization was derived from the concept of a commons as a meeting ground.

DEBORA A. SLEE is an attorney and writer with experience in managed care organization and licensure, healthcare law, medical staff affairs, and quality and resource management. She received her BA from the

---

2. CPHA's initial computer system had to be lifted by crane to the second floor of an old office building in downtown Ann Arbor, Michigan. The building had been overhauled to reinforce the floor, add a two-foot depth to run cables and ducts through, and add the air conditioning critical to keeping the machines cool. It required the entire second floor to accommodate the computers, which used magnetic tape on large rolls. Today, most laptops have more performance capability.

University of Michigan and her JD from William Mitchell College of Law. Ms. Slee developed quality assurance tools for ambulatory care at the University of Minnesota in the 1970s, and in the 1980s created a quality management system for nonclinical services at an acute care hospital in New Hampshire. She is contributing author to *The Law of Hospital and Health Care Administration, Second Edition,* by Arthur F. Southwick, and coauthor of *Health Care Terms, Fourth Comprehensive Edition.* She works today as a consultant with the Tringa Group, which specializes in information management systems and healthcare communications.

H. JOACHIM SCHMIDT ("HJ") is a retired farmer and lawyer who has spent the past two decades being immersed in the tidal wave of information technology. He has a BA from Yale University and JD from William Mitchell College of Law. A veteran software applications engineer, he is now a consultant with the Tringa Group, where he specializes in making information more accessible and useful by taking advantage of new technology. He is also a coauthor of the *Slee's Health Care Terms* series of reference works.

Colophon

Work on this book began in about 1990, just before the last push for healthcare reform appeared. The dynamic nature of the decade from the healthcare perspective required a work platform that would allow three authors — one working twelve-hundred miles from the others — to work their way through mountains of information and ideas without getting mired down. The approach used by the authors was to have all writing and editing done on PCs using a software program called Folio Views® 4.11, and to then use Adobe's FrameMaker® 5.5.6 to format the text and graphics for final printing. Graphics were manipulated primarily with CorelDraw® 8.0. Adobe Acrobat® Exchange™ 3.0, with its annotations feature, was extremely helpful in passing edits around among the authors.

The Folio software serves the needs of having an editor ("word processor"), a research repository ("free-form database"), and an organizing tool ("to-do lists," etc.) all in one program. Its multi-user capability allows all authors to be working on the book at the same time. A special "filter" program written by one of the authors (HJ Schmidt) translated the book from its Folio® "infobase" format into the FrameMaker® format. Once formatted for its final book form, the content was then converted into a PostScript file as a preliminary step to "distilling" it into a "PDF" file. This single PDF file was then transmitted to the book manufacturer for the actual printing process.

The book is typeset in Sabon, Sabon SC, and Formata typefaces. Book and cover design and execution are by Debora Slee.

Index